Implementing Pediatric Integrative Medicine in Practice

Implementing Pediatric Integrative Medicine in Practice

Special Issue Editor
Hilary McClafferty

MDPI • Basel • Beijing • Wuhan • Barcelona • Belgrade

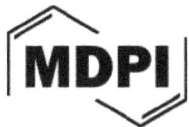

Special Issue Editor
Hilary McClafferty
University of Arizona
USA

Editorial Office
MDPI
St. Alban-Anlage 66
4052 Basel, Switzerland

This is a reprint of articles from the Special Issue published online in the open access journal *Children* (ISSN 2227-9067) from 2018 to 2019 (available at: https://www.mdpi.com/journal/children/special_issues/integrative_medicine_practice)

For citation purposes, cite each article independently as indicated on the article page online and as indicated below:

LastName, A.A.; LastName, B.B.; LastName, C.C. Article Title. *Journal Name* **Year**, *Article Number*, Page Range.

ISBN 978-3-03897-762-9 (Pbk)
ISBN 978-3-03897-763-6 (PDF)

© 2019 by the authors. Articles in this book are Open Access and distributed under the Creative Commons Attribution (CC BY) license, which allows users to download, copy and build upon published articles, as long as the author and publisher are properly credited, which ensures maximum dissemination and a wider impact of our publications.
The book as a whole is distributed by MDPI under the terms and conditions of the Creative Commons license CC BY-NC-ND.

Contents

About the Special Issue Editor vii

Preface to "Implementing Pediatric Integrative Medicine in Practice" ix

Anna Esparham, Sanghamitra Misra, Erica Sibinga, Timothy Culbert, Kathi Kemper, Hilary McClafferty, Sunita Vohra and Lawrence Rosen
Pediatric Integrative Medicine: Vision for the Future
Reprinted from: *Children* **2018**, *5*, 111, doi:10.3390/children5080111 1

Anna Esparham, Sanghamitra Misra, Erica Sibinga, Timothy Culbert, Kathi Kemper, Hilary McClafferty, Sunita Vohra and Lawrence Rosen
Correction: Esparham, A., et al., Pediatric Integrative Medicine: Vision for the Future. *Children*, 2018, 5, 111
Reprinted from: *Children* **2018**, *5*, 123, doi:10.3390/children5090123 14

Pamela Kaiser, Daniel P. Kohen, Melanie L. Brown, Rebecca L. Kajander and Andrew J. Barnes
Integrating Pediatric Hypnosis with Complementary Modalities: Clinical Perspectives on Personalized Treatment
Reprinted from: *Children* **2018**, *5*, 108, doi:10.3390/children5080108 16

Anna Esparham, Anne Herbert, Emily Pierzchalski, Catherine Tran, Jennifer Dilts, Madeline Boorigie, Tammie Wingert, Mark Connelly and Jennifer Bickel
Pediatric Headache Clinic Model: Implementation of Integrative Therapies in Practice
Reprinted from: *Children* **2018**, *5*, 74, doi:10.3390/children5060074 41

Gautam Ramesh, Dana Gerstbacher, Jenna Arruda, Brenda Golianu, John Mark and Ann Ming Yeh
Pediatric Integrative Medicine in Academia: Stanford Children's Experience
Reprinted from: *Children* **2018**, *5*, 168, doi:10.3390/children5120168 51

Marion Eckert, Catharina Amarell, Dennis Anheyer, Holger Cramer and Gustav Dobos
Integrative Pediatrics: Successful Implementation of Integrative Medicine in a German Hospital Setting—Concept and Realization
Reprinted from: *Children* **2018**, *5*, 122, doi:10.3390/children5090122 71

Marion Eckert and Melanie Anheyer
Applied Pediatric Integrative Medicine: What We Can Learn from the Ancient Teachings of Sebastian Kneipp in a Kindergarten Setting
Reprinted from: *Children* **2018**, *5*, 102, doi:10.3390/children5080102 80

Seema Kumar, Ivana T. Croghan, Bridget K. Biggs, Katrina Croghan, Rose Prissel, Debbie Fuehrer, Bonnie Donelan-Dunlap and Amit Sood
Family-Based Mindful Eating Intervention in Adolescents with Obesity: A Pilot Randomized Clinical Trial
Reprinted from: *Children* **2018**, *5*, 93, doi:10.3390/children5070093 87

Nicholas Chadi, Elli Weisbaum, Catherine Malboeuf-Hurtubise, Sara Ahola Kohut, Christine Viner, Miriam Kaufman, Jake Locke and Dzung X. Vo
Can the Mindful Awareness and Resilience Skills for Adolescents (MARS-A) Program Be Provided Online? Voices from the Youth
Reprinted from: *Children* **2018**, *5*, 115, doi:10.3390/children5090115 97

Avneet K. Mangat, Ju-Lee Oei, Kerry Chen, Im Quah-Smith and Georg M. Schmölzer
A Review of Non-Pharmacological Treatments for Pain Management in Newborn Infants
Reprinted from: *Children* **2018**, *5*, 130, doi:10.3390/children5100130 . . . . **109**

Anava A. Wren, Alexandra C. Ross, Genevieve D'Souza, Christina Almgren, Amanda Feinstein, Amanda Marshall and Brenda Golianu
Multidisciplinary Pain Management for Pediatric Patients with Acute and Chronic Pain: A Foundational Treatment Approach When Prescribing Opioids
Reprinted from: *Children* **2019**, *6*, 33, doi:10.3390/children6020033 . . . . **121**

Genevieve D'Souza, Anava A Wren, Christina Almgren, Alexandra C. Ross, Amanda Marshall and Brenda Golianu
Pharmacological Strategies for Decreasing Opioid Therapy and Management of Side Effects from Chronic Use
Reprinted from: *Children* **2018**, *5*, 163, doi:10.3390/children5120163 . . . . **144**

Missy Hall, Susanne M. Bifano, Leigh Leibel, Linda S. Golding and Shiu-Lin Tsai
The Elephant in the Room: The Need for Increased Integrative Therapies in Conventional Medical Settings
Reprinted from: *Children* **2018**, *5*, 154, doi:10.3390/children5110154 . . . . **155**

Megan E. Voss and Mary Jo Kreitzer
Implementing Integrative Nursing in a Pediatric Setting
Reprinted from: *Children* **2018**, *5*, 103, doi:10.3390/children5080103 . . . . **168**

Hilary McClafferty, Audrey J. Brooks, Mei-Kuang Chen, Michelle Brenner, Melanie Brown, Anna Esparham, Dana Gerstbacher, Brenda Golianu, John Mark, Joy Weydert, Ann Ming Yeh and Victoria Maizes
Pediatric Integrative Medicine in Residency Program: Relationship between Lifestyle Behaviors and Burnout and Wellbeing Measures in First-Year Residents
Reprinted from: *Children* **2018**, *5*, 54, doi:10.3390/children5040054 . . . . **176**

About the Special Issue Editor

Hilary McClafferty, MD, FAAP is board-certified in pediatrics, pediatric emergency medicine, and integrative medicine. She writes and speaks nationally on pediatric integrative medicine, physician wellbeing, resiliency, and whole physician wellness. She has authored two books: Mind-Body Medicine in Clinical Practice and Integrative Pediatrics: Art, Science, and Clinical Application, and is the editor of two published Special Editions in Children, MDPI on integrative medicine in pediatric practice. She is Founding Director of the Pediatric Integrative Medicine in Residency program, University of Arizona, and Medical Director, Pediatric Emergency Medicine at Tucson Medical Center, Tucson, Arizona.

Preface to "Implementing Pediatric Integrative Medicine in Practice"

Building on two published Special Issues, Introduction to Pediatric Integrative Medicine, and Mind-Body Medicine in Children and Adolescents, this Edition explores the implementation of integrative medicine by pediatricians and nurses in a rich array of venues and applications. Written by experts in their respective fields, the edition pushes open a door that was previously simply ajar, educating us on research advances and practical clinical applications in this emerging field, demonstrating the power and range of pediatric integrative medicine.

Many, if not all, of the contributing authors have faced significant challenges in program start-up, acquisition of funding sources, administrative support, and program sustainability. Their persistence gives us hope and their hard-earned insights pave the way for those blazing their own trails in the field. It is no exaggeration to say that the pediatric community pursuing this work is extraordinarily creative and resourceful.

The Edition opens with an overview of the field's evolution in an article by national leaders to provide background and perspective for those less familiar with its history. It is followed by in-depth articles on clinical hypnosis; development and implementation of a ground-breaking integrative headache clinic in an academic children's hospital; development of a comprehensive integrative medicine program at Lucille Packard's Children's Hospital at Stanford University; description of the successful embedding of a pediatric integrative medicine curriculum into a German pediatric residency—accompanied by an inspiring description of one of the group's educational outings. These excellent articles are followed by a description of a randomized trial of mindfulness in obese adolescents and an exploration of the effectiveness of an online course to teach mindfulness and resilience to adolescents.

The pressing need for non-pharmacologic approaches to pain is explored in three separate articles, one addressing the topic in newborns, an underrepresented population in the national research in this critical area. A case-based article describing interdisciplinary collaboration with a wide range of integrative therapies provides examples and creative ideas for immediate use. An article by Voss and Kreitzer, leaders in the field of nursing education, gives us a forward-looking view of the implementation of integrative nursing in a pediatric setting and emphasizes the importance of a highly collaborative approach to the pediatric patient. The Edition closes with an article describing the need for ongoing attention to the health and wellbeing of our pediatric trainees—reminding us to care for ourselves as well as those who look to us as teachers and mentors.

As this Special Edition took shape I was struck by how far the field has come in a relatively short time, and I am intensely curious to see what its future holds. I feel confident speaking for the contributors in saying that the motivation to advance the field comes from a deep desire to improve the health and well-being of children around the world, to make measurable strides towards more effective preventive pediatric care, and to reduce pain, stress, and suffering for all children and adolescents, especially those living with chronic illness.

I encourage readers to explore this issue with an open mind and to allow sparks from these contributor's creative work to catalyze new ideas and initiatives. I hope you learn as much as I did while working on this issue. Finally, thank you to all who contributed to the Edition, including the patients and families that took part in the programs and studies with the shared goal of helping the next child's experience in health care be that much smoother.

Hilary McClafferty
Special Issue Editor

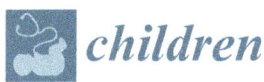

Brief Report

Pediatric Integrative Medicine: Vision for the Future

Anna Esparham [1,*], Sanghamitra M. Misra [2], Erica Sibinga [3], Timothy Culbert [4], Kathi Kemper [5], Hilary McClafferty [6], Sunita Vohra [7] and Lawrence Rosen [8]

1. Division of Child Neurology-Headache Section, Children's Mercy Hospital, University of Missouri School of Medicine-Kansas City, Kansas City, MO 64108, USA
2. Mobile Clinic Program, Texas Children's Hospital, Baylor College of Medicine, Houston, TX 77054, USA; smisra@bcm.edu
3. Department of Pediatrics, Johns Hopkins School of Medicine, Baltimore, MD 21205, USA; esibinga@jhmi.edu
4. Integrative Medicine, Prairie Care, University of Minnesota Medical School, Chaska, MN 55318, USA; tculbert@prairie-care.com
5. Department of Pediatrics, College of Medicine, Ohio State University, Columbus, OH 43210, USA; kathi.kemper@osumc.edu
6. Department of Medicine, Arizona Center for Integrative Medicine, University of Arizona, Tucson, AZ 85724, USA; hmcclafferty@email.arizona.edu
7. Integrative Health Institute, CARE Program, PedCAM Network, Department of Pediatrics, Medicine, and Psychiatry, Faculty of Medicine and Dentistry, University of Alberta, Edmonton, AB T6G 2C8, Canada; svohra@ualberta.ca
8. Whole Child Center, Oradell, NJ 07649, USA; ldrdoc@alum.mit.edu
* Correspondence: aeesparham@cmh.edu; Tel.: +816-302-3320

Received: 26 July 2018; Accepted: 16 August 2018; Published: 20 August 2018

Abstract: Pediatric integrative medicine (PIM) is of significant interest to patients, with 12% of the general pediatric population and up to 80% of children with chronic conditions using PIM approaches. The field of PIM has evolved over the past 25 years, approaching child health with a number of guiding principles: preventive, context-centered, relationship-based, personalized, participatory, and ecologically sustainable. This manuscript reviews important time points for the field of PIM and reports on a series of meetings of PIM leaders, aimed at assessing the state of the field and planning for its future. Efforts in the first decade of the 2000s led to increased visibility in academic and professional pediatric organizations and through international listservs, designed to link those interested in and practicing PIM, all of which continue to flourish. The PIM leadership summits in recent years resulted in specific goals to advance PIM further in the following key areas: research, clinical practice, professional education, patient and family education, and advocacy and partnerships. Additionally, goals were developed for greater expansion of PIM professional education, broader support for pediatric PIM research, and an expanded role for PIM approaches in the provision of pediatric care.

Keywords: pediatric integrative medicine; vision; clinical practice; education; advocacy; complementary therapies

1. Introduction

Integrative medicine is defined as relationship-centered care that focuses on the whole person, is informed by evidence, and makes use of all appropriate therapeutic approaches, healthcare professionals and disciplines to achieve optimal health and healing, including evidence-based complementary and alternative medicine. Pediatric integrative medicine (PIM) develops and promotes this approach within the field of pediatrics [1,2].

The field of pediatrics is at a crossroads. The health of our children—our future—is at stake. The prevalence rates of myriad chronic pediatric health conditions continue to rise at an unprecedented pace [3,4]. Chronic health conditions contribute to the global burden of disability [5]. Historically, the conventional solution has favored a 'disease-treatment system' that often incentivizes more invasive care at higher cost, an approach poorly aligned with the needs of today's children. Health care transformation is no longer optional; it is an absolute imperative. Advocates and stakeholders in search of better health care require new approaches to meet the complex health challenges faced by children. We are searching for safer and more cost-effective paradigms to optimize the health and well-being of children everywhere. Multidisciplinary healthcare models that implement integrative and complementary therapies for patients with chronic illness have shown improved clinical outcomes and quality of life [6,7]. In addition, health outcomes are improved through patient empowerment [8,9]. Integrative medicine promotes relationship-centered care and empowers individuals to incorporate wellness strategies such as improving nutrition, physical activity, and sleep hygiene.

Pediatric integrative medicine (PIM) represents an evolution in pediatric care, a paradigm that embodies a philosophy consistent with long-standing holistic principles of quality medical care. As Dr. Kathi Kemper noted in her Presidential Address to the Ambulatory Pediatric Association nearly 20 years ago, "Holistic medicine is really just good medicine. It means caring for the whole child in the context of that child's values, their family's beliefs, their family system, and their culture in the larger community, and considering a range of therapies based on the evidence of their benefits and cost" [10] (p. 214).

PIM is defined by several core guiding principles [2,11]:

- Preventive: True primary care pediatrics is proactive rather than reactive. Prescribing lifestyle solutions to prevent disease is generally preferable to costly and potentially risky treatments. Lifestyle prescriptions may include food, activity, nature, creativity, rest, mindfulness, and connection with others.
- Context-centered: Children must be nurtured within the context of healthy families, communities, and schools. Health in mind, body, and spirit depends on how suitable the environment is for the child.
- Relationship-based: Only through open communication and building trust are we best able to work together to ensure each child's optimal health. The connection between health professionals and families has its own healing potential.
- Personalized: Health is not a one-size-fits-all proposition. Each child carries a unique potential based on a complex interplay of genetic and environmental factors. There is no medical treatment that can be guaranteed as safe for 100% of any population. Each family has the inherent right to make health care decisions for their children, keeping in mind the best interests of the child as well as legitimate public health concerns that ethically inform these decisions.
- Participatory: Creating health should be a collaborative process, actively encouraging participation and putting children and families back in control of their own health. Patient-centered care creates hope and empowers families to make sustainable changes, inspiring children to create the future they deserve.
- Ecologically sustainable: How we practice healthcare affects the environment, which has a measurable and cyclical impact on our health. The health and well-being of all the Earth's inhabitants are intimately tied to the health of our planet.
- Evidence-informed: Therapies that are evidence-informed while using the safety-effectiveness rubric (Figure 1) are considered as part of the treatment plan.

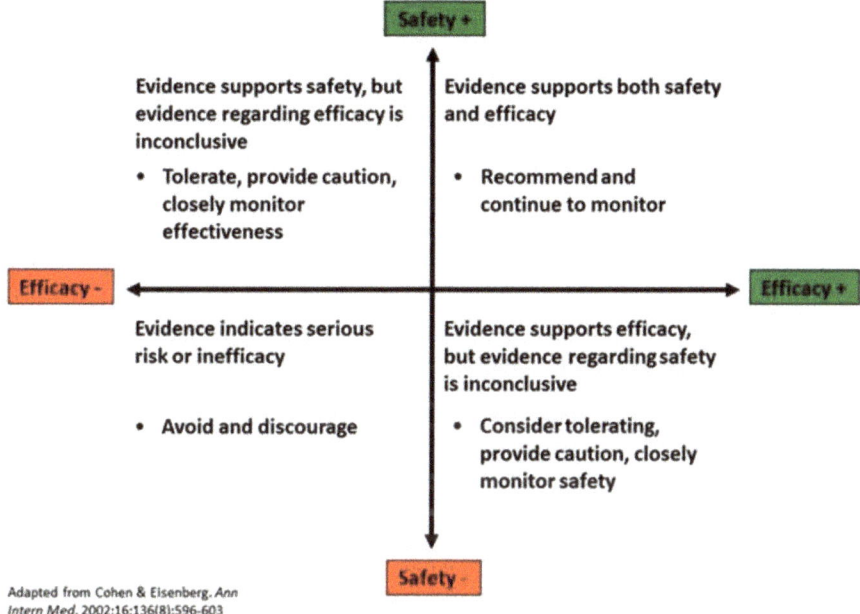

Figure 1. Safety–effectiveness therapy evaluation rubric.

2. Background

The field of PIM has developed organically over the last 25 years owing to pressing need and interest from pediatric health professionals, parents, and children. We have clear and compelling data that complementary therapies are of great interest to parents [12]. Use of these therapies in pediatrics is significant, as the 2012 National Health Interview Survey revealed that 12% of children use complementary therapies [13]. Studies in specific chronically ill populations have reported complementary therapy use in up to 80% of study participants [14,15]. We use the term "complementary" specifically to delineate these therapies from those offered within conventional Western medical care systems. PIM, by definition, embodies the integration of complementary therapies with conventional pediatric health care in a way that is informed by best available evidence and centered on the individual patient and family. Truly effective and safe patient-centered care demands that we talk with our patients about therapies of interest to them and know where to find evidence to inform these conversations.

Critics maintain that integrative therapies do not have sufficient evidence to support their use in pediatric populations. We recognize that all health interventions would benefit from more high quality pediatric research to assess both effectiveness and safety. We do not agree that, by definition, all conventional care is evidence-based and that complementary therapies, by definition, lack evidence, or else they would be incorporated as part of conventional care. Research published in reputable journals has shown over the last 30 years that myriad complementary therapies are safe and effective for a variety of pediatric conditions and symptoms. Pediatric health professionals are encouraged to ask their patients and families about complementary therapy use [12]. In a national survey sent to members of the American Academy of Pediatrics (AAP), most pediatric healthcare professionals (87%) had been asked about complementary and alternative (CAM) therapies by a patient/parent within three months of the survey [16]. In addition, over 80% of the pediatric healthcare professionals desired additional information on CAM, with fewer than 5% reporting being knowledgeable about individual CAM therapies [16]. Of the whether or not professionals 'believe' in these therapies is immaterial;

patient-centered care and patient safety demand that professionals know what health approaches are being used and considered. Health professionals must remember that evidence-informed medicine is a triad: best available evidence, clinical experience, and patient preference [17]. Dr. Kathi Kemper and Mr. Cohen, JD, MBA, MFA published a now well-established rubric to evaluate the use of therapies [18], see Figure 1.

As demonstrated in the graphic, use of therapies should be recommended if the intervention is known to be safe and effective based on best available evidence. If the therapy is known to be safe but efficacy has not yet been conclusively established, it is reasonable to tolerate use while monitoring response. If a therapy is known to be effective but its safety is questionable, after a careful informed consent discussion, use may be considered if monitored closely. Finally, a therapy is to be avoided and discouraged if it has no proven efficacy and known adverse effects. Relative risks and benefits should always be considered in light of best available evidence, and professionals can use the graphic to help guide decision-making in collaboration with patients and families. It is important to note that this rubric applies to all therapies—not just those deemed complementary—as complementary therapies may not apply to all pediatric conditions.

We recognize there are pediatric health professionals who would like to know how to discuss and apply these therapies in clinical practice, where to seek further training, and when to refer patients for these therapies. In addition, several barriers may exist for both professionals and families, such as adequate coverage of therapies and availability of PIM resources for the underserved or for those living in resource-poor locations [19,20]. The PIM Leadership Initiative (PIMLI) has developed this position statement to provide a unified vision for PIM to meet the needs of professionals in the service of pediatric patients and families. As PIM is still growing, although 20 years old, providing structure and vision is imperative for the continued, sustainable development of the field.

3. Evolution of Pediatric Integrative Medicine

The field of PIM has evolved tremendously over the past two decades. The sentinel events that have shaped the current PIM landscape are noted below.

Pediatric integrative medicine timeline, 1995–2017:

- 1995 Ambulatory Pediatric Association establishes Holistic Pediatrics Special Interest Group
- 1996 "The Holistic Pediatrician" published (Kemper)
- 1998 Boston Children's Hospital establishes Center for Holistic Pediatric Education and Research
- 1999 First PIM Conference hosted by University of Arizona; Dr. Kemper's APA Presidential Address (*Holistic Pediatrics = Good Medicine*)
- 2000 Second PIM Conference hosted by Children's Hospitals and Clinics (Minneapolis) and University of Minnesota, AAP Task Force on CAM established and AAP NCE CAM sessions start
- 2004 First PIMLI Summit in St. Paul, MN; Pediatric Complementary and Alternative Medicine Research & Education (PedCAM) Network (Vohra) and International Pediatric Integrative Medicine (IPIM) Network (Rosen) started
- 2005 AAP Provisional Section on Complementary, Holistic, and Integrative Medicine (CHIM) and Integrative Pediatrics Council (IPC) established
- 2005–2008 International PIM/Pangea conferences hosted by IPC
- 2006 *Pediatrics in Review* series on PIM debuts (Vohra, editor)
- 2007 *Pediatric Clinics of North America* volume on PIM published (Rosen, Riley ed.)
- 2008 AAP Section on CHIM official (name later changed to Section on Complementary and Integrative Medicine, or SOCIM); *The Use of Complementary and Alternative Medicine in Pediatrics* AAP Clinical Report published in *Pediatrics*, IPC dissolves
- 2009 "Textbook on Integrative Pediatrics" published (Culbert, Olness ed.)
- 2012 PIM program survey published (*Pediatric integrative medicine: pediatrics' newest subspecialty?* Vohra S, et al.); University of Arizona Center for Integrative Medicine launches Pediatric

Integrative Medicine in Residency (PIMR) curriculum; AAP SOCIM name changed to Section on Integrative Medicine (SOIM)
- 2014 *Physician Health and Wellness* AAP Clinical Report published in *Pediatrics*; inaugural AAP SOIM Pioneer Award given to Dr. Kemper; "A Guide to Integrative Pediatrics" textbook published (Misra, Verissimo)
- 2015 PIMLI Summit II in Boston, MA
- 2016 PIMLI Summit III in Hackensack, NJ; "The Holistic Pediatrician, 20th Anniversary Edition" published (Kemper); *Mind-Body Therapies in Children and Youth* AAP Clinical Report published in *Pediatrics*
- 2017 "Integrative Pediatrics: Art, Science, and Clinical Application" textbook published (McClafferty)

All events are listed to the best of the PIMLI's Summit collective knowledge and may not include all international PIM events.

As noted, the first official meeting of PIM leaders in the United States was held in 2004 and termed the Pediatric Integrative Medicine Leadership Initiative (PIMLI) Summit. The first PIMLI Summit spawned several major initiatives: A Section on Integrative Medicine within the AAP, an interprofessional PIM nonprofit (the IPC), and two international online resources (the IPIM-Network and PedCAM). These entities spearheaded numerous educational programs, including (1) PIM content at the AAP's National Conferences and Pangea PIM Conferences; (2) publication of key PIM books and scholarly articles; and (3) the establishment of the PIM in Residency (PIMR) training program. The decade of significant progress following this first PIMLI Summit coupled with the desire to nurture sustainable growth in the field prompted PIM leaders to systemically revisit the vision for the future of PIM [2,21,22].

4. 2015 PIMLI Summit

Supported by a generous grant from the Marino Health Foundation, Drs. Kathi Kemper and Lawrence Rosen—in partnership with the AAP—developed the second PIMLI Summit held in Boston, MA in June 2015 to accomplish the following objectives: (1) develop a long-term vision for PIM addressing gaps and future needs for clinical, educational, research, and advocacy domains; and (2) develop future PIM leaders who can achieve the vision through practical strategies and partnerships.

A group of fifteen PIM leaders from the United States and Canada were invited to attend the Summit. These physicians had a varying range of expertise in PIM with different stages of career development, and practiced in a variety of settings. They also represented the AAP Section on Integrative Medicine, Academy of Integrative Health and Medicine, University of Arizona Pediatric Integrative Medicine in Residency program, various North American pediatric academic programs, and the PedCAM and IPIM Networks. An intentional effort was made to incorporate a balance of early career and established leaders. Representatives from many other professions and partner organizations were consulted during meeting preparation to optimize long-term sustainability and success and to embody the interprofessional philosophy inherent in integrative care. Specifically, with organizational support by John Weeks, a pioneer in collaborative interprofessional IM efforts over several decades, representatives from the Academic Collaborative for Integrative Health (ACIH) participated in a comprehensive pre-Summit survey.

4.1. Professional Pre-Summit Survey Summary

In May 2015, more than 30 integrative health professionals provided feedback on the definition of integrative medicine, the state of child health, and a vision for PIM through a pre-Summit survey developed by Drs. Kemper and Rosen (unpublished data). In addition to pediatricians, these professionals represented expertise in Ayurvedic Medicine, botanical medicine, chiropractic, education, energy medicine, family medicine, health policy, massage therapy, mental health, naturopathy, Traditional Chinese Medicine, and yoga. Drs. Kemper and Rosen coordinated a conference call with John Weeks and a specially-designed 15-member interprofessional task force to discuss the survey and provide guidance for the Summit. A wordcloud (Figure 2) was created from stakeholder comments about what integrative medicine meant to them (unpublished data).

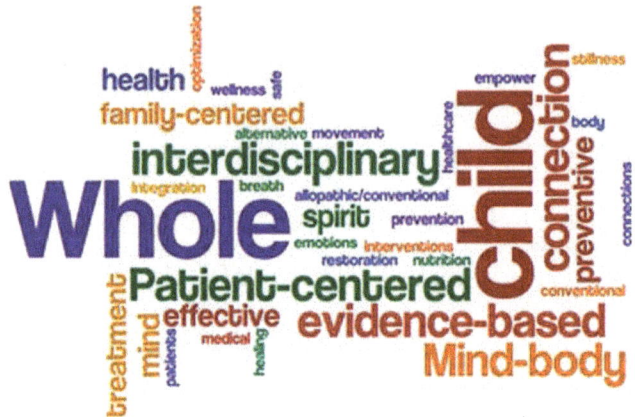

Figure 2. What does integrative medicine mean to you?

Regarding the current state of children's health, respondents noted that while pediatric acute care is 'good', both the quality and quantity of medical care for children and youth with chronic conditions often is not optimal. Survey participants felt the current conventional health care system is failing to adequately address the rising prevalence of chronic illnesses in children. They believed there is a need for a larger workforce of PIM health professionals to meet the challenges of complex childhood conditions while also promoting wellness. They also highlighted the importance of educating families about lifestyle approaches including healthy nutrition, physical activity, sleep, and stress coping skills. A need for more effective advocacy for improving children's health globally was mentioned, including a push for healthier modes of transportation, sustainable agriculture and food sources, and addressing health related environmental factors.

When asked how pediatricians can more effectively work with other stakeholders to best serve children's needs, survey participants responded that collaboration with other health professionals, parent groups, third-party payers, and community organizations is key. PIM stakeholders' vision for what pediatric integrative medicine would look like in 10 years included the wish that "decisions regarding a child's healthcare would be made from an integrative perspective, taking all possible healthcare options into account". Pediatric clinics would provide integrative care as part of the medical home with respect for all members of the patient's health care team. In addition, schools that train health professionals will incorporate integrative medicine training and provide interprofessional learning environments to build trust and facilitate patient-centered collaborative care. Finally, increased public and private funding would be available to support the investigation of all evidence-informed approaches that are personalized to the individual, given their health, preferences, and goals.

4.2. Parent Survey Summary

Parents are key PIM stakeholders and, therefore, a national parent online survey was conducted just prior to the PIMLI Summit to guide the meeting, with the logistical support of Kiwi Magazine, a publication focused on healthy lifestyle approaches for families. A sample of 1500 parents solicited through Kiwi's Moms Meet network (https://momsmeet.com, unpublished data) answered questions regarding their knowledge of PIM, PIM therapies they'd like to see offered in pediatric practices, and their willingness to advocate for insurance coverage of PIM therapies. Of note, even in this sample of natural health oriented parents, nearly one in four respondents were not familiar with IM. Fewer than one in seven definitively consider their pediatrician integrative while approximately 60% of parents believe having an integrative pediatrician for their children is important. Information about therapies is most commonly found online, and the two most desired in-office therapies are nutritional counseling and behavioral/mental health services. Key survey findings are shown in Figure 3a–d below.

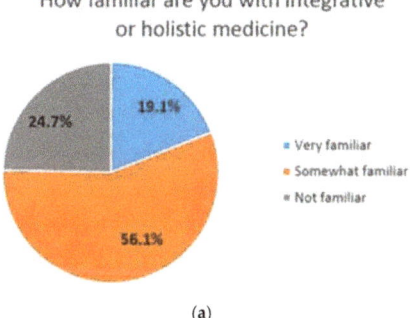

(a)

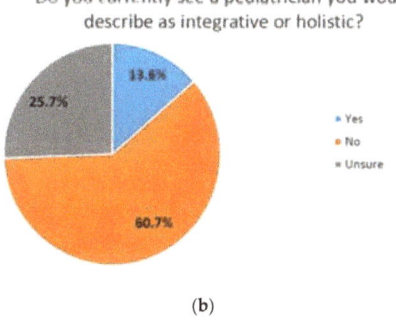

(b)

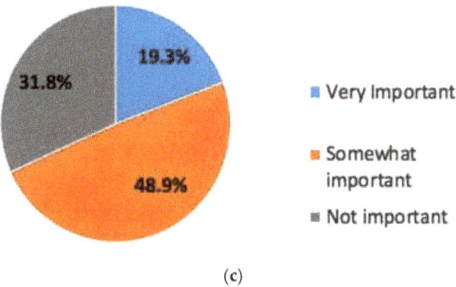

(c)

Figure 3. *Cont.*

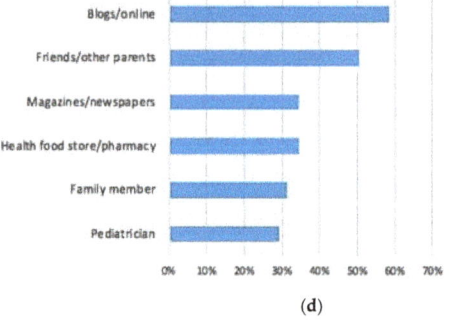

Figure 3. (**a**) Parent response to question "how familiar are you with integrative or holistic medicine?" Answer options included: very familiar, somewhat familiar, and not familiar; (**b**) Parent response to question "do you currently see a pediatrician you would describe as integrative or holistic?" Answer options included: yes, no, and unsure; (**c**) Parent response to question "how important is it to you to be able to find an integrative pediatrician for your child/children?" Answer options included: very important, somewhat important, and not important; (**d**) Parent response to question "where do you get information about natural or holistic therapies?" Answer options included all options that applied to parents: blogs/websites, friends/other parents, magazines/newspapers, health food store/pharmacy, family member, pediatrician, and other (as outlined above).

4.3. 2015 PIMLI Summit Summary

At the opening of the 2015 Summit, the 15 PIM leaders in attendance reviewed the professional survey as well as the evolution of the field to date. Using a World Café meeting paradigm, participants explored five strategic domains critical to the sustainable growth of the PIM field: research, clinical practice, professional education, patient and family education, and advocacy and partnerships [23]. Small groups were tasked with describing the existing gaps for each domain with specific strategies to address those gaps. The whole group then worked to clarify gaps and strategies to identify realistic and specific action steps to address each domain.

The following strategies were ultimately identified within each domain:

Research

- Expand the AAP Section on Integrative Medicine research and education grant program.
- Explore the development of a multi-center PIM research network.
- Publish PIM research articles in mainstream academic journals.

Clinical practice

- Promote use of existing quality clinical resources such as *Pediatrics in Review* articles, special issues in professional journals, well-designed research trials on complementary therapies, and integrative pediatrics textbooks.
- Compile and distribute sample encounter forms, handouts, and smart phrases for electronic health records to support PIM clinical care.
- Develop an interprofessional online clinical resource repository.

Professional education

- Maximize distribution and utilization of PIM residency curriculum and fellowship programs.

- Facilitate a regularly occurring interprofessional conference to advance PIM education, leadership development, and to embrace and grow the PIM community.
- Present PIM content at pediatric subspecialty meetings and other health professional conferences, including those targeting the underserved.
- Participate in initiatives to address policy development for modern health problems such as chronic pain and opioid addiction that significantly impact children.

Patient and Family Education

- Develop multilingual descriptions of PIM therapies in child-friendly language.
- Increase PIM content on the AAP's parent information website (healthychildren.org) by adapting existing *Pediatrics in Review* articles.
- Develop an online video series featuring children and families discussing integrative care success stories.
- Develop a robust library of PIM patient handouts for widespread use in the clinical setting.

Advocacy and Partnerships

- Establish an online presence to serve as a strong independent voice advocating for PIM as mainstream pediatric healthcare, including a repository for research, clinical, and educational resources.
- Partner with disease-specific organizations to spread knowledge of PIM therapies that may improve quality of life for their stakeholders.
- Cultivate strong relationships with specialties also serving children, such as family medicine, medicine/pediatrics, and obstetrics/gynecology.
- Work with federal and state organizations to develop and promote preventive lifestyle policies for children and families.
- Contribute to resource development and advocacy efforts that support payment for PIM services and models of care.
- Explore sustainable resources for philanthropy to support ongoing growth of the field.

The group noted that these are considerable tasks and that an organization does not currently exist to oversee and coordinate all of these strategies. Meeting participants unanimously expressed a strong desire to explore the creation of an ongoing, sustainable PIMLI leadership group to coordinate this work. Immediate next steps were debated, leading to the development of specific action plans related to the above strategies and the delegation to participants. Finally, meeting participants prioritized the following activities most needing financial support:

- Sustainable support for the AAP SOIM research and education grant program.
- Re-printing and redistribution of the "Talk with Your Doctor" PIM poster (http://www.cpsp.cps.ca/uploads/publications/Posters-CAM.pdf) to pediatricians.
- Establishment of a new organization as the independent voice advocating for PIM as mainstream pediatric health care, engaging and nurturing current and future leaders of the PIM movement.

The first two activities were delegated to the AAP SOIM Executive Committee. A PIMLI steering committee was formed to pursue the third priority.

5. 2016 PIMLI Summit

With additional generous funding by the Marino Health Foundation, members of the PIMLI steering committee met in July 2016 at the Hackensack University Medical Center in New Jersey to further discuss the establishment of a new organization to coordinate PIM initiatives. In preparation for this meeting, key PIM stakeholders were consulted via an online survey to assess current community needs (unpublished data). Survey participants were recruited from two professional listservs: the IPIM Network and the AAP Section on Integrative Medicine listserv.

2016 Professional Survey Highlights

- A total 93 health professionals completed the survey.
- Approximately 75% identified as pediatricians (MD/DO) with a total of 17 professional disciplines represented.
- Approximately 50% had been in practice more than 20 years, and more than 80% had been in practice more than 10 years.
- Over 75% stated that currently available PIM resources online are not sufficient to support their pediatric practice.
- The top two most valuable current online PIM resources were the two listservs noted above; no current website was rated as valuable by more than 25% of respondents.

Conversations with key stakeholders and advisors confirmed the need and desire for an independent organization focused specifically on PIM education and advocacy, directed at the broad 'middle' of the professional and consumer populations. Challenges identified included: (1) prioritizing PIM both within a larger pediatric organization and within a larger integrative organization; (2) securing funding for administrative support given the significant ongoing clinical, research, and educational commitments of PIM leadership—creating a balanced interprofessional leadership group; and (3) nurturing leadership development to ensure sustainability of the organization. Understanding these obstacles, the PIMLI steering committee evaluated and debated potential partners to host this initiative, concluding that no existing group ideally met our needs. They proposed exploration of hosting an independent nonprofit organization as the first option. Paramount to the success of this organization would be the design and launch of a robust multimedia website that serves as a hub for all PIM activities, including:

- Membership for pediatric healthcare professionals providing specialized access to educational and community-building resources, including integrating existing interprofessional and international PIM networks (IPIM Network, PedCAM network).
- Consumer and policymaker engagement via media tools and the development of short promotional videos profiling PIM "success stories".
- Educational and Research Resource Repository, including professional presentations and a searchable PIM publication bibliography.
- Continuing education online conferences and webinars.
- Professional consultative service assisting the development of academic PIM centers and clinical practices.
- Coordination of PIM efforts with the AAP SOIM and other reputable national/international organizations.

Organizational structure and funding needs were discussed including potential funding partners and self-sustainable sources of support and leadership. Given the huge scope of the proposed activities above and the clearly expressed needs in the 2016 professional survey, the scope was initially narrowed to online PIM professional education, because opportunities to fill the gap of online educational resources currently exist. At this time, PIM education exists through the University of Arizona Center for Integrative Medicine: Pediatric Integrative Medicine in Residency (PIMR) curriculum for pediatric resident physicians, various continuing education conferences, and online resources [24]. The PIMR program consists of a 100-h online educational curriculum initially piloted in five diverse pediatric residency training programs in the United States. In 2016, the PIMR program had grown to include more than 500 residents nationally and internationally in nine residency programs. Of note, the PIMR program is specifically limited to pediatric resident physicians. The AAP SOIM sponsors PIM educational sessions each year at the AAP National Conference to a broader group of pediatricians, though these sessions are not accessible to many other PIM professional groups nor to nonmembers of the AAP. Ultimately, collaborative efforts to reinforce interactive and online curricula at various steps during training and practice may help to meet the demand for therapeutic options that are safe, effective, and aligned with patients' values. A comprehensive, accessible online professional PIM education hub would be optimally situated to meet the needs of the larger PIM community.

6. Vision for the Future

Based on work at the 2015 and 2016 Summits, long-range visions for PIM's next decade are outlined:

- PIM exemplifies a mainstream model of comprehensive care that emphasizes a personalized, participatory, and evidence-informed approach to the whole child.
- PIM emphasizes preventive health, understanding of the etiology of underlying illness, and exploration of all appropriate treatment options to optimize health and well-being.
- PIM promotes a cohesive, respectful, and interprofessional team approach focused on the well-being of the child as a growing, developing individual in the context of the family.
- Professionals collaborate across disciplines and geographic boundaries in advocating for the needs of patients and families from all socioeconomic and cultural backgrounds.
- Integrative professionals embrace self-care as a cornerstone of health.
- Integrative professionals support identification of and access to reliable PIM educational, clinical, and research resources for all those interested in maximizing patient health and wellness.

To achieve this vision, proposed tangible outcomes include:

- Establishment of an international and interprofessional pediatric group to coordinate and advance the work of PIM in collaboration with the AAP SOIM. This two-pronged approach ultimately represents the optimal strategy to ensure the sustainable growth, evolution, and impact of PIM within the field of Pediatrics.
- Medical schools, residencies, and other professional training programs teach PIM routinely and widely.
- Hospitals, clinics, and academic centers promote co-located PIM services (e.g., credentialing nurses and/or other providers and staff in biofeedback, aromatherapy, clinical hypnosis, etc.).
- Pediatric training programs implementing the PIMR curriculum and PIM fellowship programs experience high enrollment and active participation of alumni.
- A yearly interprofessional symposium is established and brings together PIM professionals for collaborative learning.
- PIM materials (e.g., description of therapies, licensing/credentialing information, clinical guidance, patient educational materials, research summaries, and updates) are compiled and hosted on an independent website for ready access by professionals, patients, and institutions.
- PIM research is adequately funded to develop the science of utilization, safety, efficacy, and cost-effectiveness of PIM therapies, and a multi-center research network is established to facilitate the acquisition of this knowledge.
- Safe, effective, and cost-effective PIM therapies and health care systems receive endorsement from national organizations, hospital leadership, and other decision makers to judiciously expand PIM as appropriate.

Author Contributions: A.E., S.M.M., and L.R. were the authors responsible for the conceptualization and writing of this manuscript; E.S., T.C., K.K., H.M., and S.V. contributed to the writing and editing of this manuscript.

Funding: The Pediatric Integrative Medicine Leadership Initiative Summit was funded by the Marino Health Foundation.

Acknowledgments: The Pediatric Integrative Medicine Leadership Initiative would like foremost to thank the Marino Health Foundation for its generous support of the 2015 and 2016 Summits and related work. The PIMLI would also like to acknowledge the American Academy of Pediatrics, in particular Teri Salus and Anne Gramiak, for their logistical support coordinating and facilitating the 2015 PIMLI Summit. PIMLI leaders are extremely grateful to John Weeks and the ACIH committee who helped in preparation for the 2015 Summit, and to *Kiwi Magazine* and the Moms Meet Network for assistance with the 2015 Parent Survey. Finally, the PIMLI group thanks the members of the PIM community who participated in the 2015 and 2016 professional surveys. Thank you to all the PIMLI leaders involved, in addition to the authors: Michelle Bailey, David Becker, Anu French, Scott Shannon, David M. Steinhorn, Minal Vazirani, and Ana Maria Verissimo.

Conflicts of Interest: The authors declare no conflict of interest. The funders had no role in the design of the summit, in the writing of the manuscript, or in the decision to publish the manuscript.

References

1. Academic Consortium for Integrative Medicine and Health. Available online: https://imconsortium.org/about/introduction/ (accessed on 27 August 2018).
2. Vohra, S.; Surette, S.; Mittra, D.; Rossen, L.D.; Gardiner, P.; Kemper, J.K. Pediatric integrative medicine: Pediatrics' newest subspecialty? *BMC Pediatr.* **2012**, *15*, 12–123. [CrossRef] [PubMed]
3. National Center for Health Statistics. *Health United States with Chartbook on Trends in the Health of Americans*; Table 58. Md; National Center for Health Statistics: Hyattsville, MA, USA, 2006.
4. Perrin, J.M.; Bloom, S.R.; Gortmaker, S.L. The increase of childhood chronic conditions in the United States. *JAMA* **2007**, *27*, 2755–2759. [CrossRef] [PubMed]
5. GBD 2015 DALYs and HALE Collaborators. Global, regional, and National disability-adjusted life-years (DALYs) for 315 diseases and injuries and healthy life expectancy (HALE), 1990–2015: A systematic analysis for the Global Burden of Disease Study 2015. *Lancet* **2016**, *8*, 1603–1658. [CrossRef]
6. Rabin, J.; Brown, M.; Alexander, S. Update in the treatment of chronic pain with pediatric patients. *Curr. Probl. Pediatr. Adolesc. Health Care* **2017**, *47*, 167–172. [CrossRef] [PubMed]
7. Jacobs, H.; Gladstein, J. Pediatric headache: A clinical review. *Headache* **2012**, *52*, 333–339. [CrossRef] [PubMed]
8. Powers, T.L.; Bendall, D. Improving health outcomes through patient empowerment. *J. Hosp. Mark. Public Relat.* **2003**, *15*, 45–59. [CrossRef]
9. Maizes, V.; Rakel, D.; Niemiec, C. Integrative medicine and patient-centered care. *Explore* **2009**, *5*, 277–289. [CrossRef] [PubMed]
10. Kemper, K.J. Holistic pediatrics = good medicine. *Pediatrics* **2001**, *105*, 214–218.
11. Becker, D.K. Pediatric Integrative Medicine. *Prim. Care* **2017**, *44*, 337–350. [CrossRef] [PubMed]
12. Kemper, K.J.; Vohra, S.; Walls, R.; Task Force on Complementary and Alternative Medicine; Provisional Section on Complementary, Holistic, and Integrative Medicine. American Academy of Pediatrics. The use of complementary and alternative medicine in pediatrics. *Pediatrics* **2008**, *122*, 1374–1386. [CrossRef] [PubMed]
13. NCCIH Children and the Use of Complementary Health Approaches. Available online: https://nccih.nih.gov/health/children#hed1 (accessed on 31 March 2017).
14. Slader, C.A.; Reddel, H.K.; Jenkins, C.R.; Armour, C.L.; Bosnic-Anticevich, S.Z. Complementary and alternative medicine use in asthma: Who is using what? *Respirology* **2006**, *11*, 373–387. [CrossRef] [PubMed]
15. Post-White, J.; Fitzgerald, M.; Hageness, S.; Sencer, S.F. Complementary and alternative medicine use in children with cancer and general and specialty pediatrics. *J. Pediatr. Oncol. Nurs.* **2009**, *26*, 7–15. [CrossRef] [PubMed]
16. Kemper, K.J.; O'Connor, K.G. Pediatricians' recommendations for complementary and alternative medical (CAM) therapies. *Ambul Pediatr.* **2004**, *4*, 482–487. [CrossRef] [PubMed]
17. Sackett, D.L.; Rosenberg, W.M.; Gray, J.A.; Haynes, R.B.; Richardson, W.S. Evidence-based medicine: What it is and what it isn't. *BMJ* **1996**, *13*, 71–72. [CrossRef]
18. Kemper, K.J.; Cohen, M. Ethics meet complementary and alternative medicine: New light on old principles. *Contem. Pediatr.* **2004**, 482–487.
19. Cost. Use of Complementary Health Approaches in U.S. Available online: https://nccih.nih.gov/research/statistics/NHIS/2012/cost (accessed on 13 August 2018).
20. Birdee, G.S.; Phillips, R.S.; Davis, R.B.; Gardiner, P. Factors associated with pediatric use of complementary and alternative medicine. *Pediatrics* **2010**, *125*, 249–256. [CrossRef] [PubMed]

21. Highfield, E.S.; McLellan, M.C.; Kemper, K.J.; Risko, W.; Woolf, A.D. Integration of complementary and alternative medicine in a major pediatric teaching hospital: An initial overview. *J Altern. Complement Med.* **2005**, *11*, 373–380. [CrossRef] [PubMed]
22. Lin, Y.C.; Lee, A.C.; Kemper, K.J.; Berde, C.B. Use of complementary and alternative medicine in pediatric pain management service: A survey. *Pain Med.* **2005**, *6*, 452–458. [CrossRef] [PubMed]
23. World Café Method. Available online: http://www.theworldcafe.com/key-concepts-resources/world-cafe-method (accessed on 31 March 2017).
24. McClafferty, H.; Dodds, S.; Brooks, A.J.; Brenner, M.G.; Brown, M.L.; Fraizer, P.; Mark, J.D.; Weydert, J.A.; Wilcox, G.M.G.; Lebensohn, P.; et al. Pediatric Integrative Medicine in Residency (PIMR): Description of a New Online Educational Curriculum. *Children* **2015**, *17*, 98–107. [CrossRef] [PubMed]

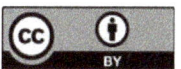

© 2018 by the authors. Licensee MDPI, Basel, Switzerland. This article is an open access article distributed under the terms and conditions of the Creative Commons Attribution (CC BY) license (http://creativecommons.org/licenses/by/4.0/).

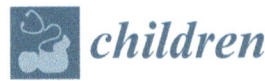

Correction

Correction: Esparham, A., et al., Pediatric Integrative Medicine: Vision for the Future. *Children*, 2018, 5, 111

Anna Esparham [1,*], Sanghamitra M. Misra [2], Erica Sibinga [3], Timothy Culbert [4], Kathi Kemper [5], Hilary McClafferty [6], Sunita Vohra [7] and Lawrence Rosen [8]

1. Division of Child Neurology-Headache Section, Children's Mercy Hospital, University of Missouri School of Medicine-Kansas City, Kansas City, MO 64108, USA
2. Mobile Clinic Program, Texas Children's Hospital, Baylor College of Medicine, Houston, TX 77054, USA; smisra@bcm.edu
3. Department of Pediatrics, Johns Hopkins School of Medicine, Baltimore, MD 21205, USA; esibinga@jhmi.edu
4. Integrative Medicine, Prairie Care, University of Minnesota Medical School, Chaska, MN 55318, USA; tculbert@prairie-care.com
5. Department of Pediatrics, College of Medicine, Ohio State University, Columbus, OH 43210, USA; kathi.kemper@osumc.edu
6. Department of Medicine, Arizona Center for Integrative Medicine, University of Arizona, Tucson, AZ 85724, USA; hmcclafferty@email.arizona.edu
7. Integrative Health Institute, CARE Program, PedCAM Network, Department of Pediatrics, Medicine, and Psychiatry, Faculty of Medicine and Dentistry, University of Alberta, Edmonton, AB T6G 2C8, Canada; svohra@ualberta.ca
8. Whole Child Center, Oradell, NJ 07649, USA; ldrdoc@alum.mit.edu
* Correspondence: aeesparham@cmh.edu; Tel.: +1-816-302-3320

Received: 29 August 2018; Accepted: 30 August 2018; Published: 5 September 2018

The authors wish to make the following corrections to their paper [1]:

The middle initial has been added to the name of co-author Sanghamitra Misra. The correct name is Sanghamitra M. Misra.

The citation website link to the first reference in the original paper is now unavailable. The correct reference is as follows:

1. Academic Consortium for Integrative Medicine and Health. Available Online: https://imconsortium.org/about/introduction/ (accessed on 27 August 2018).

In addition, we found that the organization name listed in Section 4 (p. 5) and in the acknowledgments section is incorrect—the reference to the Academic Consortium for Integrative Medicine and Health (ACIHM) is incorrect. The correct organization name is the Academic Collaborative for Integrative Health (ACIH). The corrected last sentence of the second paragraph in Section 4 is as follows:

Specifically, with organizational support by John Weeks, a pioneer in collaborative interprofessional IM efforts over several decades, representatives from the Academic Collaborative for Integrative Health (ACIH) participated in a comprehensive pre-summit survey.

The corrected acknowledgments are as follows:

Acknowledgments: The Pediatric Integrative Medicine Leadership Initiative would like foremost to thank the Marino Health Foundation for its generous support of the 2015 and 2016 summits and related work. The PIMLI would also like to acknowledge the American Academy of Pediatrics, in particular Teri Salus and Anne Gramiak, for their logistical support coordinating and facilitating the 2015 PIMLI Summit. PIMLI leaders are extremely grateful to John Weeks and the ACIH committee who helped in preparation for the 2015 summit, and to Kiwi Magazine and the Moms Meet Network for assistance with the 2015 Parent Survey. Finally, the PIMLI group thanks the members of the PIM community who participated in the 2015 and 2016 professional surveys. Thank you to all the PIMLI leaders involved, in addition to the authors: Michelle Bailey, David Becker, Anu French, Scott Shannon, David M. Steinhorn, Minal Vazirani, and Ana Maria Verissimo.

The authors would like to apologize for any inconvenience caused to the readers by these changes that do not affect the scientific results. The manuscript will be updated and the original will remain on the article webpage, with a reference to this Correction.

Reference

1. Esparham, A.; Misra, S.M.; Sibinga, E.; Culbert, T.; Kemper, K.; McClafferty, H.; Vohra, S.; Rosen, L. Pediatric Integrative Medicine: Vision for the Future. *Children* **2018**, *5*, 111. [CrossRef] [PubMed]

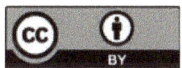

© 2018 by the authors. Licensee MDPI, Basel, Switzerland. This article is an open access article distributed under the terms and conditions of the Creative Commons Attribution (CC BY) license (http://creativecommons.org/licenses/by/4.0/).

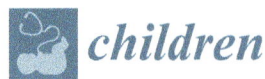

Review

Integrating Pediatric Hypnosis with Complementary Modalities: Clinical Perspectives on Personalized Treatment

Pamela Kaiser [1,*], **Daniel P. Kohen** [1,2,3], **Melanie L. Brown** [3,4], **Rebecca L. Kajander** [1] **and Andrew J. Barnes** [1,3]

1. National Pediatric Hypnosis Training Institute (NPHTI), 29 Western Terrace, Minneapolis, MN 55426, USA; dpkohen@umn.edu (D.P.K.); rebeccakajander@gmail.com (R.L.K.); drbarnes@umn.edu (A.J.B.)
2. Partners-in-Healing, 10505 Wayzata Blvd #200, Minnetonka, MN 55305, USA
3. Department of Pediatrics, University of Minnesota, 717 Delaware St SE #353, Minneapolis, MN 55414, USA; melanie.brown@childrensmn.org
4. Children's Hospitals and Clinics of Minnesota, 2525 Chicago Ave, Minneapolis, MN 55404, USA
* Correspondence: drpkaiser@gmail.com; Tel.: +1-650-323-2222

Received: 15 June 2018; Accepted: 31 July 2018; Published: 7 August 2018

Abstract: While pediatric integrative medicine (PIM) emphasizes an "evidence-based practice using multiple therapeutic modalities"; paradoxically, literature reviews examining the prevalence and/or efficacy of such mind–body approaches often address PIM modalities separately. Such contributions are relevant, yet documentation of how to deliver combined complementary approaches in children and youth are scarce. Nevertheless, integrative practitioners in clinical practice routinely mix approaches to meet the individual needs of each patient. Best practices are flexible, and include blending and augmenting services within the same session, and/or connecting modalities sequentially for an incremental effect, and/or referring to outside resources for additional interventions. Resonating with integrative medicine's definition, this article's goal is to demonstrate paradigms that "bring together complementary approaches in a coordinated way within clinical practice" by linking clinical hypnosis, the trail-blazer modality in PIM's history, with mindfulness, biofeedback, acupuncture, and yoga. Following the consideration of the overlap of guided imagery with hypnosis and an abridged literature report, this clinical perspective considers the selection of modalities within a collaborative relationship with the child/teen and parents, emphasizing goodness-of-fit with patients' contexts, e.g., symptoms, resources, interests, goals, and developmental stage. Case vignettes illustrate practical strategies for mixing approaches.

Keywords: integrative medicine; hypnosis; mindfulness; biofeedback; acupuncture; yoga; guided imagery; self-regulation; complementary; education

1. Introduction

1.1. Clinical Hypnosis: The Roots of Pediatric Integrative Medicine (PIM)

The cornerstone of pediatric mind–body approaches is clinical hypnosis—i.e., positive, mastery-oriented suggestions coupled with imagery to optimize individualized goals related to health, well-being, self-regulation, and resilience [1,2]—which supports a family [3] and preventative [4] perspective [5]. This approach is unified by utilization of the child's internal resources, interests, context, and capacity for healthy dissociation and imaginative involvement [6,7].

Although pediatric integrative medicine (PIM) is one of the newest recognized academic subspecialties [8], the clinical utility of hypnosis has long been recognized as an approach complementary to conventional medicine and has been cited in the medical literature within the past two centuries [9]. Fundamental to PIM's growth and credibility, the field of pediatric hypnosis (see overviews of research [5] and training [10]) began to distinguish itself as a mind–body modality in the 1960s–1980s.

Clinical hypnosis helped set the standard for the broad applications of pediatric integrative health. Groundbreaking publications addressed its efficacy in combination with or in lieu of conventional medical approaches for a remarkable range of pediatric health issues. These have included hypnosis for pediatric learning problems [11–13], anesthesia [14], asthma [15], drug abuse [16], burns [17], enuresis [18–20], functional megacolon [21], warts [22], sleep disorders [23,24], habit disorders [1], autism [25], pelvic exams [26], cancer [2], pain and procedure-related anxiety [27], psychoneuroimmunology [28,29], healing [30], refractory irritable bowel syndrome [31], hemophilia [32], chronic illness [33], hospitalization [34], emergencies [35], aphasia [36], Tourette's syndrome [37–39], migraine [40,41], sickle cell disease [42], chemotherapy-related nausea and vomiting [43], and behavioral issues [44].

Current reviews highlight further evidence- and empirically-based incorporation of hypnosis for children's health care [5,45–48]. Applications to specific behavioral and physical concerns and contexts include anxiety [49,50], asthma [51], cystic fibrosis [52], dental issues [53], enuresis [54], habits [55], headaches [56], vocal cord dysfunction [57], pain [58,59], palliative care [60], primary care [61], psychoneuroimmunology [62], and the potential value in pediatric inflammatory bowel disease [63].

One particularly exciting area of research is the work of Vlieger's team in the Netherlands showing strong efficacy of pediatric hypnosis as the sole treatment for gut disorders. For example, in double-blind study gut-directed hypnotherapy (HT) was shown to be highly effective for pain frequency and intensity in pediatric patients (ages 8–18) with diagnoses of functional abdominal pain or irritable bowel syndrome compared to standard medical therapy (SMT), with continued efficacy at one year follow-up (85% for HT group compared to 25% for SMT group) [64]. Subsequent studies by the same group showed similar results [65–67].

Going forward, hypnosis' cutting-edge research includes the work of Amir Raz, Ph.D., Canada Research Chair in the Cognitive Neuroscience of Attention at the Department of Psychiatry at McGill University. The thrust of his team's and colleagues' cognitive neuroscience and neuroimaging studies is to expand the understanding of hypnosis' underlying mechanisms related to attention, self-regulation, expectation, and consciousness [68].

1.2. Guided Imagery vs. Hypnosis

Definitive conclusions about the value of pediatric guided imagery (GI) are obscured by a muddle of inaccurate and contradictory differentiations from clinical hypnosis [69,70], the overlap of the two approaches, and GI's low methodological quality of research to date [71–73]. It is difficult to find a clear definition of GI distinguishing it from clinical hypnosis, given mistaken assertions—e.g., that pediatric hypnosis does not involve imagery [73–75]. Even professional organizations (and many GI websites) struggle with accurate differentiation [76,77].

While there is some evidence for the efficacy of GI scripts [71], the literature suggests that this modality—infused with hypnotic elements—could be analogous to the clinician-designed hypnotic experience. Congruence between hypnosis and GI include the involvement of the child's senses, incorporation of their imagination, focus on attention, and enhancement of well-being and self-regulation. Like GI, combining imagery while tapping the child's senses is routinely used in pediatric hypnosis [78] and both often incorporate relaxation. Further support for this hypothesis is the literature's repeated recognition of these overlapping elements. Martin Rossman, MD (a student of hypnosis and early advocate of GI) borrowed from Ericksonian hypnosis and other popular modalities to delineate key GI steps for 'healing' various health conditions. In point of fact, all but one are hypnotic elements [69]. We can only speculate that perhaps the 1970s origins of this modality stem, even if only in part, from a purposeful disengagement from the myths and other negative preconceived notions associated with the term 'hypnosis'. The inter-relation between the two continues: a current review of high-quality studies of gut-directed hypnotherapy for children included guided imagery with the rationale that GI "is a technique that is highly comparable to hypnotherapy, because both are using relaxation and imageries and both aim to change mental and physical experiences with the use of suggestions" (p. 223) [79]. Beyond this blended/overlapping view, some authors explicitly consider the two modalities as completely equivalent [80–82].

It is important to clarify the mistaken assumption of some authors that hypnosis does not include imagery. Experts from the 1800s to recent times note "the importance of imagery and its integral role in hypnosis, particularly in children" (p. 21) [44]. In a 1984 seminal article entitled "Use of Relaxation-Mental Imagery (Self-Hypnosis) in the Management of 505 Pediatric Behavioral Encounters", the protocol included the "cultivation of natural imaginative skills" (p. 22) [44]. Another key paper described hypnosis "as a process of 'cultivation of imagination' for the patient's own benefit" [44].

One clear disparity between hypnosis and GI is the required intensive training in pediatric hypnosis for licensed clinicians with advanced degrees to design tailor-made, individualized sessions vs. the abundant, ready-made GI scripts available to clinicians and lay people. The non-profit National Pediatric Hypnosis Training Institute (www.NPHTI.org) offers the only recurring pediatric-specific clinical hypnosis skills training workshops in North America. NPHTI provides extensive, supervised experiential learning practice of skills as well as to become adept with careful monitoring of each patient's psychophysiological phenomena and responses; checking in as needed and adjusting the pacing, content, delivery, and prosody (voice speed, cadence, etc.) of the thoughtfully planned, goal-related suggestions, rich imagery, and metaphoric stories.

By contrast, the author of GI scripts imposes his/her own imagery onto the child/teen which could be inferred incorrectly that children prefer that sensory modality and type of imagery. Such scripts written for "every patient" are read-aloud by the clinician or lay people who must look at their paper rather than attending to the content's impact on their patient. A recent study found that the use of a home-based CD-script vs. a therapist-read script (followed by the same home-based CD) for students with IBS, FAP, or FAPS had comparably very favorable results [67]. Based on the article's description of the delivery of these approaches, it appears that this was a comparison of *two ways of delivering an identical GI script.* Furthermore, there were a number of qualified subjects dropped due to insufficient motivation, either due to preference for a therapist-led intervention or lack of interest in protocol requirements. Clearly, the researchers are to be commended for an otherwise exquisitely designed study, including controlling for relevant confounders (e.g., anxiety and depression) in this demonstration of a cost-effective intervention for a large group of children. Because it is our opinion that a personalized approach optimizes the potential for a meaningful therapeutic outcome, hopefully, future studies will contrast the individually designed intervention of pediatric hypnosis with these two different modes of script delivery.

1.3. Integrating Hypnosis with PIM

Other pediatric mind–body approaches also share some elements with hypnosis: mindfulness, biofeedback, yoga (and perhaps to a lesser degree) acupuncture also utilize the child/teen's unfolding curiosity for novelty and learning; overall motivation for mastery; capacity for focused, narrowed attention; openness to positive suggestions and expanding internal resources; and willingness to practice emerging skills. Breath is often incorporated and patients learn the easily accessible value of slowed, diaphragmatic ('belly') breathing to activate the parasympathetic nervous system (aka the 'calming control center'). It may be safe to say that the over-arching intent of mind–body modalities is to offer these "gifts" to maximize one's own health, well-being, self-regulation, self-confidence, and self-efficacy.

Following a brief synopsis of the literature, the following sections offer clinical perspectives from clinicians on *how* to interlink hypnosis with four distinct complementary mind–body approaches (mindfulness, biofeedback, acupuncture, and yoga). The additional case vignettes illustrate ways to blend PIM approaches, highlighting the importance of context for goodness-of-fit as well as practical points and considerations when personalizing PIM treatment.

2. Integrating Mindfulness and Hypnosis

2.1. Background

A specific form of meditative practice called "mindfulness" was popularized by Jon Kabat-Zinn [83,84] who defined mindfulness as "the awareness that emerges through paying attention on purpose, in the present moment, and non-judgmentally to the unfolding of experience moment by moment" [85]. Early works by Kabat-Zinn summarized the history of mindfulness as well as its emergence into clinical contexts as a broadened approach to mind–body interventions.

Mindfulness continues to gain popularity, with an increasing presence in school curricula, workplace wellbeing initiatives, and health care settings. In clinics and hospitals, mindfulness-based stress reduction is prototypical of such practices in health care, first developed as a program to relieve suffering among adults with chronic conditions [86]. Similar practices have been used in other therapies (albeit not necessarily called 'mindfulness') including acceptance and commitment therapy, dialectical-behavioral therapy, and mindfulness-based cognitive therapy [87].

Experience-based practice with formal meditative approaches (such as the body scan, moving meditation, and sitting meditation) and informal meditation during everyday activities (such as eating) are called "guided mindfulness meditations" because they use in-person or recorded instructions. Collectively, these guided experiences and self-directed practices are called mindfulness-based practices (MBPs) [87]. Some MBPs are delivered in a group format, others individually, and others a combination. A number of apps, recordings, and lay-press books detail mindfulness activities for children and adolescents, and these very frequently include developmentally-tailored exercises and therapeutic metaphors (e.g., Sitting Still Like a Frog [88] and Breathe, Think, Do with Sesame [89]).

Guided mindfulness and other MBPs differ from clinical hypnosis in that the former is rooted within a contemplative philosophy with historical roots that did not include therapeutic goals. The hallmark of hypnosis is the use of specific therapeutic suggestions oriented towards one or more health-related goals. However, as therapist Michael Yapko, Ph.D. points out in his seminal book, *Mindfulness and Hypnosis: The Power of Suggestion to Transform Experience* [90], mindfulness applied in a clinical context always implies goal-oriented changes in one's health or experience of health (as opposed to mindfulness practiced for spiritual contemplation). Thus, both mindfulness and hypnosis training done with a health professional require some level of interactional suggestions that, at the very least, facilitate a patient's focus, absorption, and awareness to achieve therapeutic outcomes. For these reasons, Yapko advocates for clinicians using MBPs to develop a deep understanding of hypnotic suggestion, verbal and nonverbal communication, and inter- and intra-personal processes. Furthermore, the precise terminology used in clinical practice (mindfulness, hypnosis, et al.) is perhaps less important than gaining an appreciation for both hypnosis and mindfulness as processes that lead to self-regulation and associated neurobiological changes.

In fact, therapeutic goals are now a common component of mindfulness and simple MBPs as part of an integrative approach for children with psychological and mind–body issues, including those with chronic worries; rumination or being too 'in their heads'; many 'what-ifs' who seek frequent reassurance; frequent over-estimation of the potential for negatives such as risk, threat, or danger; generalized anxiety disorder; major depression; and/or sleep-onset or sleep-maintenance insomnia. This modality is perfect to help these children and youth quiet their minds and be more fully present in the current moment (instead of being 'stuck' in the imagined negative future). This can be practiced and summarized with children and adolescents briefly with these simple steps developed by the first author (P.K.):

- Focus your attention on being present, in this very moment ... now THIS very moment ... now THIS very moment ...

- Amplify this moment-to-moment awareness by focusing on your five senses: be aware of what you hear NOW, what you see NOW, what you feel NOW, what you smell NOW, and what you taste NOW ... and integrate that to being just present in this very moment ...
- NOW, the final of the three steps: Create a feeling of deep Appreciation ... it could be for your pet, your friend or another wonderful person, the shower, your favorite food, the sunset, your bed, or anything else that you really truly are grateful for.

Pediatric well-being can be improved through guided mindfulness and other MBPs in other contexts. A recent meta-analysis of MBPs in children and adolescents showed positive effects on academic achievement, school functioning, negative emotionality, subjective distress, internalizing symptoms, and a number of physical health indicators [91]. For example, in a randomized controlled trial, African-American teens with elevated blood pressure were taught to sit "upright in a comfortable position with eyes closed ... focus on diaphragm movements while breathing ... acknowledge and accept [unwanted thoughts, ideas or images] without making judgments about them and shift attention back to diaphragmatic breathing", and encouraged to practice this for 10 min before and after school for three months. The MBP group had significant reductions in systolic blood pressure during the school day and at night, as well as decreased urinary excretion of sodium and resting heart rate [92]. MBPs are also being investigated to help reverse the impact of trauma and adversity during childhood [93] and to help parents of children with intellectual and developmental differences to decrease parenting stress and indirectly promote behavioral competence in their children [94]. Some of the MBPs studied in children have shown benefits with just one session of guided mindfulness, whereas others have used multiple guided sessions with active home practice.

Other elements now thought to be important to such mindfulness-based programs that strikingly overlap with the inherent phenomena, process, and purposes of hypnosis include (a) dissociating from, and letting go of reactive or distressing thoughts and feelings and (b) cultivating absorbed attention, intention, and evoking curiosity to foster emotional-behavioral self-regulation [87]. Further, mental imagery a mainstay of clinical hypnosis, is now commonly used within various MBPs, e.g., by suggesting that feelings or thoughts are like moving ants on a log floating down a river in order to help shift from ruminative or perseverative thinking to more flexible thinking or positive alterative thoughts.

Ongoing research aims to better specify the ways in which mindfulness and hypnosis work, including the extent to which they affect the central nervous system [95,96]. One example of the practical overlap between hypnosis and mindfulness can be seen in a series of studies in which four-to-six-year-olds were instructed to pretend to be "an exemplar other [such as Batman]". These young children performed better on tasks of executive function and perseverance than did their peers who were instructed to take either a first-person or third-person perspective on themselves [97,98]. The utilization of the hero as a figure in play is also a classic developmental marker of preschool- and early-school-aged children's beneficial use of imagination. Thus, the imaginative suggestions to embody a powerful hero are commonly employed in self-hypnosis with children at this developmental stage, and the resulting 'self-distancing' is often part of mindfulness-based approaches. The outcome of this hero-role-play—improved executive function—demonstrates how self-regulation can be promoted in children, tailored to their developmental level, through the integration of mindfulness and hypnosis.

In a similar way, "jettison" techniques [5] blend mindful awareness with hypnotic phenomena, and are particular well-suited to school-age and adolescent patients—these strategies use self-generated imagery (e.g., picturing a distressful emotion as a shape, color, or other metaphor such as a liquid in the body) and focused sensorimotor action (e.g., to allow the pictured emotion to 'flow' or 'move' gradually down an arm into a fist that clenches to hold the emotional imagery until it is 'released' as the fisted fingers release and relax as if a faucet opening) to 'externalize' and self-regulate emotions—clearly blending mindfulness with hypnosis.

To further underline the commonalities between pediatric clinical hypnosis and MBPs, children and adolescents who learn self-hypnosis in clinical settings will frequently and spontaneously refer to their home practice as 'meditation'. Indeed, when invited to demonstrate their self-hypnosis to the clinician or parent, some young people will adopt a stereotypical meditative posture such as the index fingers touching the thumbs while the dorsum of each hand rests upon each knee (which is itself a yogic pose called 'gyan mudra', symbolizing attunement with higher power, wisdom, and knowledge).

Regardless of whether it is called mindfulness, meditation, hypnosis, or something else made up like "that thing the doctor showed me how to do", such child-generated language is to be encouraged and built upon, not only as hypnotic ego-strengthening and utilization of a child's individual strengths and talents, but also as post-hypnotic suggestions that empower children to apply therapeutic strategies across contexts. Because of the powerful self-regulation that can result from mindfulness-based hypnotic approaches as summarized above, clinical applications can include decreasing ruminative cognitions among vulnerable children [99], and preventive care and general health promotion from infancy through adolescence [9].

Best practices for mindfulness-based hypnosis [100] in pediatrics include a strong relationship (rapport and therapeutic resonance) with the patient and family, in addition to a thorough understanding of the patient's developmental level, history, and temperament. For children with a cognitive level of 8–10 years or less, it is often helpful to help parents learn these approaches for themselves and also how to best incorporate them into their daily routine with their child (either as something each person does individually or as a collective experience). For older children and adolescents, having a recording with which to practice can also be useful, especially for children who are just learning. At times, mindfulness-based approaches can be taught first, and hypnotic approaches added to this later—this can work especially well for children with shorter attention spans or who do not enjoy or have facility with mental imagery, because such children can benefit from brief mindfully-oriented strategies to re-orient their awareness (i.e., 1-to-5-min practices). With practice, these children can utilize more complex and longer hypnotic strategies with or without imagery (e.g., with cognitively-behaviorally oriented suggestions). For children with longer attention spans, or who enjoy physical activity or more kinesthetic experiences, active/alert hypnosis can be taught first (e.g., with eyes open, standing/moving) and mindfulness added over time through activity-based practices (such as moving a hula hoop gradually up the body as a 'body scan' to engage somatic awareness). For children who are very imaginative, imagery-oriented, and/or have average-to-high executive function or attention spans, hypnosis and mindfulness can be seamlessly woven together from the outset for sessions of 5–20 min in length—some children will make their preferences for various approaches known over time, so longitudinal dialogue and debriefing with each individual patient and family about how they do their ongoing practice is essential for the clinician to learn how and when to blend approaches or lean more heavily on one approach.

2.2. Case Example

M. was first referred to the developmental-behavioral pediatrician at age 10 by his psychiatrist for recurrent abdominal pain. The psychiatrist had previously diagnosed M. with attention-deficit/hyperactivity disorder, inattentive type, co-occurring with generalized anxiety disorder, each treated with appropriate medications that had somewhat improved his ability to manage the symptoms of these conditions. These medications did not seem to affect his abdominal pain for better or worse, and a thorough medical evaluation by his primary care physician had confirmed the diagnosis of recurrent abdominal pain. His mother said that at home he would often cry in the morning due to the pain, and many nights he would "work himself up" worrying about the pain recurring the next day. His mother also indicated in private that he had experienced high levels of family dysfunction and maltreatment in early childhood. He presented as a thin, somewhat disheveled-appearing boy who was distracted, inattentive, and behaviorally inhibited. He spoke tentatively and with much elaboration about the characteristics of the pain, saying only "it hurts a lot sometimes" in the periumbilical region and could be "dull", occurring most often before school.

The first visit's goals were to establish therapeutic resonance and to help M develop new ways of discriminating various levels of comfort. To do so, after acknowledging the reality of M.'s physical pain, the clinician reframed it as "discomfort" and affirming his "strength ... shown so well already ... because that's what it means to get to school every morning even if we're feeling uncomfortable". The clinician 'wondered' with M. about "what else (he) might notice between today and the next visit about how the body feels or what the brain is thinking right before, or during, or even after, the discomfort shows up" to evoke M.'s curiosity and enlist his ability to be mindful, i.e., "pay attention on purpose", of his experiences. At the following visit, M. said he had noticed that his "heart beat differently, like not faster but weird" right before an episode of abdominal discomfort. The clinician affirmed this new awareness, then began to teach M. about mindfulness: being aware of bodily sensations and perceptions when "the heart started to beat differently, and if the breathing changed or the chest changed in other ways, and when that abdomen began to feel any change in its level of comfort, and when any other parts had other differences in how they felt" (this language was also chosen to help him learn to distance himself from his bodily sensations when in pain, also known as hypnotic dissociation).

The clinician then got out his stethoscope and offered to teach M. how to use it, and M. responded with interest. As M. began to listen to his heartbeat, the clinician suggested that he "just notice the little or big differences" in his heart rate when inhaling vs. exhaling vs. holding his breath vs. hyperventilating. As he did so, he became very attentionally absorbed, and gradually began to smile. When he took off the stethoscope, the clinician asked him what else he noticed physically at that moment, and he responded that his entire body felt "relaxed" and that his abdominal area felt "calm and cool". He was instructed to become more and more aware of sensory changes, in the tradition of a mindful body scan, i.e., "just take a few moments, or a few minutes, one or two or more times every day for the next two week, to check in with your body and notice how every part is feeling ... like changes in temperature, or changes in how heavy or light a part feels, or tingly, or bigger or smaller, or differences between one side or area and another, or even colors that might look different on the skin if any part needs calming or cooling or comfort, then you can make that happen, because you discovered how to do that just now." He was instructed to do this practice in the manner of alert hypnosis (i.e., eyes open with focused attention) although no specific name was given to him for this practice.

Several visits later, M. reported that he had been regularly practicing his "noticing" (his word for the body scan) and his abdominal pain had completely abated. Over the next five years, his abdominal pain remained in full remission. He had transient, intermittent episodes of milder somatic complaints as well as mood difficulties, usually during times of life transition such as starting at a new school. Over time, with the clinician's guidance, he discussed the traumatic events and adversity he had faced earlier in his childhood and connected these experiences to "stress ... and stress makes me have more (aches and pains) and be crabby".

At this time (a bit more than five years after the initial visit) the clinician invited him to learn self-hypnosis to address the long-term goal of handling stress more effectively, and he said he was motivated to do so. To begin, he was simply asked to do the "noticing" body scan that he had previously found helpful; as he did so, he spontaneously closed his eyes and the clinician suggested he talk aloud to himself as he noticed each part of his body felt. The clinician then suggested he could "change any of those (sensations) now if they're not yet comfortable, or just allow them to be how they are until they change themselves to be more comfortable". Suggestions for self-paced stress reduction were then permissively offered, included metaphoric imagery such as letting go of one or more balloons filled with stress and watching them slowly rise, the stress getting smaller and smaller as the balloons went higher and higher into the sky, as well as imagery for strength such as pulling a heavy load of stress and watching it get smaller and eventually fade away to nothing as he got stronger and pulled it further. It was further suggested that by pulling that heavy load so far, he had become so strong that most stressors would bounce off of him and the few that did not bounce off would be easy for him to move around or transform into something harmless. He was then offered post-hypnotic suggestions, i.e., suggestions given during the hypnotic experience to be recalled and used with automaticity within the context of the patient's everyday life, for a "power word" of M's choosing, that he could use every time he would be practicing self-hypnosis at home which would then allow him to quickly and easily engage this "inner-strength stress-relief system" during times of distress or recovery from stressors. M. continues to do this self-hypnosis practice several times per week and uses his "power word" to deal effectively with life's ups and downs, including interpersonal relationships, family transitions, and school.

2.3. Summary

In the case of M., the session with the stethoscope integrated a mindfulness-based approach (i.e., body scan and nonjudgmental awareness of, and ability to distance himself from (dissociate), unpleasant physical sensations) to promote M. orienting towards (instead of avoiding) his somatic experiences in a neutral manner, and as a hypnotic and post-hypnotic suggestion for self-regulation of neurophysiology (e.g., pain perception and stress reactivity). His subsequent use of these strategies on his own demonstrates the enduring value of mindfulness-oriented self-hypnotic approaches that empower young people who have faced chronic 'toxic' stress.

3. Integrating Biofeedback and Hypnosis

3.1. Background

Similar to hypnosis—and hypnosis with children [9,101–103]—biofeedback has had fluctuating definitions in its extensive literature [104–106]. Most theorists would agree that biofeedback utilizes technology typically with computer-based equipment to monitor a patient's various physiologic functions and in real time relay this to the patient, i.e., feed these measurements back to the patient for their use in acknowledging and then manipulating/altering the physiologic variable in the direction of a pre-determined, agreed-upon therapeutic direction and outcome [104,107,108]. Modern advances in computer technology commonly display the feedback in sophisticated, colorful, and engaging visual and/or auditory modes. This feedback is also used by the clinician to assess and monitor the patient's responses to events during the session (e.g., to specific suggestions for relaxation and/or mental imagery).

It is common, appropriate, and effective to invite children to consider and learn computerized biofeedback by presenting it as a "video game for your body". With the everyday, even constant availability and prevalence of videogames, high tech formats are relevant and syntonic with popular culture, so much so that 'apps' on smart-phones and 'smart watches' and other portable devices now can and do provide multiple biofeedback options to children and adults alike, not to mention comparable resources on social media. Indeed, they are even promoted as therapeutic devices (e.g., Inner Balance from Heartmath [109], Elvira Lang's "My Comfort Talk" [110], Ben Furman's "KIDS SKILLS" [111]). Types of feedback modalities commonly and typically utilized are heart rate variability for children with anxiety, stress, positional orthostatic tachycardia syndrome (POTS), and a host of other conditions (www.heartmath.com); or EMG (electromyography) and peripheral skin temperature for migraine headaches [112,113].

It has been our experience that most, if not all, biofeedback with children includes hypnotic suggestions whether or not 'named' and/or intended as such. Increasingly, even more extensive hypnotherapeutic procedures are commonly and often elegantly integrated with the electronic feedback information and re-structuring of that information in the direction of the collaboratively agreed upon (between children, parents, and clinician) therapeutic outcomes. In clinical as well as research studies, reference to, or identification of, the hypnotic elements are barely mentioned in passing if at all. For example, in most scientific paper describing biofeedback research, several paragraphs are often devoted to a description of the electronic monitoring equipment and the nature of the electrodes and operating systems, before a one- or two-line statement almost blithely states something like "and the child was instructed to relax and imagine a favorite activity". This obvious hypnotic invitation/suggestion is rarely characterized as such though it seems it is integral to the clinical experience and, we believe, to the success of the therapeutic intervention. To our knowledge, no one has sought to discriminate the differential influence of the biofeedback process vs. the hypnotic suggestions per se.

As the biofeedback experience proceeds, and particularly as the clinician observes the 'results' of improving physiologic regulation, the clinician commonly offers 'ego-strengthening' suggestions including compliments and verbal feedback that the subject is 'doing well', doing it 'right', and 'the more you do it the better you get'. These reinforcing hypnotic suggestions are often used to provide future-oriented (i.e., 'post-hypnotic') suggestions for continued practice/rehearsal of the hypnotic-biofeedback strategy at home as a self-empowerment approach. Because anxious children typically experience exaggerated psychophysiological stress reactivity, they benefit from learning relaxation skills and self-regulation strategies to reduce over-arousal [5]. Examples include "as you notice on the computer how well you have slowed your breathing ... "; or "while your skin temperature is going up in your fingertips, it's great to notice how much your headache is going away"; or "the more you notice how relaxed your muscles are, just realize and notice how happy and proud you feel, and how those worries are disappearing ... and the more you do this every day for 5 or 10 min, the more and sooner you'll be successful (in resolving that (problem) or eliminating that (pain, anxiety, worry)".

We have come to understand that biofeedback is a form of self-hypnosis and self-hypnosis is the ultimate form of biofeedback [108]. More than 40 years ago, the late Psychologist, Beata Jencks, Ph.D. published Your Body-Biofeedback at its Best [114] reflecting her initial training in the art of J.H. Schultz's "Standard Autogenic Training" and her emphasis on Mind–body integration. Jencks' work had substantial influence in a study applying hypnosis and pulmonary function biofeedback in a preschool family asthma education program [15].

Writing in the first textbook on Integrative Pediatrics in the chapter "A Pediatric Perspective on Mind–body Medicine" Kohen wrote about the hypnosis/biofeedback interface:

> Hypnosis and biofeedback are strategies directed at evoking innate experiential resources to alter psycho-physiologic responses which have become maladaptive. Hypnosis relies on the resonance and rapport of a therapeutic relationship and the language of positive expectancy to (help the child to) cultivate the imagination. Biofeedback provides an external somatic focus as a proxy for internal psycho-physiological change. BOTH involve narrowly focused, intensified attention and heightened responsiveness to new ideas and associations. This 'trance' state can be reinforced by the clinician's therapeutic language AND by the nature of the electronic/computerized information being received in the feedback. [115] (p. 287)

3.2. Case Example

A 12-year-old boy, F., was referred to the developmental-behavioral pediatrician by his primary care pediatrician for the presenting complaint of school phobia. Though his school refusal had begun soon after the beginning of his first semester in 6th grade in his first year at the Junior High School, most of his elementary school peers were in the same school and as a good student he did not find the classes difficult or the teachers challenging, intimidating, or otherwise problematic. In fact, as is often the case, academic or peer-related anxiety was not the concern.

He reportedly had "difficulty falling asleep" though this too was a function of underlying separation anxiety and not insomnia or other sleep disorder. He spoke of being afraid of the dark, not liking it, and being upset that his parents and siblings were asleep before he was, i.e., that he was the one awake and, "What if something happens?!" His mother noted that even when he told his parents he was "feeling fine now" and would "baby-sit" his younger six-year-old sister when the parents were going out for dinner for 2 h before dark, as soon as they would begin to back the car down the driveway, he would run after the moving car, crying and not wanting to be left alone. On occasion when they would go out and he and his sister stayed with a "baby-sitter" he frequently called his parents every 5–10 min at the restaurant to find out when they would come home.

After developing rapport during the initial visit, F. was willing to acknowledge that he had a lot of "worry" and "nervousness"; and that this made him afraid to go to school, to be away from his parents, and to do stuff. When he thought about this he said he said he thought it was "dumb" and that he wished it would go away. He was especially embarrassed about having hyperventilation and crying "so easily, like a baby" when he was anxious.

He was intrigued by the idea that with self-hypnosis he could learn to use his mind to be "the boss of his body". He quickly learned the self-hypnotic technique of "three and six" [116], focusing on his own body's biofeedback by paying careful attention to his respiratory cycle, i.e., slowly breathing in to a slow count to three, then slowly breathing out to a slow count to six. A "second" three and six would be identical along with eye closure. The next breath (also three and six) would keep eyes closed and begin to imagine favorite place imagery, and the next three and six would begin to add progressive relaxation linked to each successive out-breath.

Though F.'s anxiety improved, and he was able to more easily make it to school, he continued to call his mother frequently from school, with varying complaints that he "didn't feel well" or "needed to come home", and frequent visits to the nurse's office. Despite his mother's effectiveness in being sensitive in listening to F., she followed guidance to not pick him up early from school, and the School Nurse was equally collaborative in offering comfort and reassurance while dispatching F. back to class. As this continued, and in the context of knowing that F. also found comfort in successfully immersing himself in video games he could WIN, it was decided to introduce him to biofeedback by offering to show him "a computer-game for your body". He was immediately intrigued by the graphics and the easy-to-understand process of the Emwave PRO computerized biofeedback (Heartmath Inc., Boulder Creek, CA). As children commonly do, as he became focused and absorbed in attending to the images on the computer screen (monitoring and measuring his heart rate variability), he spontaneously moved into a hypnotic state, evidenced by his body stillness in his chair, fixed gaze stare at the computer screen (with infrequent blinking), and spontaneous slowing of respirations, along with slowing of heart rate, without any verbal hypnotic suggestion to do any of those behaviors.

He quickly became proficient at 'winning' the various games available in this program through control of his heart rate variability (HRV); and his pride and confidence in his growing competence were natural by-products of the process. As he enjoyed these biofeedback sessions, hypnotic suggestions were brief and focused upon suggestions directed at strengthening inner resources such as self-confidence (such as "you're doing this exactly right!" or "wonderful!") and post-hypnotic suggestions to foster competence and control over target symptoms (such as "the more you do this, the better you get", and "pretty soon you'll be so good at this that you'll hardly notice any of that anxiety or worry or nervous feelings that used to be there before . . . "). After two biofeedback sessions he and his family were encouraged to consider obtaining a personalized, portable version of the Emwave program, the Emwave PSR (Personal Stress Reliever), which monitors and gives visual and auditory feedback of pacing and slowing of breathing, signaling when HRV is in a positive 'coherence' state.

F. continued to improve. One day he came in for an appointment after school and was eager to report, "You won't believe what happened today!" He said that at lunchtime he was on the playground and three older boys began bullying him. He said he did not know why, but they were pushing him around and he was getting sad and nervous and he began to cry and ran away. Luckily, they did not follow him. He ran to his locker, planning to get his Emwave PSR from his backpack and find a private place he could practice his Emwave and calm himself ("I didn't want to cry more or call my Mom or go to the Nurse."). He got his backpack, found a place in a corner where he could be in private. All set to practice his Emwave he discovered that it was not in his backpack! Hearing this, the clinician said "Oh, no! What did you DO to SOLVE this?" (Note the suggestions of the clinician regarding their confidence to help himself). F. said "Well, I decided all that I could do was "just pretend and imagine that I did have the Emwave, so I pretended to attach it (the HRV monitoring electrode) to my earlobe, and then I imagined I was holding it in my hand, and I closed my eyes and was doing the imagination and my breathing got slower and I was fine and didn't feel like crying any more. I realized then that actually I am the Emwave, and the Emwave is me!" Beyond complimenting F., the clinician asked if it was okay to tell that story to other students, of course without mentioning his name ... and he too was thrilled that his experience could be of help to others in that way.

It was clearly a combination of self-hypnosis and biofeedback that allowed F. to develop mastery over his symptoms, and to cope with parental separation and stressful situations at school.

3.3. Summary

In the foregoing, it was critical to identify a biofeedback system and modalities within that system that would be concordant with the abilities, interests, and maturation and cognitive developmental style of the child, 12-year-old F. Rapport with F. and knowledge of his facility and interest in videogames were identified as key resources that made this easy to accomplish, in part because the HRV biofeedback system selected has games that appeal to various ages and interests in childhood and adolescence. Just as we emphasize the importance of tailoring hypnotic approaches to the developmental level and capacity of the young [9,102], so it is essential that biofeedback approaches be selected that appeal to the interests and developmental capacity of the patient.

As reflected in the described case of F, hypnosis and biofeedback share similar (if not identical) characteristics, including:

- positive expectations for therapeutic outcomes;
- absorption/concentration/focused, narrowed attention;
- spontaneous relaxation in association with vigilant attention;
- concurrent psychophysiological changes (used to give feedback to the subject that they are "doing this 'exactly right'"—biofeedback clinicians may simply refer to these as encouragement or positive verbal feedback).

4. Integrating Acupuncture and Hypnosis

4.1. Background

Acupuncture is a form of eastern medicine that originated in China over 2000 years ago. The traditional concept of acupuncture is that Qi, the basic life force, travels along channels, i.e., meridians, which can be accessed by fine instruments (traditionally acupuncture needles) to balance and remove obstructions to its flow in order to treat mental and physical ailments and improve health. Acupuncture is one of the most popular complementary medicine modalities in the US [117] according to a 2008 survey [118], with 20% of children in the US having used it. Acupuncture has been used to treat several conditions [119] and is gaining particular attention for its usefulness in treating pain. The mechanism of acupuncture is not completely known, but acupuncture can cause an endogenous opioid response that is blunted by naloxone in a dose dependent fashion [120].

The unity between mind and body, i.e., an interactive relationship between the two, is an important component of Eastern medicine. As a result of this interaction, hypnosis and acupuncture may be uniquely suited to complement each other as therapies [121]. Numerous studies have supported the use of hypnosis for both procedural and chronic pain. Kemper [122] previously reported that acupuncture is well tolerated in pediatrics with many patients identifying it as "helpful and pleasant". Others note that acupuncture is safe and well tolerated in the pediatric population when carried out by appropriately trained individuals [123,124]. Zeltzer et al.'s [125] study provided further support for the feasibility and acceptability of acupuncture in the pediatric population and illustrated its utility in combination with hypnosis. In this study of over 31 children with chronic pain at the UCLA pain center, acupuncture was combined with a standardized hypnosis program using a pain dial technique in which the children imagined being in a plane cockpit with a dial connected to the area of pain. Rather than using the word pain, but they suggested using the phrase "altering the feeling as needed". The 28 children completing the study reported decreased symptoms [125,126].

Acupuncture is well tolerated in patients from infancy to adulthood [127]. The management of commons symptoms such as pain, nausea, and other GI distress are particularly good fits for a combination of hypnosis and acupuncture. Recommended ages for the combination of the two include any child who is of appropriate age for hypnosis. Hypnosis may help in the tolerability of painful acupoints and augment the response to acupuncture in painful conditions such as headache [128]. Acupuncture may be useful in facilitating and augmenting hypnotic suggestion in patients who are preparing for dental and surgical procedures and have a history of phobias and panic attacks [129]. In a study of 108 adults with history of panic attacks and dental/surgical phobias, the acupuncture point GV-24 (the "third eye" point on the forehead) was found to enhance hypnotic induction [129]. GV-20 (the "governing vessel" point on the scalp vertex) and surrounding points have been used to decrease anxiety associated with dental procedures [130]. Though more research is needed, the combined use of hypnosis with acupuncture appears to be beneficial for pediatric patients.

4.2. Case Example

J. is a 14-year-old adolescent with sickle cell disease who was referred to an outpatient integrative medicine clinic by her hematologist for assistance with pain management. J.'s sickle cell symptoms had been relatively well controlled until about a year ago when she began to present with painful crises requiring hospitalization every two months. She was receiving a number of medications for pain as needed including: acetaminophen, ibuprofen, gabapentin, and oxycodone. The hematologist had recommended hydroxyurea. The family was considering the addition of hydroxyurea but had some concerns about side effects.

The initial integrative medicine visit was 90 min. Considerable time was spent listening to J's story and how her sickle cell disease affected her life including her relationships and interactions with friends and family. We also discussed her goals for this session and for management of her pain in general, including the potential benefits of adding hydroxyurea as recommended by her hematologist. After development of rapport, J. was able to recognize that her fear of the pain, or of pain coming, was interfering with the enjoyment of her daily life. J.'s main goal was to be able to fully participate in the activities that she enjoyed with her friends. Her parents were concerned that she was beginning to isolate herself and hoped that when her pain was controlled that she would be able to continue to participate in the afterschool activities that she used to enjoy. Though she did continue to attend school despite the pain, she was worried about being too active—that doing so would cause the pain to return and that she would need to go back to the hospital for pain management. J. and her parents were very interested in acupuncture for pain management, but J. said that she was afraid of needles and too scared to have acupuncture.

The clinician and J. discussed using her imagination to help her relax and explained that when she was in a more relaxed state she might be surprised to find that she does not mind having acupuncture at all and that she may find the experience to be pleasant and helpful (all of these were alert hypnotic suggestions to enlist her cooperation). It was explained that some people also call this way of using your imagination hypnosis and that hypnosis is about using the mind and imagination to give her the power to be able to do the things that she wants such as having acupuncture and spending time with her friends without worry. She was curious about the process and agreed to proceed with reassurance that she was in control and could stop whenever she liked. This provided the safe space to allow her to more fully experience the trance state.

The clinician proceeded with hypnosis using favorite place imagery for calming and relaxation during the acupuncture session. The clinician began with a conversational induction, speaking to J. in a calm and soothing voice about what we were planning to do. Reassurance was provided that she would remain in control and the discussion centered around 'wondering' what this experience would be like for her. It was also suggested that she would be able to speak and interact while maintaining a calm and relaxed state. Her gaze became fixed and her breath elongated as she began to deepen into trance, she then was invited her to close her eyes. Her eyelids closed. A few moments later rapid movement of her eyes beneath her closed lids was noted. Then, she was invited to imagine a door beyond which was her favorite place with all of her senses. As she explored her favorite place, she was able to report that her favorite place was her grandmother's house. She was encouraged her to fully imagine being there, including paying particular attention to the look, the feel, sounds, and the smells. As she explored her favorite place, she became comfortable enough to accept the acupuncture needles. Encouragement and praise were provided for her continuing to fully experience her favorite place during acupuncture. She was able to share that in her favorite place she felt, "warm", "safe", and "loved". It was suggested that she could continue to maintain those feelings.

At that time, it was asked if she was ready to proceed with the treatment. She nodded that she was. With her permission, a needle was placed in GV-20 for deeper relaxation and then auricular acupuncture was performed using the battlefield technique for pain management [131]. J. did not appear to notice when the needles were placed. After the needles were placed, she was invited to bring her awareness back to the room. As she brought her awareness back to the room, she maintained a calm and relaxed state and was pleasantly surprised to find that in her experience, "the needles don't hurt at all!" We completed the acupuncture treatment and the needles were removed. There were no complications. She tolerated the procedure well and requested to continue acupuncture and hypnosis at future visits. Weekly acupuncture was recommended for six weeks and she tolerated all future treatments well. The family decided to start hydroxyurea. J. continued to use self-hypnosis with favorite place imagery at home for pain and anxiety and her hospital admissions decreased. The combination of acupuncture and hypnosis allowed J. to fully explore treatment options that she initially feared. Had it not been for the combination of acupuncture and hypnosis, J. would not have been relaxed and comfortable enough to allow the needles. It is also likely that needling at GV-20 allowed for deeper relaxation and deepening of the trance state. In addition, J. also developed the skill of self-hypnosis which provided another tool in her toolbox to help her better manage her pain.

4.3. Summary

Acupuncture and hypnosis are useful tools on their own, but when used in combination can work synergistically. In the case presented above, hypnosis allowed for relaxed state that provided an opening for the acceptance of the acupuncture needles. Acupuncture to GV-20 likely assisted with deepening which may have augmented the hypnotic state and experience.

5. Integrating Yoga and Hypnosis

5.1. Background

The practice of yoga, an ancient mind–body, "moving meditation" modality originating from India, traditionally involved a set of beliefs and rituals with an over-arching goal of a person's union with Supreme Reality or the Universal Self [132]. Various yoga systems emphasized different paths toward that goal. By contrast, the version used by adults in the United States primarily focuses on combining various exercises involving postures ('asanas'), regulation of breathing ('pranayama'), and, at times, meditation to achieve emotional balance [133].

Moving beyond the one-on-one tradition, group instruction became the norm. In recent years a plethora of yoga programs for children and teens has propagated across the U.S. In 2012, 3.1% of U.S. children (1.7 million) used some form of yoga [118]. Parents, teachers, professionals and others with no yoga experience can become certified to teach youth in groups by completing an online (webinars and home-study) or live program. Some may pursue an optional registration as a registered children's yoga teacher (RCYT) with Yoga Alliance, a non-profit organization with a mission to foster "integrity and diversity of teaching yoga" [134]. The RCYT designation is accomplished by fulfilling their requirements, i.e., the equivalent of over 40 days of training acquired over time, and an annual fee. YogaKids, a registered children's yoga school offers such training through a sequence of levels [135].

Of note, YogaKids describes that future teachers of YogaKids learn how to combine yoga with other activities involving music, books, games, art, reading, writing, and science for a group of children. Thus, perhaps not surprisingly, yoga has found its way into the classroom [136]. On the one hand, this combination seems developmentally on target to facilitate children's learning and enjoyment; on the other, it begs the research question whether such confounders are controlled or measured in studies. One would be hard pressed to conclude that benefits of yoga group classes of this nature are solely due to learning yoga poses, postures, and breathing. Clearly, learning yoga in a more narrowed sense (postures, breathing, with or without meditation) or on a one-on-one basis would offer a very different learning environment.

Yoga Calm is another child- and family-oriented yoga program that incorporates "mindfulness" and "relaxation and reflection activities" with a goal of "self-regulation" and "social-emotional learning" [137]. Parents and professionals seeking certification and instructor training must complete the required 40 h of online courses and 40 h of practicum. This training is distinguished by providing graduate level college credits and continuing education units from many colleges and organizations. Further, efforts to ground their program with science is evident by their listing of research in these related domains (i.e., self-regulation, etc.) and their active engagement in research projects in collaboration with the University of Minnesota, a public-school system, and a children's hospital.

Early reviews of yoga focusing on the physical and mental health for children and teens expressed caution in making conclusions, citing only preliminary benefits due to methodological limitations [133,138,139]. More recently, some clinicians writing about yoga vary in their interpretation about potential benefits for children/teens' physical [140,141] and mental health [142,143]. Further, randomly chosen websites and blogs about this topic frequently reveal far-reaching conclusions, with minimal mention of the still preliminary conclusions. Hopefully correcting this trend is a 2017 Clinical Report by the AAP about pediatric integrative medicine that noted that while recent studies suggest benefits of yoga for children, the committee advocated for more systematic studies to ferret out this inquiry [144].

While PIM research has progressed remarkably, to date, research reviews of yoga focusing on outcomes of physical and mental health for children/teens have not yet examined differences based on many variables that complicate the comparison and contrast of findings and obscure conclusions about efficacy. As this area of study continues to unfold, investigators surely will begin to examine such variables as content (yoga type, elements, exercises, and other activities); format (e.g., session number, frequency, and time frame); context (individual vs. group (and size) vs. home); age range; home practice expectations and adherence; teacher's expertise; and long-term outcomes.

Exciting, fresh lines of research about the neuroscience underpinnings of therapeutic yoga are very promising and adds credibility to this PIM modality. Similarly, sound exploration of theoretical models for potential self-regulatory mechanisms of yoga for psychological and physical health is expanding. An article by researchers from Harvard and other institutions [145] provide evidence of yoga's top-down (cognitive) and bottom-up (emotions generated by the limbic system) pathways for self-regulation of cognition, emotions, behavior, and physiology. They also propose an intriguing model whereby these yoga-based processes may influence self-regulation of physical and emotional stress.

A complementary article by a group of University of California researchers offers a comprehensive, scholarly literature review, including a unique, methodical deconstruction of yoga's main components, i.e., "posture or movement sequences, conscious regulation of the breath, and techniques to improve attentional focus" [146]. Cogent hypotheses are laid out regarding how the neurocircuitry and physiological processes promoted by yoga may explain the mechanisms for change. They propose that yoga's main components may directly activate the vagal afferent system and other circuits, possibly resulting in enhanced autonomic, emotional, and cognitive regulation. Building on these neurophysiological frameworks, a recent paper connects therapeutic yoga to polyvagal theory (PVT), developed by Porges in 2011, to further explain the patterns of autonomic regulation related to emotional expression and social behavior and relationships [147].

Information about combining traditional yoga with hypnosis is scarce. Dalal and Barber's 2008 chapter (a modestly revised version of a 1969 paper) on this topic is the notable exception with its discussion and challenge of the purported similarities, i.e., an altered state of consciousness (trance states) with associated unusual phenomena [148]. Like some of the other PIM modalities, the shared elements of pediatric hypnosis and westernized yoga include the pre-requisite building of trust and alliance or rapport; goals toward self-regulation, health, well-being, and emotional balance; narrowed attention and inner absorption; frequent use of the breath; reduced psychophysiological reactivity via activation of the parasympathetic nervous system with vagal tone to evoke calmness; and varying degrees of dissociation. The latest theories on hypnosis emphasize its top-down neurophysiological components [68,95].

5.2. Case Example

S. is a 14-year-old female referred for integrative therapies to help her manage physical symptoms of headache and body aches, difficulty with sleep onset, and a history of generalized anxiety disorder. S.'s anxiety problems began at eight years of age with separation anxiety and specific phobia symptoms. On the first day of ninth grade, she had a panic episode with multiple symptoms including racing heartbeat, shaking, sweating, cold extremities, and fear of "losing it". Subsequently, she developed recurrent headaches due to clenching her teeth and general increased muscle tension of her neck, shoulders and back. In addition to being an excellent student, she was also an accomplished dancer but had become unable to participate in recitals due to performance anxiety.

At her first appointment, considerable time was spent developing rapport by listening closely to her story, learning about her family, her interests, and her goals for this intervention. She specifically said she wished to learn skills to avoid taking more "anti-anxiety pills", feel more comfortable in the classroom, and be able to dance in recitals with her friends. The clinician discussed with S. how she might learn to help herself achieve these goals by learning about the brain/body connections, combining yoga and hypnosis.

Yoga was defined for S. as "uniting the mind, body and spirit." It includes using the breath ('pranayama'), physical poses ('asanas'), and conscious awareness to create balance. She had done a little of this in a physical education class. She was more unsure of hypnosis, so the clinician talked about how it is "using your imagination on purpose", which she already knew how to do since she practiced her dance routines in her mind. S. also described how she occasionally reminds herself (to reframe worries) that she "can do it!" The clinician suggested she might reframe her worries and fears to experiencing herself as strong, competent and successful. Hypnosis was further defined as beginning with focused attention on the breath, the body, or an image and may be intensified with greater sensory, or imagery awareness. The process then shifts to using specific goal-oriented suggestions to change one's symptoms, perceptions, or behavior. The clinician emphasized that it is important to be certain that the use of hypnosis is appropriate for the desired outcome. S. and the clinician collaboratively planned for S. to spend time before the next visit simply noticing how she felt physically and emotionally when she was doing something she really enjoyed.

At the second visit, S. could more easily describe how her heart raced, her muscles tightened, her hands got sweaty and she forgot what she wanted to say when anxious, in contrast to how she felt when she was calm. The clinician again reviewed the possibilities of S. learning to help herself by using interventions such as yoga and hypnosis to help her become more aware of her ability to be in control in healthy, positive ways. The clinician invited S. to begin with heart/belly breathing because all these modalities use breathing as a means of inducing calmness, relaxation, increasing body awareness, and being in the present moment. The clinician then gently put one hand over her own heart and the other hand over her own abdomen. The clinician further suggested that S focus her attention on her breath as it moved through her body and simply say to herself, "I breathe in (in breath) and I breathe out (out breath)". As she did this she naturally elongated the exhalation and commented on feeling relaxed. After this invitation of narrowed attention to induce the hypnotic experience, the clinician then suggested that S. continue breathing in this easy and natural way while she imagined herself in her favorite place—laying in a hammock in her back yard. Utilizing this classic imagery technique to intensify the hypnotic experience, she visualized her mother's colorful flower garden, felt the warm sun on her arms and legs and the gentle sway of the hammock. The clinician suggested that S allow herself to be absorbed inside her mind by these images and sensations and say to herself, "I am safe and calm" while doing so. Her assignment following this visit was to practice her self-hypnosis (i.e., breathing, favorite place imagery, and positive suggestions to herself) daily for approximately 10 min as well as any time she began to feel anxious.

At the next visit she wanted to learn more about yoga. The clinician invited her to stand in "mountain pose" with her feet about hip width apart, imagining her feet reaching deep into the roots of the earth. During this heightened focus on her body's position and posture, S. was then offered hypnotic suggestions of self-efficacy and self-regulation, to repeat phrases in her mind, such as "I am strong" and "I can do this". She then brought her hands to her heart and energetically pushed her hands and arms above her head—like an exploding volcano releasing worries, fears, negative self-talk, and anything that she no longer needed. This hypnotic metaphor, imagery, and suggestions were combined with the "releasing" process (movement and pose) in yoga that needs to occur before someone can calm down. Using her love of dance, she then created a routine that included using her breath to calmly sustain her while she gracefully moved her body—stretching forward/backward, and side to side releasing tension while imagining strength and courage to move further out into her world with confidence and success.

After this introduction to combining hypnosis with yoga, S. found a class in her community where she could practice yoga with the support of others. She continued to interweave the practice the hypnotic phenomena of intentional breathing, focused attention, and absorption in mental imagery of favorite activities and rehearsal of future successes (as post-hypnotic suggestions).

5.3. Summary

This case illustrates that hypnosis and yoga can work well together to manage physical symptoms, anxious thoughts and negative self-perceptions and are readily accepted by children and teens as a means of improving self-care and resilience. They can easily build on patients' knowledge and experiences.

6. Discussion

PIM touts a growing array of approaches that initially were considered to be solely adjunctive interventions. For several years now, diligent efforts have preliminarily documented the efficacy and safety of separate integrative strategies that improve quality of care in order to recognize PIM as credible and viable by mainstream pediatrics. In spite of the epic history and groundwork of hypnosis as a common root of mind–body PIM, hypnosis may be overlooked as an integrative approach. There is confusion in the PIM literature where hypnosis 'belongs', as it has variably been considered a conventional [149], complementary [118,150], or cast-aside [8] approach. Yet a 2016 article published on the website of the National Center for Complementary and Integrative Health (NCCIH) includes hypnosis as a complementary approach [151]. Might this diminished inclusion be partially due to the recognition that some other PIM modalities (e.g., aromatherapy (essential oils) and nutritional supplements) perhaps sound more acceptable, are simpler to teach, are quicker to grasp, or are easier to incorporate—thus, hypnosis has become out of sight and out of mind?

A related question concerns guided imagery (GI): despite both its heritage and oft-revealed overlapping ingredients with hypnosis as discussed above in this article, might this more neutral name (guided imagery) and its scripts similarly be preferred by some institutions, journals, and clinicians?

It is our reasoning that GI bypasses the investment of time, effort, and cost needed to acquire skills that characterize the uniquely therapeutic communication of hypnosis.

Beyond these two thorny questions, we have highlighted three key themes throughout this paper: (1) common components shared by pediatric hypnosis with GI as well as other mind–body techniques form the core of PIM, i.e., mindfulness, biofeedback, acupuncture, and yoga; and (2) permutations of combined PIM modalities reveal that individual PIM modalities are actually evolving by 'borrowing' elements from one another. Just like the 'blending trend' of integrative approaches with CBT, e.g., "cognitive hypnotherapy" [152,153] and "mindfulness-based cognitive therapy" [154], emerging new terms in integrative health publications further illustrate this trajectory, such as "mindful self-hypnosis" [155]. Research is needed to document the efficacy of combining these multi-modal approaches [156].

A third key theme of this paper is the value and importance of designing personalized treatments in PIM. Health professionals new to PIM modalities quickly discover the range of responses among children/teens, driven by underlying developmental, learning, experiential, and other individual differences. While some clinicians choose to deliver the same 'procedure' to every patient, others are embracing the critical importance of establishing rapport and solidifying trust and attunement in order to maximize each patient's receptivity, cooperation, and adherence to acquiring new skills. As clinicians become more seasoned and secure in their use of PIM modalities, they invite and incorporate the child/teen's own specific goals while contemplating goodness-of-fit between each patient and the potpourri of PIM approaches. The case vignettes we chose for this paper illustrated the additive value of incorporating hypnosis as well as numerous practical strategies and clinical acumen as guidelines for integrating PIM modalities to achieve this goal of individualized care. Honing one's sensitivity to and flexibility in the selection, timing, and presentation of integrative approaches completes the criteria toward a new PIM benchmark for designing personalized treatment with each patient. Beyond the *sequential* use of integrative approaches, future research may find that a more refined delivery model [156], of 'mingling modalities' as illustrated in the case vignettes, could potentially offer a synergistic effect that might become PIM's new norm.

Acquiring expertise in such a practice model takes time, mentoring, and ongoing training. PIM approaches vary widely in terms of effort, time, and cost to achieve competence or mastery, and differ in terms of complex skill development (e.g., hypnosis, biofeedback, and acupuncture) vs. knowledge attainment (e.g., nutritional supplements, essential oils). Obviously, such variations differentially lend themselves to hands-on learning, intensive supervised practice, and ongoing mentoring [10] vs. online webinars and lectures. The phenomenal launches of the online pediatric integrative medicine in residency (PIMR) curriculum [157] and the first pediatric integrative medicine fellowship (under the direction of Ann Ming Yeh, M.D., at Stanford) are ground-breaking contributions to medical education. While the PIMR curriculum includes some on-site activities, hopefully residency program directors (and future iterations of PIMR) will include opportunities for clinicians-in-training to have access to skills training in hypnosis as a fundamental principle and core construct underlying many PIM modalities that prioritize goals relating to children's self-regulation.

While the current integrative medicine board-certification exam in the US includes hypnosis as an area of core content [158], more work remains to incorporate hypnosis into formal curricula. For the thematic reasons outlined in this paper, we recommend that clinical hypnosis be more deeply and broadly promoted as a fundamental root of PIM. Basically, pediatric hypnosis combines imagery with nuanced verbal and nonverbal suggestions to promote therapeutic change from within. As such, curricula in PIM will be strengthened by specific, detailed training in hypnosis in order to develop the nuanced capacities of creating a design (in collaboration with the child/teen) of multi-sensorial imagery and of formulating therapeutic suggestions including an awareness and use of voice prosody, including the speaker's word selection, phrasing, rate, stress, loudness, pitch, and quality [159]. Further, research on clinicians' training in purposeful word choice to design positive suggestions shows substantial evidence of the positive benefits for patients undergoing surgery and procedures, as well as for those experiencing chronic pain, somatization, warts, etc. [160,161]. Creating 'therapeutic presence' via prosodic vocalizations, facial expressions, and gestures has shown to enhance a child and parent's sense of safety within the clinician–patient encounter [162]. Thus, learning such refined details in delivering suggestions speaks to the pragmatic utility of including hypnosis in training for all pediatric professionals to better address physical, mental, and behavioral health issues in an integrative manner.

Author Contributions: Conceptualization, P.K.; Methodology, P.K. and A.J.B.; Writing—Original Draft Preparation, P.K., D.P.K., M.L.B., R.L.K., and A.J.B.; Writing—Review & Editing, P.K. and A.J.B.

Funding: This research was funded by Maternal & Child Health Bureau (MCHB) of the US Department of Health and Human Services grant numbers T73MC12835 and T20MC07469 to the University of Minnesota.

Conflicts of Interest: The authors declare no conflict of interest.

References

1. Olness, K.; Gardner, G.G. Some guidelines for uses of hypnotherapy in pediatrics. *Pediatrics* **1978**, *62*, 228–233. [PubMed]
2. Olness, K. Hypnosis in pediatric practice. *Curr. Probl. Pediatr.* **1981**, *12*, 1–47. [CrossRef]
3. Gardner, G.G. Hypnosis with children. *Int. J. Clin. Exp. Hypn.* **1974**, *22*, 20–38. [CrossRef] [PubMed]
4. Olness, K.N.; Conroy, M.M. A Pilot Study of Voluntary Control of Transcutaneous PO$_2$ by Children: A Brief Communication. *Int. J. Clin. Exp. Hypn.* **1985**, *33*, 1–5. [CrossRef] [PubMed]
5. Kohen, D.P.; Kaiser, P. Clinical hypnosis with children and adolescents—What? Why? How?: Origins, applications, and efficacy. *Children* **2014**, *1*, 74–98. [CrossRef] [PubMed]
6. Erickson, M.H. Pediatric hypnotherapy. *Am. J. Clin. Hypn.* **1958**, *1*, 25–29. [CrossRef]
7. Hilgard, J.R. *Personality and Hypnosis: A Study of Imaginative Involvement*, 2nd ed.; University of Chicago Press: Chicago, IL, USA, 1979.
8. Vohra, S.; Surette, S.; Mittra, D.; Rosen, L.D.; Gardiner, P.; Kemper, K.J. Pediatric integrative medicine: Pediatrics' newest subspecialty? *BMC Pediatr.* **2012**, *12*, 123. [CrossRef] [PubMed]
9. Kohen, D.P.; Olness, K.O. *Hypnosis and Hypnotherapy with Children*, 4th ed.; Routledge, Taylor & Francis Group: New York, NY, USA, 2011.
10. Kohen, D.P.; Kaiser, P.; Olness, K. State-of-the-art pediatric hypnosis training: Remodeling curriculum and refining faculty development. *Am. J. Clin. Hypn.* **2017**, *59*, 292–310. [CrossRef] [PubMed]
11. Krippner, S. The use of hypnosis with elementary and secondary school children in a summer reading clinic. *Am. J. Clin. Hypn.* **1966**, *8*, 261–266. [CrossRef] [PubMed]
12. Jampolsky, G.; Haight, M. Hypnosis and sensory motor stimulation to aid children with learning problems. *J. Learn. Disabil.* **1970**, *3*, 570–575. [CrossRef]
13. Johnson, L.S.; Johnson, D.L.; Olson, M.R.; Newman, J.P. The uses of hypnotherapy with learning disabled children. *J. Clin. Psychol.* **1981**, *37*, 291–299. [CrossRef]
14. Antitch, J.L. The use of hypnosis in pediatric anesthesia. *J. Am. Soc. Psychosom. Dent. Med.* **1967**, *14*, 70–75. [PubMed]
15. Kohen, D.P.; Wynne, E. Applying hypnosis in a preschool family asthma education program: Uses of storytelling, imagery, and relaxation. *Am. J. Clin. Hypn.* **1997**, *39*, 169–181. [CrossRef] [PubMed]
16. Baumann, F. Hypnosis and the adolescent drug abuser. *Am. J. Clin. Hypn.* **1970**, *13*, 17–21. [CrossRef] [PubMed]
17. Labaw, W.L. Adjunctive trance therapy with severely burned children. *Int. J. Child Psychother.* **1973**, *2*, 89–92.
18. Olness, K. The use of self-hypnosis in the treatment of childhood nocturnal enuresis. A report on forty patients. *Clin. Pediatr.* **1975**, *14*. [CrossRef] [PubMed]
19. Edwards, S.D.; Van der Spuy, H.I. Hypnotherapy as a treatment for enuresis. *J. Child Psychol. Psychiatry.* **1985**, *26*, 161–170. [CrossRef] [PubMed]
20. Friman, P.C.; Handwerk, M.L.; Swearer, S.M.; McGinnis, J.C.; Warzak, W.J. Do children with primary nocturnal enuresis have clinically significant behavior problems? *Arch. Pediatr. Adolesc. Med.* **1998**, *152*, 537–539. [CrossRef] [PubMed]
21. Olness, K. Autohypnosis in functional megacolon in children. *Am. J. Clin. Hypn.* **1976**, *19*, 28–32. [CrossRef] [PubMed]

22. Clawson, T.A.; Swade, R.H. The hypnotic control of blood flow and pain: The cure of warts and the potential for the use of hypnosis in the treatment of cancer. *Am. J. Clin. Hypn.* **1975**, *17*, 160–169. [CrossRef] [PubMed]
23. Porter, J. Guided fantasy as a treatment for childhood insomnia. *Aust. N. Z. J. Psychiatry* **1975**, *9*, 169–172. [CrossRef] [PubMed]
24. Kohen, D.P.; Mahowald, M.W.; Rosen, G.M. Sleep-terror disorder in children: The role of self-hypnosis in management. *Am. J. Clin. Hypn.* **1992**, *34*, 233–244. [CrossRef] [PubMed]
25. Gardner, G.G.; Tarnow, J.D. Adjunctive hypnotherapy with an autistic boy. *Am. J. Clin. Hypn.* **1980**, *22*, 173–179. [CrossRef] [PubMed]
26. Kohen, D.P. Relaxation/mental imagery (self-hypnosis) and pelvic examinations in adolescents. *J. Dev. Behav. Pediatr.* **1980**, *1*, 180–186. [CrossRef] [PubMed]
27. Zeltzer, L.; LeBaron, S. Hypnosis and nonhypnotic techniques for reduction of pain and anxiety during painful procedures in children and adolescents with cancer. *J. Pediatr.* **1982**, *101*, 1032–1035. [PubMed]
28. Hall, H.R. Hypnosis and the immune system: A review with implications for cancer and the psychology of healing. *Am. J. Clin. Hypn.* **1982**, *25*, 92–103. [CrossRef] [PubMed]
29. Olness, K.; Culbert, T.; Uden, D. Self-regulation of salivary immunoglobulin A by children. *Pediatrics* **1989**, *83*, 66–71. [PubMed]
30. Hall, H.R. Hypnosis, suggestion, and the psychology of healing: A historical perspective. *Adv. Inst. Adv. Heal.* **1986**, *3*, 29–37.
31. Whorwell, P.J.; Prior, A.; Faragher, E.B. Controlled trial of hypnotherapy in the treatment of severe refractory irritable-bowel syndrome. *Lancet* **1984**, *2*, 1232–1234. [CrossRef]
32. Swirsky-Sacchetti, T.; Margolis, C.G. The effects of a comprehensive self-hypnosis training program on the use of factor VIII in severe hemophilia. *Int. J. Clin. Exp. Hypn.* **1986**, *34*, 71–83. [CrossRef] [PubMed]
33. Zeltzer, L.K.; LeBaron, S. Fantasy in children and adolescents with chronic illness. *J. Dev. Behav. Pediatr.* **1986**, *7*, 195–198. [CrossRef] [PubMed]
34. Barnes, A.J.; Kohen, D.P. Clinical hypnosis as an effective adjunct in the care of pediatric inpatients. *J. Pediatr.* **2006**, *149*, 563–565. [CrossRef] [PubMed]
35. Kohen, D.P. Applications of relaxation/mental imagery (self-hypnosis) in pediatric emergencies. *Int. J. Clin. Exp. Hypn.* **1986**, *34*, 283–294. [CrossRef] [PubMed]
36. Thompson, C.K.; Hall, H.R.; Sison, C.E. Effects of hypnosis and imagery training on naming behavior in aphasia. *Brain Lang.* **1986**, *28*, 141–153. [CrossRef]
37. Kohen, D.P.; Botts, P. Relaxation-imagery (self-hypnosis) in Tourette syndrome: Experience with four children. *Am. J. Clin. Hypn.* **1987**, *29*, 227–237. [CrossRef] [PubMed]
38. Young, M.H.; Montano, R.J. A new hypnobehavioral method for the treatment of children with Tourette's disorder. *Am. J. Clin. Hypn.* **1988**, *31*, 97–106. [CrossRef] [PubMed]
39. Culbertson, F.M. A four-step hypnotherapy model for Gilles de la Tourette's syndrome. *Am. J. Clin. Hypn.* **1989**, *31*, 252–256. [CrossRef] [PubMed]
40. Olness, K.; MacDonald, J.T.; Uden, D.L. Comparison of self-hypnosis and propranolol in the treatment of juvenile classic migraine. *Pediatrics* **1987**, *79*, 593–597. [PubMed]
41. McGrath, P.J.; Humphreys, P.; Goodman, J.T.; Keene, D.; Firestone, P.; Jacob, P.; Cunningham, S.J. Relaxation prophylaxis for childhood migraine: a randomized placebo-controlled trial. *Dev. Med. Child Neurol.* **1988**, *30*, 626–631. [CrossRef] [PubMed]
42. Dinges, D.F.; Whitehouse, W.G.; Orne, E.C.; Bloom, P.B.; Carlin, M.M.; Bauer, N.K.; Gillen, K.A.; Shapiro, B.S.; Ohene-Frempong, K.; Dampier, C.; et al. Self-hypnosis training as an adjunctive treatment in the management of pain associated with sickle cell disease. *Int. J. Clin. Exp. Hypn.* **1997**, *45*, 417–432. [CrossRef] [PubMed]
43. Jacknow, D.S.; Tschann, J.M.; Link, M.P.; Boyce, W.T. Hypnosis in the prevention of chemotherapy-related nausea and vomiting in children: a prospective study. *J. Dev. Behav. Pediatr.* **1994**, *15*, 258–264. [CrossRef] [PubMed]
44. Kohen, D.P.; Olness, K.N.; Colwell, S.O.; Heimel, A. The use of relaxation-mental imagery (self-hypnosis) in the management of 505 pediatric behavioral encounters. *J. Dev. Behav. Pediatr.* **1984**, *5*, 21–25. [CrossRef] [PubMed]
45. Wingert, A.; Ali, S. The Cochrane Library and procedural pain in children: an overview of reviews. *Evidence-Based Child Heal. A Cochrane Rev. J.* **2012**, *7*, 1363–1399.

46. Uman, L.S.; Birnie, K.A.; Noel, M.; Parker, J.A.; Chambers, C.T.; McGrath, P.J.; Kisely, S.R. Psychological interventions for needle-related procedural pain and distress in children and adolescents. *Cochrane Database Syst. Rev.* **2013**, *10*, CD005179. [CrossRef] [PubMed]
47. Olness, K.O. Pediatrics. In *Handbook of Medical and Psychological Hypnosis: Foundations, Applications, and Professional Issues*; Elkins, G.R., Ed.; Springer Publishing Company, LLC: New York, NY, USA, 2017; pp. 371–378.
48. Sawni, A.; Breuner, C.C. Clinical hypnosis, an effective mind-body modality for adolescents with behavioral and physical complaints. *Children* **2017**, *4*, 19. [CrossRef] [PubMed]
49. Kaiser, P. Childhood anxiety, worry, and fear: individualizing hypnosis goals and suggestions for self-regulation. *Am. J. Clin. Hypn.* **2011**, *54*, 16–31. [CrossRef] [PubMed]
50. Kaiser, P. Anxiety in Children and Teens. In *Handbook of Medical and Psychological Hypnosis: Foundations, Applications, and Professional Issues*; Elkins, G.R., Ed.; Springer Publishing Company, LLC: New York, NY, USA, 2017; pp. 477–484.
51. Anbar, R.D. Asthma. In *Handbook of Medical and Psychological Hypnosis: Foundations, Applications, and Professional Issues*; Elkins, G.R., Ed.; Springer Publishing Company, LLC: New York, NY, USA, 2017; pp. 161–168.
52. Anbar, R.D. Cystic Fibrosis. In *Handbook of Medical and Psychological Hypnosis: Foundations, Applications, and Professional Issues*; Elkins, G.R., Ed.; Springer Publishing Company, LLC: New York, NY, USA, 2017; pp. 199–204.
53. Hogg, F. Hypnosis. In *Dental Fear and Anxiety in Pediatric Patients*; Campbell, C., Ed.; Springer International Publishing: Basel, Switzerland, 2017; pp. 153–172.
54. Lazarus, J.E. Enuresis. In *Handbook of Medical and Psychological Hypnosis: Foundations, Applications, and Professional Issues*; Elkins, G.R., Ed.; Springer Publishing Company, LLC: New York, NY, USA, 2017; pp. 225–234.
55. Kohen, D.P. Nail Biting. In *Handbook of Medical and Psychological Hypnosis: Foundations, Applications, and Professional Issues*; Elkins, G.R., Ed.; Springer Publishing Company, LLC: New York, NY, USA, 2017; pp. 321–325.
56. Kohen, D.P. Headaches—Children. In *Handbook of Medical and Psychological Hypnosis: Foundations, Applications, and Professional Issues*; Elkins, G.R., Ed.; Springer Publishing Company, LLC: New York, NY, USA, 2017; pp. 259–271.
57. Anbar, R.D.; Fernandez, B.A. Vocal Cord Dysfunction. In *Handbook of Medical and Psychological Hypnosis: Foundations, Applications, and Professional Issues*; Elkins, G.R., Ed.; Springer Publishing Company, LLC: New York, NY, USA, 2017; pp. 429–434.
58. Kuttner, L. *A Child in Pain: What Health Professionals Can Do to Help*; Crown House Publishing: Camarthen, UK, 2010.
59. Saadat, H. Clinical Hypnosis in Children. In *Handbook of Pediatric Chronic Pain: Current Science and Integrative Practice (Perspectives on Pain in Psychology)*; McClain, B.C., Suresh, S., Eds.; Springer-Verlag: New York, NY, USA, 2011.
60. Friedrichsdorf, S.J.; Kohen, D.P. Integration of hypnosis into pediatric palliative care. *Ann. Palliat. Med.* **2018**, *7*, 136–150. [CrossRef] [PubMed]
61. Pendergrast, R.A. Incorporating hypnosis into pediatric clinical encounters. *Children* **2017**, *4*, 18. [CrossRef] [PubMed]
62. Hall, H.R.; Olness, K.O. Hypnosis, imagery, self-regulation and immune activity. In *Psychoneuroimmunology and Psychotherapy*; Schubert, C., Ed.; Schattauer-Verlag: Stuttgart, Germany, 2014.
63. Yeh, A.M.; Wren, A.; Golianu, B. Mind-body interventions for pediatric inflammatory bowel disease. *Children* **2017**, *4*, 22. [CrossRef] [PubMed]
64. Vlieger, A.M.; Menko-Frankenhuis, C.; Wolfkamp, S.C.; Tromp, E.; Benninga, M.A. Hypnotherapy for children with functional abdominal pain or irritable bowel syndrome: A randomized controlled trial. *Gastroenterology* **2007**, *133*, 1430–1436. [CrossRef] [PubMed]
65. Vlieger, A.M.; Rutten, J.M.T.M.; Govers, A.M.A.P.; Frankenhuis, C.; Benninga, M.A. Long-term follow-up of gut-directed hypnotherapy vs. standard care in children with functional abdominal pain or irritable bowel syndrome. *Am. J. Gastroenterol.* **2012**, *107*, 627–631. [CrossRef] [PubMed]

66. Rutten, J.M.; Vlieger, A.M.; Frankenhuis, C.; George, E.K.; Groeneweg, M.; Norbruis, O.F.; Tjon a Ten, W.; Van Wering, H.; Dijkgraaf, M.G.; Merkus, M.P.; et al. Gut-directed hypnotherapy in children with irritable bowel syndrome or functional abdominal pain (syndrome): a randomized controlled trial on self exercises at home using CD versus individual therapy by qualified therapists. *BMC Pediatr.* **2014**, *14*, 140. [CrossRef] [PubMed]
67. Rutten, J.M.T.M.; Vlieger, A.M.; Frankenhuis, C.; George, E.K.; Groeneweg, M.; Norbruis, O.F.; Tjon a Ten, W.; van Wering, H.M.; Dijkgraaf, M.G.W.; Merkus, M.P.; et al. Home-based hypnotherapy self-exercises vs individual hypnotherapy with a therapist for treatment of pediatric irritable bowel syndrome, functional abdominal pain, or functional abdominal pain syndrome. *JAMA Pediatr.* **2017**, *171*, 470. [CrossRef] [PubMed]
68. Terhune, D.B.; Cleeremans, A.; Raz, A.; Lynn, S.J. Hypnosis and top-down regulation of consciousness. *Neurosci. Biobehav. Rev.* **2017**, *81*, 59–74. [CrossRef] [PubMed]
69. Rossman, M. *Guided Imagery for Self-Healing: An Essential Resource for Anyone Seeking Wellness*; H.J. Kramer, Inc.: Tiburon, CA, USA, 2000.
70. Fung, E. Relaxation, guided imagery and hypnosis training not just for the Olympic athletes. In *NASW Child Welfare, Section Connection*; National Association of Social Workers: Chicago, IL, USA, 2008; Issue 2.
71. Roffe, L.; Schmidt, K.; Ernst, E. A systematic review of guided imagery as an adjuvant cancer therapy. *Psychooncology.* **2005**, *14*, 607–617. [CrossRef] [PubMed]
72. Hadjibalassi, M.; Lambrinou, E.; Papastavrou, E.; Papathanassoglou, E. The effect of guided imagery on physiological and psychological outcomes of adult ICU patients: A systematic literature review and methodological implications. *Aust. Crit. Care* **2018**, *31*, 73–86. [CrossRef] [PubMed]
73. Weydert, J.A.; Shapiro, D.E.; Acra, S.A.; Monheim, C.J.; Chambers, A.S.; Ball, T.M. Evaluation of guided imagery as treatment for recurrent abdominal pain in children: A randomized controlled trial. *BMC Pediatr.* **2006**, *6*, 29. [CrossRef] [PubMed]
74. Gruzelier, J.H. A review of the impact of hypnosis, relaxation, guided imagery and individual differences on aspects of immunity and health. *Stress* **2002**, *5*, 147–163. [CrossRef] [PubMed]
75. Dormoy, M. *Imagery Work with Kids: Essential Practices to Help Them Manage Stress, Reduce Anxiety & Build Self-Esteem*; W.W. Norton & Company: New York, NY, USA, 2016.
76. American Psychological Association. Want Better Health? Use Your Head! Available online: http://www.apa.org/research/action/head.aspx (accessed on 24 July 2018).
77. Vohra, S.; McClafferty, H.; Becker, D.; Bethell, C.; Culbert, T.; King-Jones, S.; Rosen, L.; Sibinga, E.; Bailey, M.; Weydert, J.; et al. Mind-body therapies in children and youth. *Pediatrics* **2016**, *138*, e20161896.
78. Huynh, M.E.; Vandvik, I.H.; Diseth, T.H. Hypnotherapy in child psychiatry: The state of the art. *Clin. Child Psychol. Psychiatry* **2008**, *13*, 377–393. [CrossRef] [PubMed]
79. Rutten, J.M.; Reitsma, J.B.; Vlieger, A.M.; Benninga, M.A. Gut-directed hypnotherapy for functional abdominal pain or irritable bowel syndrome in children: A systematic review. *Arch. Dis. Child.* **2013**, *98*, 252–257. [CrossRef] [PubMed]
80. Lambert, S.A. The effects of hypnosis/guided imagery on the postoperative course of children. *J. Dev. Behav. Pediatr.* **1996**, *17*, 307–310. [CrossRef] [PubMed]
81. Brown, J.L. Imagination training: A tool with many uses. *Contemp. Pediatr.* **1995**, *12*, 22–26, 29–30. [PubMed]
82. Van Tilburg, M.A.; Chitkara, D.K.; Palsson, O.S.; Turner, M.; Blois-Martin, N.; Ulshen, M.; Whitehead, W.E. Audio-recorded guided imagery treatment reduces functional abdominal pain in children: a pilot study. *Pediatrics* **2009**, *124*, e890–e897. [CrossRef] [PubMed]
83. Kabat-Zinn, J. *Full Catastophe Living*; Delacorte Press: New York, NY, USA, 1990.
84. Kabat-Zinn, J. *Full Catastrophe Liviing: Using the Wisdom of Your Body and Mind to Face Stress, Pain, and Illness*; Bantam Dell: New York, NY, USA, 2013.
85. Kabat-Zinn, J. Mindfulness-based interventions in context: Past, present, and future. *Clin. Psychol. Sci. Pract.* **2003**, *10*, 144–156. [CrossRef]
86. Kabat-Zinn, J.; Lipworth, L.; Burncy, R.; Sellers, W. Four-year follow-up of a meditation-based program for the self-regulation of chronic pain: Treatment outcomes and compliance. *Clin. J. Pain* **1986**, *3*, 60. [CrossRef]
87. Crane, R.S.; Brewer, J.; Feldman, C.; Kabat-Zinn, J.; Santorelli, S.; Williams, J.M.G.; Kuyken, W. What defines mindfulness-based programs? The warp and the weft. *Psychol. Med.* **2017**, *47*, 990–999. [CrossRef] [PubMed]
88. Snel, E. *Sitting Still Like a Frog: Mindfulness Exercises for Kids (and Their Parents)*; Shambhala Publication: Boulder, CO, USA, 2013.

89. Breathe, Think, Do with Sesame. Available online: https://sesamestreetincommunities.org/activities/breathe-think-do/ (accessed on 3 August 2018).
90. Yapko, M. *Mindfulness and Hypnosis: The Power of Suggestion to Transform Experience*; W.W. Norton & Company: New York, NY, USA, 2011.
91. Klingbeil, D.A.; Renshaw, T.L.; Willenbrink, J.B.; Copek, R.A.; Chan, K.T.; Haddock, A.; Yassine, J.; Clifton, J. Mindfulness-based interventions with youth: A comprehensive meta-analysis of group-design studies. *J. Sch. Psychol.* **2017**, *63*, 77–103. [CrossRef] [PubMed]
92. Barnes, V.A.; Pendergrast, R.A.; Harshfield, G.A.; Treiber, F.A. Impact of breathing awareness meditation on ambulatory blood pressure and sodium handling in prehypertensive African American adolescents. *Ethn. Dis.* **2008**, *18*, 1–5. [PubMed]
93. Ortiz, R.; Sibinga, E. The role of mindfulness in reducing the adverse effects of childhood stress and trauma. *Children* **2017**, *4*, 16. [CrossRef] [PubMed]
94. Crnic, K.A.; Neece, C.L.; McIntyre, L.L.; Blacher, J.; Baker, B.L. Intellectual disability and developmental risk: Promoting intervention to improve child and family well-being. *Child Dev.* **2017**, *88*, 436–445. [CrossRef] [PubMed]
95. Wark, D.M. Traditional and alert hypnotic phenomena: Development through anteriorization. *Am. J. Clin. Hypn.* **2015**, *57*, 254–266. [CrossRef] [PubMed]
96. Tang, Y.Y.; Hölzel, B.K.; Posner, M.I. The neuroscience of mindfulness meditation. *Nat. Rev. Neurosci.* **2015**, *16*, 213–225. [CrossRef] [PubMed]
97. White, R.E.; Carlson, S.M. What would Batman do? Self-distancing improves executive function in young children. *Dev. Sci.* **2016**, *19*, 419–426. [CrossRef] [PubMed]
98. White, R.E.; Prager, E.O.; Schaefer, C.; Kross, E.; Duckworth, A.L.; Carlson, S.M. The "Batman Effect": Improving perseverance in young children. *Child Dev.* **2017**, *88*, 1563–1571. [CrossRef] [PubMed]
99. Lyons, L. *Using Hypnosis with Children: Creating and Delivering Effective Interventions*; W.W. Norton & Company: New York, NY, USA, 2015.
100. Alladin, A. Mindfulness-based hypnosis: Blending science, beliefs, and wisdoms to catalyze healing. *Am. J. Clin. Hypn.* **2014**, *56*, 285–302. [CrossRef] [PubMed]
101. Lynn, S.J.; Rhue, J.W. (Eds.) *Theories of Hypnosis: Current Models and Perspectives*; Guilford Press Inc.: New York, NY, USA, 1988.
102. Sugarman, L.I.; Wester, W.C., II (Eds.) *Therapeutic Hypnosis with Children and Adolescents*; Crown House: Carmarthen, UK, 2013; Volume 2.
103. Yapko, M.D. *Trancework: An Introduction to the Practice of Clinical Hypnosis*, 5th ed.; Guilford Press Inc.: New York, NY, USA, 2018.
104. Schwartz, M. *Biofeedback: A Practitioner's Guide*; Guilford Press Inc.: New York, NY, USA, 1987.
105. Sugarman, L.I. Hypnosis and Biofeedback. In *Pediatric Primary Care*; Hoekelman, R.A., Friedman, S.R., Nelson, N.M., Seidel, H.M., Weitzman, M.L., Eds.; Mosby: St Louis, MO, USA, 2000.
106. Shaffer, F.; Moss, D. Biofeedback. In *Textbook of Complementary and Alternative Medicine*; Yuan, C.S., Bieber, E.J., Bauer, B.A., Eds.; Taylor & Francis Group: New York, NY, USA, 2005.
107. Barowsky, E. The use of biofeedback in the treatment of disorders of childhood. *Ann. N. Y. Acad. Sci.* **1990**, *602*, 221–233. [CrossRef] [PubMed]
108. Culbert, T.P.; Reaney, J.B.; Kohen, D.P. "Cyberphysiologic" strategies for children: The clinical hypnosis/biofeedback interface. *Int. J. Clin. Exp. Hypn.* **1994**, *42*, 97–117. [CrossRef] [PubMed]
109. Heartmath Inner Balance. Available online: www.heartmath.com (accessed on 3 August 2018).
110. Lang, E.V. My Comfort Talk. Available online: www.comforttalk.com (accessed on 3 August 2018).
111. Furman, B. Kids' Skills App. Available online: http://www.kidsskillsapp.com (accessed on 3 August 2018).
112. Dikel, W.; Olness, K. Self-hypnosis, biofeedback, and voluntary peripheral temperature control in children. *Pediatrics* **1980**, *66*, 335–340. [PubMed]
113. Culbert, T.P.; Banez, G. Pediatric Applications of Biofeedback Other than Headache. In *Biofeedback: A Practitioner's Guide*; Schwartz, M., Andrasik, F., Eds.; Guilford Press Inc.: New York, NY, USA, 2003.
114. Jencks, B. *Your Body—Biofeedback at Its Best*; Nelson-Hall Company: Chicago, IL, USA, 1977.
115. Kohen, D.P. Pediatric Perspective on Mind-Body Medicine. In *Integrative Pediatrics*; Culbert, T.P., Olness, K.O., Eds.; Oxford University Press: New York, NY, USA, 2010; pp. 267–301.

116. Kohen, D.P. The "3 and 6" Hypnotic Induction Technique for Children and Adolescents. In *The Art and Practice of Hypnotic Induction: Favorite Methods of Master Clinicians*; Jensen, M.P., Ed.; Denny Creek Press: Kirkland, WA, USA, 2017.
117. Lu, D.P.; Lu, G.P. A Historical Review and Perspective on the Impact of Acupuncture on US Medicine and Society. *Med. Acupunct.* **2013**, *25*, 311–316. [CrossRef] [PubMed]
118. Black, L.I.; Clarke, T.C.; Barnes, P.M.; Stussman, B.J.; Nahin, R.L. Use of complementary health approaches among children aged 4-17 years in the United States: National Health Interview Survey, 2007–2012. *Natl. Health Stat. Report.* **2015**, *78*, 1–19.
119. Lee, M.S.; Ernst, E. Acupuncture for pain: An overview of Cochrane reviews. *Chin. J. Integr. Med.* **2011**, *17*, 187–189. [CrossRef] [PubMed]
120. Pomeranz, B.; Chiu, D. Naloxone blockade of acupuncture analgesia: Endorphin implicated. *Life Sci.* **1976**, *19*, 1757–1762. [CrossRef]
121. Schiff, E.; Gurgevich, S.; Caspi, O. Potential synergism between hypnosis and acupuncture—Is the whole more than the sum of its parts? *Evid. Based. Complement. Alternat. Med.* **2007**, *4*, 233–240. [CrossRef] [PubMed]
122. Kemper, K.J.; Sarah, R.; Silver-Highfield, E.; Xiarhos, E.; Barnes, L.; Berde, C. On pins and needles? Pediatric pain patients' experience with acupuncture. *Pediatrics* **2000**, *105*, 941–947. [PubMed]
123. Jindal, V.; Ge, A.; Mansky, P.J. Safety and efficacy of acupuncture in children. *J. Pediatr. Hematol. Oncol.* **2008**, *30*, 431–442. [CrossRef] [PubMed]
124. Slover, R.; Neuenkirchen, G.L.; Olamikan, S.; Kent, S. Chronic pediatric pain. *Adv. Pediatr.* **2010**, *57*, 141–162. [CrossRef] [PubMed]
125. Waterhouse, M.; Stelling, C.; Powers, M.; Levy, S.; Zeltzer, L.K. Acupuncture and hypotherapy in the treatment of chronic pain in children. *Clin. Acupunct. Orient. Med.* **2000**, *1*, 139–150. [CrossRef]
126. Zeltzer, L.K.; Tsao, J.C.I.; Stelling, C.; Powers, M.; Levy, S.; Waterhouse, M. A phase I study on the feasibility and acceptability of an acupuncture/hypnosis intervention for chronic pediatric pain. *J. Pain Symptom Manage.* **2002**, *24*, 437–446. [CrossRef]
127. Golianu, B.; Krane, E.; Seybold, J.; Almgren, C.; Anand, K.J.S. Non-pharmacological techniques for pain management in neonates. *Semin. Perinatol.* **2007**, *31*, 318–322. [CrossRef] [PubMed]
128. Samuels, N. Integration of hypnosis with acupuncture: Possible benefits and case examples. *Am. J. Clin. Hypn.* **2005**, *47*, 243–248. [CrossRef] [PubMed]
129. Lu, D.P.; Lu, G.P. A comparison of the clinical effectiveness of various acupuncture points in reducing anxiety to facilitate hypnotic induction. *Int. J. Clin. Exp. Hypn.* **2013**, *61*, 271–281. [CrossRef] [PubMed]
130. Rosted, P.; Bundgaard, M.; Gordon, S.; Pedersen, A.M.L. Acupuncture in the management of anxiety related to dental treatment: A case series. *Acupunct. Med.* **2010**, *28*, 3–5. [CrossRef] [PubMed]
131. Tsai, S.-L.; Fox, L.M.; Murakami, M.; Tsung, J.W. Auricular acupuncture in emergency department treatment of acute pain. *Ann. Emerg. Med.* **2016**, *68*, 583–585. [CrossRef] [PubMed]
132. Barber, T.X. *LSD, Marijuana, Yoga and Hypnosis*; Aldine Transaction Publishing: New Brunswick, NJ, USA, 2008.
133. Sibinga, E.M.S.; Kemper, K.J. Complementary, holistic, and integrative medicine: Meditation practices for pediatric health. *Pediatr. Rev.* **2010**, *31*, e91–e103. [CrossRef] [PubMed]
134. Yoga Alliance. Yoga Alliance Home Page. Available online: www.yogaalliance.org (accessed on 3 August 2018).
135. Yoga Kids. Yoga Kids Training and Certificiation. Available online: www.yogakids.com/training-and-certification (accessed on 3 August 2018).
136. Butzer, B.; Ebert, M.; Telles, S.; Khalsa, S.B.S. School-based yoga programs in the United States: A survey. *Adv. Mind. Body. Med.* **2015**, *29*, 18–26. [PubMed]
137. Yoga Calm. Yoga Calm Home Page. Available online: https://www.yogacalm.org/ (accessed on 3 August 2018).
138. Birdee, G.S.; Yeh, G.Y.; Wayne, P.M.; Phillips, R.S.; Davis, R.B.; Gardiner, P. Clinical applications of yoga for the pediatric population: A systematic review. *Acad. Pediatr.* **2009**, *9*, 212–220. [CrossRef] [PubMed]
139. Kaley-Isley, L.C.; Peterson, J.; Fischer, C.; Peterson, E. Yoga as a complementary therapy for children and adolescents: A guide for clinicians. *Psychiatry* **2010**, *7*, 20–32. [PubMed]

140. Telles, S. Iyengar Yoga for Adolescents and Young Adults with Irritable Bowel Syndrome. In *Child and Adolescent Mental Health*; Nayar, U., Ed.; SAGE Publications: Thousand Oaks, CA, USA, 2012; pp. 219–227.
141. Evans, S.; Lung, K.C.; Seidman, L.C.; Sternlieb, B.; Zeltzer, L.K.; Tsao, J.C.I. Iyengar yoga for adolescents and young adults with irritable bowel syndrome. *J. Pediatr. Gastroenterol. Nutr.* **2014**, *59*, 244–253. [CrossRef] [PubMed]
142. Noggle, J.J.; Steiner, N.J.; Minami, T.; Khalsa, S.B. Benefits of yoga for psychosocial well-being in a US high school curriculum: A preliminary randomized controlled trial. *J. Dev. Behav. Pediatr.* **2012**, *33*, 193–201. [CrossRef] [PubMed]
143. Khalsa, S.B. Yoga in schools research: Improving mental and emotional health. In Proceedings of the Second International Conference on Yoga for Health and Social Transformation, Haridwar, India, 7–10 January 2013.
144. McClafferty, H.; Vohra, S.; Bailey, M.; Brown, M.; Esparham, A.; Gerstbacher, D.; Golianu, B.; Niemi, A.-K.; Sibinga, E.; Weydert, J.; et al. Section on Integrative Medicine. Pediatric Integrative Medicine. *Pediatrics* **2017**, *140*, e20171961. [CrossRef] [PubMed]
145. Gard, T.; Noggle, J.J.; Park, C.L.; Vago, D.R.; Wilson, A. Potential self-regulatory mechanisms of yoga for psychological health. *Front. Hum. Neurosci.* **2014**, *8*, 770. [CrossRef] [PubMed]
146. Schmalzl, L.; Powers, C.; Henje Blom, E. Neurophysiological and neurocognitive mechanisms underlying the effects of yoga-based practices: towards a comprehensive theoretical framework. *Front. Hum. Neurosci.* **2015**, *9*, 235. [CrossRef] [PubMed]
147. Sullivan, M.B.; Erb, M.; Schmalzl, L.; Moonaz, S.; Noggle Taylor, J.; Porges, S.W. Yoga therapy and polyvagal theory: The convergence of traditional wisdom and contemporary neuroscience for self-regulation and resilience. *Front. Hum. Neurosci.* **2018**, *12*, 67. [CrossRef] [PubMed]
148. Dalal, A.; Barber, T.X. Yoga and Hypnotism. In *LSD, Marijuana, Yoga, and Hypnosis*; Aldine Transaction Publishing: New Brunswick, NJ, USA, 2008; pp. 117–132.
149. Landier, W.; Tse, A.M. Use of complementary and alternative medical interventions for the management of procedure-related pain, anxiety, and distress in pediatric oncology: an integrative review. *J. Pediatr. Nurs.* **2010**, *25*, 566–579. [CrossRef] [PubMed]
150. Bethell, C.; Kemper, K.J.; Gombojav, N.; Koch, T.K. Complementary and conventional medicine use among youth with recurrent headaches. *Pediatrics* **2013**, *132*, e1173–e1183. [CrossRef] [PubMed]
151. National Institutes of Health/National Center for Complementary and Integrative Health. Complementary, Alternative, or Integrative Health: What's In a Name? NCCIH. Available online: https://nccih.nih.gov/health/integrative-health (accessed on 12 June 2018).
152. Robertson, D. *Cognitive Hypnotherapy: An Integrated Approach to the Treatment of Emotional Disorders*; Karnac: London, UK, 2012.
153. Alladin, A. Cognitive hypnotherapy for accessing and healing emotional injuries for anxiety disorders. *Am. J. Clin. Hypn.* **2016**, *59*, 24–46. [CrossRef] [PubMed]
154. Semple, R.J.; Lee, J. Mindfulness-based cognitive therapy for children. In *Mindfulness-Based Treatment Approaches: Clinician's Guide to Evidence Base and Applications*; Baer, R., Ed.; Elsevier: Amsterdam, The Netherlands, 2014; pp. 161–188.
155. Elkins, G.R.; Roberts, R.L.; Simicich, L. Mindful self-hypnosis for self-care: An integrative model and illustrative case example. *Am. J. Clin. Hypn.* **2018**, *61*, 45–56. [CrossRef] [PubMed]
156. Kemper, K.J. Integrative medicine is becoming mainstream: Research on multimodal interventions needs to catch up. *Complement. Ther. Med.* **2018**, in press. [CrossRef] [PubMed]
157. McClafferty, H.; Dodds, S.; Brooks, A.; Brenner, M.; Brown, M.; Frazer, P.; Mark, J.; Weydert, J.; Wilcox, G.; Lebensohn, P.; et al. Pediatric Integrative Medicine in Residency (PIMR): Description of a new online educational curriculum. *Children* **2015**, *2*, 98–107. [CrossRef] [PubMed]
158. American Board of Physician Subspecialties Integrative Medicine Exam Description. Available online: http://www.abpsus.org/integrative-medicine-description (accessed on 15 June 2018).
159. Shriberg, L.D.; Kwiatkowski, J. Developmental phonological disorders. I: A clinical profile. *J. Speech Hear. Res.* **1994**, *37*, 1100–1126. [CrossRef] [PubMed]
160. Kekecs, Z.; Varga, K. Positive suggestion techniques in somatic medicine: A review of the empirical studies. *Interv. Med. Appl. Sci.* **2013**, *5*, 101–111. [CrossRef] [PubMed]

161. Lang, E.V.; Hatsiopoulou, O.; Koch, T.; Berbaum, K.; Lutgendorf, S.; Kettenmann, E.; Logan, H.; Kaptchuk, T.J. Can words hurt? Patient-provider interactions during invasive procedures. *Pain* **2005**, *114*, 303–309. [CrossRef] [PubMed]
162. Geller, S.M.; Porges, S.W. Therapeutic presence: Neurophysiological mechanisms mediating feeling safe in therapeutic relationships. *J. Psychother. Integr.* **2014**, *24*, 178–192. [CrossRef]

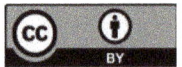

© 2018 by the authors. Licensee MDPI, Basel, Switzerland. This article is an open access article distributed under the terms and conditions of the Creative Commons Attribution (CC BY) license (http://creativecommons.org/licenses/by/4.0/).

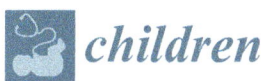

Review

Pediatric Headache Clinic Model: Implementation of Integrative Therapies in Practice

Anna Esparham *, Anne Herbert, Emily Pierzchalski, Catherine Tran, Jennifer Dilts, Madeline Boorigie, Tammie Wingert, Mark Connelly and Jennifer Bickel

Children's Mercy Hospital, University of Missouri-Kansas City School of Medicine, Division of Child Neurology, 2401 Gillham Rd., Kansas City, MO 64108, USA; ajherbert@cmh.edu (A.H.); ecpierzchalski@cmh.edu (E.P.); ctq44@mail.umkc.edu (C.T.); jjdilts@cmh.edu (J.D.); meboorigie@cmh.edu (M.B.); twingert@cmh.edu (T.W.); mconnelly1@cmh.edu (M.C.); jlbickel@cmh.edu (J.B.)
* Correspondence: aeesparham@cmh.edu; Tel.: +1-(816)-302-3320

Received: 22 May 2018; Accepted: 8 June 2018; Published: 12 June 2018

Abstract: The demand for integrative medicine has risen in recent years as research has demonstrated the efficacy of such treatments. The public has also become more conscientious of the potential limitations of conventional treatment alone. Because primary headache syndromes are often the culmination of genetics, lifestyle, stress, trauma, and environmental factors, they are best treated with therapies that are equally multifaceted. The Children's Mercy Hospital, Kansas City, Missouri Headache Clinic has successfully incorporated integrative therapies including nutraceuticals, acupuncture, aromatherapy, biofeedback, relaxation training, hypnosis, psychology services, and lifestyle recommendations for headache management. This paper provides a detailed review of the implementation of integrative therapies for headache treatment and discusses examples through case studies. It can serve as a model for other specialty settings intending to incorporate all evidenced-based practices, whether complementary or conventional.

Keywords: headache; migraine; integrative medicine; complementary therapies; pediatric; mind-body; clinic model; multidisciplinary; implementation

---

1. Introduction

Headaches are one of the most common disorders in childhood, with 60–75% of children reporting that they have had a significant headache by the age of 15 [1,2]. Headache disorders in children are truly a biopsychosocial phenomenon, best addressed with a holistic approach utilizing multidisciplinary therapeutic strategies [3,4]. Integrative medicine aims to make use of all evidence-based therapies, whether complementary or conventional, especially when treating chronic conditions [5,6]. Integrative medicine fosters optimal team dynamics, supports interdisciplinary providers and their staff, encourages healthy communication and mutual respect, and ultimately results in better care for patients [5]. As certain integrative therapies have been proven effective for certain conditions, healthcare providers may benefit from an understanding of the "how-to" of practical implementation of these integrative therapies into their practice [3,4].

Several studies have demonstrated that integrative therapies such as acupuncture, biofeedback, relaxation and stress coping skills, nutraceuticals/supplements, and aromatherapy are efficacious for headaches [7–14]. The use of complementary and integrative therapies in children with headaches may be as high as 76% in some populations [15]. Non-pharmacologic therapies implemented in practice with conventional medicine may prevent medication overuse and chronification of headaches. Because medical prophylaxis alone may often be insufficient, integrative approaches optimize clinical outcomes and provide patients with the best treatment experience [3,16]. Integrative therapies also increase patient self-care and empowerment by taking steps toward better health [17].

Much of the literature on integrative and complementary treatment modalities focuses on the public's use of such therapies as well as their efficacy and safety. There is a paucity of literature on the various ways in which integrative therapies can be implemented in clinical practice. We describe how integrative therapies have been incorporated into a pediatric headache clinic in a Midwest academic medical center, Children's Mercy Hospital and Clinics, Kansas City, Missouri (CMH). In this descriptive article, we outline integrative therapies and the evidence to support their use. Utilizing case studies, we describe how integrative therapies have been successfully incorporated into an academic headache practice. The case studies were deemed exempt by the CMH institutional review board.

2. Integrative Approaches and Their Implementation in Practice

2.1. Nutraceuticals/Dietary Supplements

Magnesium, riboflavin, and coenzyme Q10 are dietary supplements that are more commonly used for migraine headaches, based on the American Academy of Neurology and American Headache Society (AHS/AAN) guidelines [7]. Magnesium is involved in over 300 enzymatic reactions and participates in neuronal homeostasis through antagonizing the N-methyl-D-aspartate (NMDA) receptor, blocking calcium channels, and decreasing neurogenic inflammation [18]. Riboflavin plays a role in membrane stability, energy-related cellular function, and mediation of oxidative stress. Coenzyme Q10 (CoQ10) is involved in healthy mitochondrial function and acts as an antioxidant [19]. Butterbur exhibits anti-inflammatory effects by inhibiting leukotriene synthesis and regulating calcium channels [20]. Magnesium and riboflavin are considered by the AHS and AAN as Level B evidence: Probably effective for migraine prevention [7]. CoQ10 is considered Level C: Possibly effective for migraine prevention [7]. The American Academy of Neurology withdrew butterbur from their 2012 migraine prevention guidelines due to the associated risk of hepatotoxicity, as butterbur may contain petazolides [21]. The dietary supplement industry does not regulate the removal of petazolides, so caution is required.

In the CMH pediatric headache clinic, providers typically initiate a preventive supplement and/or medication for patients having four or more headaches per month. Preventive supplements or medications are each trialed one at a time for three months in order to determine therapeutic effect with the goal of decreasing headache severity and frequency. Potential risks, benefits, and side effects of supplements and medications are discussed with patients and their families to determine which preventive option is the best fit.

2.2. Acupuncture

Acupuncture's mechanisms of action include activating the endorphin-enkephalin system, inhibiting pain pathways in the spinal cord and midbrain through neurotransmitter release, and cell-to-cell signaling through connective tissue manipulation [22–25]. Acupuncture has demonstrated efficacy for prevention of both episodic migraines and episodic tension-type headaches [8,9]. A 2016 Cochrane review demonstrated that acupuncture may be more effective at reducing migraine frequency compared to prophylactic drug treatment (Standard Mean Deviation (SMD) −0.25; 95% Confidence Interval (CI) −0.39–−0.10: 3 trials, 739 participants), but not at long-term follow-up [8]. Migraine frequency decreased by 50% in 41% of participants receiving acupuncture versus 17% of those not receiving acupuncture (Risk Ratio (RR) 2.40; 95% CI 2.08–2.76; 4 studies; 2519 participants) [8].

One large trial of 1265 participants in a Cochrane review, comparing acupuncture to routine care in the treatment of tension type headaches, showed a 50% reduction of headache frequency in 48% of acupuncture recipients versus 19% of those with routine treatment (RR 2.52; 95% CI 2.11–3.02; number needed to treat 3; 95% CI 3–5) [9]. A second trial of 207 participants, comparing acupuncture to routine care found 45% versus 4% improvement, respectively; (RR 11.36; 95% CI 3.69–34.98; number needed to treat 2; 95% CI 1–9) [9].

Acupuncture began to be utilized for our headache patients in 2015. Dr. Jennifer Bickel, MD, a neurologist and medical acupuncturist, developed the acupuncture program, which now includes three medical acupuncturists, all trained via a 300 h medical acupuncture course. According to a market data report by the CMH de-identified information database approved by CMH, the majority of patients treated with acupuncture included older adolescents, predominantly female, and of white race. One hundred and thirty patients received acupuncture between October 2015 and November 2017. The average number of acupuncture visits per patient was 4.1. The number of new and total acupuncture visits increased in relation to the addition of medical acupuncturists. Patients with refractory headaches were more likely to receive acupuncture, compared to patients with less frequent headaches. A significant proportion of acupuncture patients had also tried more aggressive treatments, such as OnabotulinumtoxinA injections (16%) and valproic acid (10%), suggesting that the patients receiving acupuncture had complex and intractable headaches.

CMH marketed the acupuncture program by developing a page on their website that launched in April 2017. The acupuncture page has received nearly 200 views and is currently ranked second in Google searches for the keyword phrase "acupuncture for headaches in children". The acupuncture clinic has expanded to include referrals from other CMH providers, predominantly from general neurology, pain management, rehabilitation, gastroenterology, and physical therapy. Acupuncture training privileges for acute pain protocols have also recently been approved by the CMH credentialing committee. The acupuncture training program will target physicians in the acute care setting (i.e., emergency department, urgent care) teaching two acute pain protocols.

2.3. Aromatherapy

Aromatherapy refers to the medicinal or therapeutic use of essential oils derived from plant sources [26]. Lavender essential oil has been commonly used for its anxiolytic and mood stabilizing properties. It has been evaluated for migraines in a placebo-controlled clinical trial. Inhaling lavender essential oil for 15 min reduced headache severity on the Visual Analogue Scale (VAS) from 3.6 ± 2.8 to 1.6 ± 1.6 and was statistically significant compared to the control group [10].

Aromatherapy started in the CMH Headache Clinic as a nurse-driven project, utilized as an adjunctive therapy with acupuncture. CMH provided training to personnel on aromatherapy through an online module course. Acupuncture patients were offered a hospital-approved lavender essential oil patch and asked to evaluate their experience. The survey asked if "using the essential oil patch enhanced my acupuncture experience" on a Likert scale of 1 (not at all) to 5 (very much). Twelve respondents completed the survey with an average Likert scale score of 3.5. All respondents unanimously responded "yes" to "I would like to use essential oil patches in the future". On the basis of the positive responses, lavender essential oil patches continue to be utilized during acupuncture.

2.4. Evidence-Based Behavioral and Self-Regulation Interventions

The United States Headache Consortium Guidelines has recommended (grade A evidence) that relaxation, biofeedback, and cognitive behavioral therapies may be considered as options for the prevention of migraines [27].

2.4.1. Biofeedback

Biofeedback teaches self-regulation of autonomic functions related to stress and pain, including heart rate, respiratory rate, and skin temperature. A meta-analysis, including five studies with 137 participants, found that biofeedback reduced pediatric migraine frequency (Mean Difference (MD) -1.97 (95% CI, $-2.72--1.21$); $p < 0.00001$), attack duration (MD -3.94 (95% CI, $-5.57--2.31$); $p < 0.00001$), and headache intensity (MD, -1.77 (95% CI, $-2.42--1.11$); $p < 0.00001$) compared with waiting-list control patients [11].

The CMH biofeedback clinic is staffed by a clinical pain psychologist and trained nursing staff. The biofeedback approach utilizes audio-visual technology to teach regulation of heart rate, respiratory rate, and skin temperature. Additionally, the pain psychologist utilizes cognitive behavioral therapy techniques, including acceptance and commitment therapy, to facilitate generalization and application of strategies in pain management. Patients who consistently practice self-regulation skills independently see the most success with this program.

2.4.2. Relaxation Training

Relaxation training includes deep/diaphragmatic breathing, progressive muscle relaxation, guided imagery, and mindfulness/meditation. Relaxation training, like biofeedback, increases patients' control over physiological responses to headache pain, reducing stress and anxiety, and decreasing sympathetic overdrive. While little data exists on relaxation in children, progressive muscle relaxation (PMR) was shown to decrease migraine frequency in adults by up to 41% after a six-week intervention [12]. In a meta-analysis, relaxation training in adult studies demonstrated an effect size of 0.55 (CI: 0.14–0.96), representing a moderate improvement in migraine headaches [28].

The CMH headache providers utilize a website, www.headachereliefguide.com, to teach relaxation strategies to patients and families. The website, developed by Dr. Jennifer Bickel, MD and Dr. Mark Connelly, PhD, contains a "relaxation section" with videos demonstrating relaxed breathing, PMR, and guided imagery. Additionally, CMH pain psychologists teach relaxation strategies during some headache clinic visits.

2.4.3. Hypnosis

Clinical hypnosis is a self-regulation strategy using self-directed suggestions to facilitate the mind-body connection, ultimately cultivating a sense of awareness and positive well-being [29]. A clinical hypnosis case series demonstrated a therapeutic benefit for adolescents with comorbid chronic daily headaches and anxiety [13]. Mind-body strategies, including clinical hypnosis, may regulate connections in the prefrontal structures of the adolescent brain, reducing the impact of stress-related conditions [30]. Mind-body therapies also balance dysregulation of the autonomic nervous system that may occur in migraines [31,32].

A headache-trained nurse practitioner at CMH received certification in clinical hypnosis at the National Pediatric Hypnosis Training Institute. This nurse practitioner offers clinical hypnosis during clinic visits to assist children and teens in self-guided relaxation, thus optimizing resilience.

2.4.4. Psychological Services

Depression and anxiety may contribute to functional impairment in children and adolescents with migraines [33]. A 2016 meta-analysis found that cognitive behavioral therapy demonstrated clinically significant improvement (50% or greater reduction of headache activity) after treatment and at follow-up three months later (Odds Ratio (OR) 9.11 (95% CI: 5.01–16.58, $p < 0.001$) and OR 9.18 (95% CI: 5.69–14.81, $p < 0.001$), respectively) [14]. A 2014 Cochrane review demonstrated that face-to-face psychological treatments reduced pain intensity in pediatric headache patients, with long-term benefits [34].

CMH Headache Clinic patients who are missing multiple days of school due to headache and/or have comorbid psychological concerns are referred to the CMH Comprehensive Headache Clinic. In this multidisciplinary clinic, patients and their families are treated by a headache physician, a clinical pain psychologist, and a headache social worker. Pain psychologists provide education in relaxation and self-regulation, pain coping strategies, and lifestyle modification. Additionally, acceptance and commitment therapy and other cognitive behavioral strategies are utilized. Pain psychologists frequently help patients and their families to find counseling services near their homes, facilitating ongoing psychological care. The headache social worker provides parental support and headache-specific school accommodations. This often includes a school letter and, when indicated, a 504 plan.

2.4.5. Lifestyle Strategies

Nutrition, sleep, water, caffeine, and physical activity all affect headaches. Skipping meals, not getting enough sleep, and decreased physical activity have been associated with recurrent headaches in the adolescent population [35]. Modifying sleep hygiene in children may play a significant role in improving headache symptoms [36]. Caffeine and food additives including monosodium glutamate, cocoa, aspartame, cheese, citrus, and nitrites are common triggers for headaches in children [37]. Caffeine abstinence has been associated with improved headache outcomes [38]. Increasing water intake may result in increased quality of life and decreased headache duration [39,40].

CMH Headache Clinic practitioners evaluate and discuss lifestyle factors at each clinic visit, often helping patients to identify a particular lifestyle factor on which to focus their improvement efforts for the next few months. Headache Clinic nurses provide additional patient education at the end of clinic visits, and written information is also provided. Additionally, patients and families are referred to www.headachereliefguide.com to review lifestyle recommendations. Lifestyle "check-ins" are done through telephone triage by nursing staff. Parents are encouraged to call a live nurse phone line regarding questions, concerns, and updates regarding their child. Nursing staff routinely ask about lifestyle behaviors and provide education, utilizing provider recommendations and the headache relief guide website. This empowers patients and families to take ownership of their own health outcomes.

3. Case Studies

All names have been changed to protect privacy.

3.1. Case Study: Claire

Claire is an 18 year-old female with diagnoses of migraine without aura, vestibular dysfunction, and ulcerative colitis. At age 14, she sought care with a neurologist at an outside facility. At that time, headaches occurred once a week. Claire's headaches worsened at the age of 15 after sustaining three mild traumatic brain injuries within a six-week time period. Screening labs and brain MRI were normal. Claire's headaches were refractory to multiple medications including nortriptyline, propranolol, topiramate, amitriptyline, CoQ10, zolmitriptan, hydrocodone-acetaminophen, and two OnabotulinumtoxinA treatments. She had not attended school for one year (due to headaches) prior to her first appointment at the CMH Headache Clinic.

Claire began treatment with a nurse practitioner at the CMH Headache Clinic at the age of 16. At her initial visit, she reported continuous occipital headaches associated with visual scotoma, dizziness, and nausea. Her nurse practitioner noted signs of vestibular dysfunction on exam and referred Claire to vestibular therapy, in addition to initiating preventive and abortive medications. The nurse practitioner counseled Claire on the importance of good headache hygiene, specifically focusing on increasing water intake and regulating sleep. Claire was receiving counseling for stress, which her nurse practitioner recommended continuing. Claire received occipital nerve blocks twice after that visit without headache improvement. She tried several preventives including tizanidine, cyproheptadine, atenolol, and lisinopril. She practiced vestibular exercises consistently and the dizziness partially improved.

Claire's nurse practitioner ordered the CMH comprehensive aggressive migraine protocol (CAMP) after nine additional months of intractable headaches despite multiple interventions. CAMP is a five-day outpatient dihydroergotamine (DHE) and magnesium infusion program. CAMP patients and their parents receive visits from a nurse practitioner, pain psychologist, and social worker. Massage, aromatherapy, hypnosis, Cefaly (an FDA-approved transcutaneous electrical nerve stimulation unit device to prevent and abort headaches), and acupuncture can also be provided during a CAMP session. Claire's headache decreased from 6 out of 10 to 1 out of 10 on the VAS by the end of the fourth day of CAMP.

Claire began monthly acupuncture sessions after CAMP. Acupuncture procedures varied at each monthly session and included electroacupuncture, scalp, auricular, neck and back, abdominal, and extremity acupoints. After each acupuncture session, she had two to three weeks of complete headache relief. She was able to wean off of preventive medication completely for several months but has since restarted daily amitriptyline and occasionally requires rizatriptan or a combination abortive treatment of ibuprofen, an antiemetic, and an antihistamine. She now attends college and is managing classes and a part time job successfully. She continues to receive monthly acupuncture for prevention of migraines and sees her nurse practitioner at regular intervals.

3.2. Case Study: Allison

Allison is an 18 year-old female with diagnoses of chronic daily headache, asthma, allergic rhinitis, and anxiety. She began treatment with a nurse practitioner at the CMH Headache Clinic at the age of 16, approximately three months after sustaining her third concussion. Her examination showed vestibular dysfunction but was otherwise normal. Allison's nurse practitioner ordered vestibular therapy, magnesium oxide daily for headache prevention, and an abortive cocktail of ibuprofen and diphenhydramine. Her abortive cocktail was limited to two to three times weekly. Lifestyle counseling on hydration, nutrition, sleep, and stress was given at the time of visit and www.headachereliefguide.com was used to teach relaxation strategies.

At her three-month follow-up visit, Allison had been compliant with her medication regimen, vestibular therapy, and lifestyle modifications. She continued to have daily headaches, but with decreased headache intensity. Additionally, she reported dizziness, fogginess, and increased anxiety. Her headache provider added a second preventive medication, amitriptyline daily, and encouraged her to initiate counseling. She was prescribed a new abortive cocktail of hydroxyzine, prochlorperazine, and ibuprofen. She was also referred for biofeedback therapy.

Allison started weekly biofeedback visits with a trained psychologist for a total of five weekly sessions. Biofeedback entailed utilizing four different sensors that measure physiologic correlates to stress or autonomic regulation: A surface electromyograph on the frontalis muscle of the forehead to measure muscle tension, a temperature sensor on pad of middle finger for thermoregulation and vascular reactivity, an electrodermal sensor on index and fourth fingers to measure skin conductance (i.e., sweat/moisture level), and a pneumograph strain gauge just below the rib cage to measure respiratory patterns. At the first visit, Allison exhibited sympathetic and vascular activation in response to stress. She was instructed to practice diaphragmatic breathing for three minutes, three times daily. At the second session, she was taught PMR. By the third session, her daily headaches had decreased to one headache per week. She completed a guided imagery exercise and was instructed to practice this in addition to diaphragmatic breathing and PMR at home. At her fourth session, she reported one headache per week, which responded well to abortive therapy. She was also taught autogenic relaxation during her fourth biofeedback session. At her fifth session, she continued to only report one headache weekly. At the end of biofeedback, she demonstrated improvement in all four biofeedback measures including reduced heart rate, reduced muscle tension on electromyography, increased skin temperature, and reduced respiratory rate. This is indicative of improvements in her ability to regulate stress or the autonomic nervous system. After biofeedback, she has continued practicing autogenic relaxation, guided imagery, PMR, and diaphragmatic breathing exercises at home.

Three months following biofeedback treatments, Allison returned for a follow-up Headache Clinic visit. Her exam, including vestibular function, was normal. Allison's headaches were still transformed from chronic daily headaches to episodic as she reported only one headache per week, alleviated by ibuprofen and sleep. She was advised to continue lifestyle recommendations and biofeedback techniques to help manage and prevent headaches, along with daily amitriptyline for prevention and an abortive cocktail as needed.

3.3. Case Study: Makayla

Makayla is a 13 year-old female with diagnoses of migraine headache, ankle pain, asthma, chronic urticaria, food allergies, and vasomotor rhinitis. She began treatment with a Headache Clinic nurse practitioner for post-concussion syndrome, after sustaining several concussions. She reported that her migraine headaches began at age seven, with worsening of headache frequency and severity after her concussions. Her post-concussive symptoms included daily continuous headaches and severe migraines three to four days per week, accompanied by light, noise, and smell sensitivity, nausea, numbness, weakness, tingling, vestibular dysfunction, daytime sleepiness, fatigue, and allodynia. She did report that school had become a major stressor for her with difficulty concentrating and not being able to keep up with the work. However, she denied suicidal ideation or poor mood. At the initial visit, she had missed 15 days of school in one semester and had discontinued sports participation after her concussions. She was referred for vestibular therapy and counseled in lifestyle factors, including nutrition, sleep, hydration, and stress management. Prior to her initial headache visit, Makayla was utilizing ibuprofen or acetaminophen on an as needed basis without relief. Her nurse practitioner initiated tizanidine and magnesium gluconate daily for headache prevention. Additionally, meloxicam daily was initiated for 30 days, and rizatriptan was prescribed as a headache abortive, limited to three times weekly.

Additional therapies included Cefaly, an occipital nerve block, and acupuncture. Cefaly was trialed at her clinic visit, with a subsequent decrease in VAS pain scores from 4 out of 10 to 3 out of 10. She trialed Cefaly during a later clinic visit, with similar results. When Makayla underwent an occipital nerve block with lidocaine and bupivacaine, she developed a delayed hypersensitivity reaction to lidocaine with worsening headaches after the nerve block. She was then prescribed prochlorperazine, diphenhydramine, and a solumedrol dosepak for the severe headache. However, these medications did not result in headache relief. Acupuncture was initiated to include scalp, auricular and extremity points, with six acupuncture sessions over eight weeks. At her first acupuncture visit, her headache decreased from 7 out of 10 to 4 out of 10 on the VAS. Additionally, she received counseling in relaxation, acupressure, and diaphragmatic breathing. The following day, she received intramuscular DHE, metoclopramide, ondansetron, and diphenhydramine along with acupuncture. Her pain decreased from 4 out of 10 to 2 out of 10 on the VAS. On subsequent acupuncture visits, she presented with 3 to 4 out of 10 headache pain, decreasing to 1 to 2 out of 10 on the VAS after acupuncture.

Makayla was also referred for clinical hypnosis with a nurse practitioner trained in pediatric clinic hypnosis. Makayla participated in several 40 min hypnosis sessions that focused on progressive muscle relaxation and imagery of a favorite place. The favorite place was a place known only to Makayla where she felt safe and calm. At the end of the visit she was taught self-hypnosis and self-relaxation techniques to trial at home, and she practiced this twice daily for 30 min. Makayla also began counseling sessions with a psychologist. At follow-up visits, she has reported that her headaches are mild and infrequent, occurring less than four times monthly.

4. Conclusions

Integrative therapies offer non-pharmacological treatment options that effectively reduce headache frequency and severity. The goal of integrative therapies is to empower individuals to take ownership of their health through a holistic patient-provider relationship that emphasizes education and at-home adherence. The CMH Headache Clinic has demonstrated positive outcomes by incorporating integrative therapies into headache treatment plans. Headache treatment in the clinic is as multifaceted as the headaches themselves. The multidisciplinary approach takes this complex etiology into account by addressing factors such as lifestyle, anxiety, and stress, through a variety of services.

Concerns about financing integrative therapies are relevant, as integrative therapies may not be covered by government or commercial insurance. CMH takes part in both government and commercial insurance for reimbursement of integrative services, such as acupuncture, biofeedback and relaxation, and psychology services. While financial sustainability is a main priority for healthcare organizations, incorporating evidenced-based treatments that improve clinical outcomes and quality measures should be prioritized.

Furthermore, future studies on integrative therapies and headaches should include larger sample sizes and randomized controlled trials specific to pediatric patients.

Author Contributions: A.E., A.H., E.P. contributed to the conceptualization of the manuscript, in addition to writing and editing the manuscript. C.T., J.D., M.B., T.W., M.C. and J.B. contributed to the writing and editing of the manuscript.

Funding: The development and writing of this manuscript did not receive external funding.

Acknowledgments: The authors would like to thank the faculty and staff in the Division of Child Neurology at Children's Mercy Hospital for their significant contributions to the success of the Headache Section and Clinics.

Conflicts of Interest: The authors declare no conflict of interest.

References

1. Steiner, T.J.; Stoverner, L.J.; Katsarava, Z.; Lainez, J.M.; Lampl, C.; Lanteri-Minet, M.; Rastenyte, D.; Ruiz de la Torre, E.; Tassorelli, C.; Barre, J.; et al. The impact of headache in Europe: Principal results of the Eurolight project. *J. Headache Pain* **2014**, *15*, 31. [CrossRef] [PubMed]
2. Bille, B. Migraine and tension-type headache in children and adolescents. *Cephalalgia* **1996**, *16*, 78. [CrossRef] [PubMed]
3. Soee, A.B.; Skov, L.; Skovgaard, L.T.; Thomsen, L.L. Headache in children: Effectiveness of multidisciplinary treatment in a tertiary pediatric headache clinic. *Cephalalgia* **2013**, *33*, 1218–1228. [CrossRef] [PubMed]
4. Kabbouche, M.A.; Powers, S.W.; Vockell, A.B.; LeCates, S.L.; Ellinor, P.L.; Segers, A.; Manning, P.; Burdine, D.; Hershey, A.D. Outcome of a multidisciplinary approach to pediatric migraine at 1, 2, and 5 years. *Headache* **2005**, *45*, 1298–1303. [CrossRef] [PubMed]
5. Maizes, V.; Rakel, D.; Niemiec, C. Integrative medicine and patient-centered care. *Explore* **2009**, *5*, 277–289. [CrossRef] [PubMed]
6. Ananth, S. Complementary and Alternative Medicine Survey of Hospitals: Summary of Results. Health Forum and Samueli Institute. 2007. Available online: http://www.samueliinstitute.org/File%20Library/Our%20Research/OHE/CAM_Survey_2010_oct6.pdf (accessed on 5 April 2018).
7. Loder, E.; Burch, R.; Rizzoli, P. The 2012 AHS/AAN guidelines for prevention of episodic migraine: A summary and comparison with other recent clinical practice guidelines. *Headache* **2012**, *52*, 930–945. [CrossRef] [PubMed]
8. Linde, K.; Allais, G.; Brinkhaus, B.; Fei, Y.; Mehring, M.; Vertosick, E.A.; Vickers, A.; White, A.R. Acupuncture for the prevention of episodic migraine. *Cochrane Database Syst. Rev.* **2016**, *28*, CD001218. [CrossRef] [PubMed]
9. Linde, K.; Allais, G.; Brinkhaus, B.; Fei, Y.; Mehring, M.; Shin, B.C.; Vickers, A.; White, A.R. Acupuncture for the prevention of tension-type headache. *Cochrane Database Syst. Rev.* **2016**, *4*, CD007587. [CrossRef] [PubMed]
10. Sasannejad, P.; Saeedi, M.; Shoeibi, A.; Gorji, A.; Abbasi, M.; Foroughipour, M. Lavender essential oil in the treatment of migraine headache: A placebo-controlled clinical trial. *Eur. Neurol.* **2012**, *67*, 288–291. [CrossRef] [PubMed]
11. Stubberud, A.; Varkey, E.; McCrory, D.C.; Pedersen, S.A.; Linde, M. Biofeedback as prophylaxis for pediatric migraine: A meta-analysis. *Pediatrics* **2016**, *138*. [CrossRef] [PubMed]
12. Meyer, B.; Keller, A.; Wöhlbier, H.; Overath, C.H.; Müller, B.; Kropp, P. Progressive muscle relaxation reduces migraine frequency and normalizes amplitudes of contingent negative variation (CNV). *J. Headache Pain* **2016**, *17*, 1–9. [CrossRef] [PubMed]
13. Kohen, D.P. Chronic daily headache: Helping adolescents help themselves with self-hypnosis. *Am. J. Clin. Hypn.* **2011**, *54*, 32–46. [CrossRef] [PubMed]
14. Ng, Q.X.; Venkatanaryanan, N.; Kumar, L. A systematic review and meta-analysis of cognitive behavioral therapy for the management of pediatric migraine. *Headache* **2017**, *57*, 349–362. [CrossRef] [PubMed]

15. Libera, D.D.; Colombo, B.; Pavan, G.; Comi, G. Complementary and alternative medicine (CAM) use in an Italian cohort of pediatric headache patients: The tip of the iceberg. *Neurol. Sci.* **2014**, *35*, 145–148. [CrossRef] [PubMed]
16. Gaul, C.; Visscher, C.M.; Bhola, R.; Sorbi, M.J.; Galli, F.; Rasmussen, A.V.; Jensen, R. Team players against headache: Multidisciplinary treatment of primary headaches and medication overuse headache. *J. Headache Pain* **2011**, *12*, 511–519. [CrossRef] [PubMed]
17. Foley, H.; Steel, A. Patient perceptions of patient-centred care, empathy and empowerment in complementary medicine clinical practice: A cross-sectional study. *Adv. Integr. Med.* **2017**, *4*, 22–30. [CrossRef]
18. Taylor, F.R. Nutraceuticals and headache: The biological basis. *Headache* **2011**, *51*, 484–501. [CrossRef] [PubMed]
19. Littaru, G.P.; Tiano, L. Clinical aspects of coenzyme Q10: An update. *Nutrition* **2010**, *26*, 250–254. [CrossRef] [PubMed]
20. Sun-Edelstein, C.; Mauskop, A. Alternative headache treatments: Nutraceuticals, behavioral and physical treatments. *Headache* **2011**, *51*, 469–483. [CrossRef] [PubMed]
21. Holland, S.; Silberstein, S.; Freitag, F.; Dodick, D.; Argoff, C.; Ashman, E. Evidence-based guideline update: NSAIDs and other complementary treatments for episodic migraine prevention in adults: [RETIRED]. *Neurology* **2012**, *78*, 1346–1353. [CrossRef] [PubMed]
22. Langevin, H.M.; Bouffard, N.A.; Badger, G.J.; Churchill, D.L.; Howe, A.K. Subcutaneous tissue fibroblast cytoskeletal remodeling induced by acupuncture: Evidence for a mechanotransduction-based mechanism. *J. Cell. Physiol.* **2006**, *207*, 767–774. [CrossRef] [PubMed]
23. Langevin, H.M.; Sherman, K.J. Pathophysiological model for chronic low back pain integrating connective tissue and nervous system mechanisms. *Med. Hypotheses* **2007**, *68*, 74–80. [CrossRef] [PubMed]
24. Langevin, H.M.; Yandow, J.A. Relationship of acupuncture points and meridians to connective tissue planes. *Anat. Rec.* **2002**, *269*, 257–265. [CrossRef] [PubMed]
25. Berman, B.M.; Langevin, H.H.; Witt, C.M.; Dubner, R. Acupuncture for chronic low back pain. *N. Engl. J. Med.* **2010**, *363*, 454–461. [CrossRef] [PubMed]
26. National Cancer Institute. Available online: https://www.cancer.gov/about-cancer/treatment/cam/hp/aromatherapy-pdq (accessed on 7 February 2018).
27. Silberstein, S.D.; Edlund, W. Practice parameter: Evidence-based guidelines for migraine headache (an evidence-based review): Report of the Quality Standards Subcommittee of the American Academy of Neurology. *Neurology* **2000**, *55*, 754–762. [CrossRef] [PubMed]
28. Goslin, R.E.; Gray, R.; McCrory, D.; Penzien, D.; Rains, J.; Hasselblad, J. Behavioral and Physical Treatments for Migraine Headache. AHRQ Technical Reviews 1999. Available online: https://www.ncbi.nlm.nih.gov/books/NBK45267/ (accessed on 16 May 2018).
29. Kohen, D.P.; Kaiser, P. Clinical hypnosis with children and adolescents—What? Why? How?: Origins, applications, and efficacy. *Children* **2014**, *1*, 74–98. [CrossRef] [PubMed]
30. Sawni, A.; Breuner, C.C. Clinical hypnosis, an effective mind-body modality for adolescents with behavioral and physical complaints. *Children* **2017**, *4*, 19. [CrossRef] [PubMed]
31. Moura, V.L.; Faurot, K.R.; Gaylord, S.A.; Mann, J.D.; Sill, M.; Lynch, C.; Lee, M.Y. Mind-body interventions for treatment of phantom limb pain in persons with amputation. *Am. J. Phys. Med. Rehabil.* **2012**, *91*, 701. [CrossRef] [PubMed]
32. Wells, R.E.; Smitherman, T.A.; Seng, E.K.; Houle, T.T.; Loder, E.W. Behavioral and Mind/Body interventions in headache: Unanswered questions and future research directions. *Headache* **2014**, *54*, 1107–1113. [CrossRef] [PubMed]
33. Kemper, K.J.; Heyer, G.; Pakalnis, A.; Binkley, P.F. Factors contribute to headache-related disability in teens? *Pediatr. Neurol.* **2016**, *56*, 48–54. [CrossRef] [PubMed]
34. Eccleston, C.; Palermo, T.M.; Williams, A.C.; Lewandowski, H.A.; Morley, S.; Fisher, E.; Law, E. Psychological therapies for the management of chronic and recurrent pain in children and adolescents. *Cochrane Database Syst. Rev.* **2014**, *5*. [CrossRef]
35. Walter, S. Lifestyle behaviors and illness-related factors as predictors of recurrent headache in U.S. adolescents. *J. Neurosci. Nurs.* **2014**, *46*, 337–350. [CrossRef] [PubMed]
36. Guidetti, V.; Dosi, C.; Bruni, O. The relationship between sleep and headache in children: Implications for treatment. *Cephalalgia* **2014**, *34*, 767–776. [CrossRef] [PubMed]

37. Taheri, S. Effect of exclusion of frequent consumed dietary triggers in a cohort of children with chronic primary headache. *Nutr. Health* **2017**, *23*, 47–50. [CrossRef] [PubMed]
38. Lee, M.J.; Choi, H.A.; Choi, H.; Chung, C.S. Caffeine discontinuation improves acute migraine treatment: A prospective clinic-based study. *J. Headache Pain* **2016**, *17*, 71. [CrossRef] [PubMed]
39. Spigt, M.G.; Kuijper, E.C.; Schayck, C.P.; Troost, J.; Knipschild, P.G.; Linssen, V.M.; Knottnerus, J.A. Increasing the daily water intake for the prophylactic treatment of headache: A pilot trial. *Eur. J. Neurol.* **2005**, *12*, 715–718. [CrossRef] [PubMed]
40. Spigt, M.; Weerkamp, N.; Troost, J.; van Schayck, C.P.; Knottnerus, J.A. A randomized trial on the effects of regular water intake in patients with recurrent headaches. *Fam. Pract.* **2012**, *29*, 370–375. [CrossRef] [PubMed]

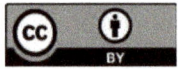

© 2018 by the authors. Licensee MDPI, Basel, Switzerland. This article is an open access article distributed under the terms and conditions of the Creative Commons Attribution (CC BY) license (http://creativecommons.org/licenses/by/4.0/).

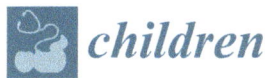

Review

Pediatric Integrative Medicine in Academia: Stanford Children's Experience

Gautam Ramesh [1], Dana Gerstbacher [2], Jenna Arruda [3], Brenda Golianu [4], John Mark [5] and Ann Ming Yeh [6],*

1. School of Medicine, University of California, San Diego, La Jolla, CA 92093, USA; gramesh@ucsd.edu
2. Division of Rheumatology, Department of Pediatrics, School of Medicine, Stanford University, Palo Alto, CA 94304, USA; gerst1@stanford.edu
3. Department of Pediatrics, School of Medicine, Stanford University, Palo Alto, CA 94304, USA; jarruda@stanford.edu
4. Division of Pediatric Anesthesia and Pain Medicine, Department of Anesthesiology, Perioperative and Pain Medicine, School of Medicine, Stanford University, Palo Alto, CA 94304, USA; bgolianu@stanford.edu
5. Division of Pulmonary Medicine, Department of Pediatrics, School of Medicine, Stanford University, Palo Alto, CA 94304, USA; jmark@stanford.edu
6. Division of Gastroenterology, Hepatology and Nutrition, Department of Pediatrics, School of Medicine, Stanford University, Palo Alto, CA 94304, USA
* Correspondence: annming@stanford.edu; Tel.: +1-650-723-5070

Received: 18 September 2018; Accepted: 29 November 2018; Published: 12 December 2018

Abstract: Pediatric integrative medicine is an emerging field which, to date, has not been described in detail in academic medical centers in the United States. Early research of pediatric integrative medicine modalities shows promise for the treatment of common pediatric conditions such as irritable bowel syndrome, acute and chronic pain, headache, and allergy, among others. In light of the growing prevalence of pediatric illnesses and patient complexity, it is crucial to emphasize the patient's overall well-being. As academic centers around the world start to develop pediatric integrative medicine programs, the aim of this manuscript is to briefly highlight evidence of effective integrative treatments in pediatric subspecialties, to describe the establishment of our integrative medicine program, to summarize its early efforts, and to discuss potential barriers and keys to success.

Keywords: pediatric; integrative medicine; academic medicine

---

1. Background

Integrative medicine (IM) is a patient-centric, evidence-based, therapeutic paradigm that coordinates the integration of all pertinent conventional and complementary approaches to achieve patient health. Integrative medicine incorporates all appropriate therapies, emphasizes the patient–provider relationship, and utilizes lifestyle changes to holistically optimize health and healing [1]. It addresses the biologic, psychosocial, spiritual, and environmental aspects of patient wellbeing. Integrative modalities range from mind–body interventions to nutrition. While current biomedical practices have made great strides in the treatment of many conditions, the addition of IM principles and practices can help restore the patient to a state of personal wellbeing and optimal function [2,3].

The National Center for Complementary and Integrative Health clarifies definitions frequently used with integrative medicine: complementary medicine refers to using non-allopathic medicine in conjunction with conventional allopathic medical treatment, and alternative medicine refers to utilizing a non-allopathic therapy instead of a conventional allopathic treatment. These two approaches are commonly referred to as complementary and alternative medicine (CAM) [4]. Throughout this article, the term "integrative medicine" (IM) or "IM practices" will be employed to refer to the concurrent use of CAM therapies in conjunction with traditional allopathic practice, in order to highlight this emerging practice paradigm in pediatric practice, except where the articles quoted have specifically employed the terminology of the terms "complementary" or "alternative" medicine.

The National Health Interview Survey results from 2012 show that 33% of adults and 12% of children used complementary health approaches [5,6]. Children with chronic illnesses are significantly more likely to use IM therapies than healthy children [7,8]. Integrative medicine is used by more than 50% of pediatric patients with chronic disease [2].

In the pediatric population, IM practices have enormous potential to reduce healthcare costs and ensure a healthier future for children by emphasizing prevention and promoting wellness [9]. The literature over the last two decades has confirmed the clinical efficacy of certain IM therapies and has demonstrated improved patient outcomes (e.g., improved quality of life, decreased cardiovascular risk factors), symptom relief, and patient satisfaction [10,11]. Large systematic reviews indicate potential cost-effectiveness and even cost savings for IM modalities in adult populations, though higher quality studies are needed [10]. Similar studies have not yet been published for pediatric patients but are currently underway [12].

By promoting healthy lifestyle practices early in the child's life, pediatric IM sets a high standard for a lifetime of disease prevention behaviors. In many instances these therapies are simple and inexpensive to implement (e.g., improved sleep hygiene, exercise) and may provide long-lasting wellbeing. Exercise and lifestyle changes can treat depression, coronary heart disease, and type II diabetes [13–18]. Consuming a myriad of fruits, vegetables, spices, and extracts have shown preventative and treatment potential [19–27]. Mindfulness meditation has undergone extensive study utilizing functional magnetic resonance imaging (fMRI), and is emerging as an effective therapy for pain, anxiety, and depression [28–33].

The majority of integrative medicine users, however, do not report usage to their primary care physician; only 34–50% disclose use to their provider [34,35]. This number is likely even lower in certain ethnic and socioeconomic groups [1]. Parents and patients may feel intimidated by clinicians' perceived negative attitudes towards alternative therapies, even though three in four pediatricians believe that parents would disclose this information [35]. Improved communication regarding IM therapies would allow for physicians to (1) understand patients' and families' priorities and values in health and illness, and (2) help avoid treatment interactions between CAM and conventional therapies [36].

It is important for pediatricians to have knowledge and facility with integrative medicine in order to initiate conversation about CAM utilization [37]. Helpful to the cause, guidelines for advising patients seeking CAM have been published [38,39]. Although clinicians have an ethical obligation to discuss treatment alternatives [40], the overwhelming majority of pediatric providers do not feel comfortable discussing CAM with their patients. Both Kemper and O'Connor [41] and Sawni and Thomas [42] found that less than 37% of pediatricians inquire regarding CAM use while taking a routine medical history; any dialogue regarding CAM is typically initiated by the family. Pediatricians have a positive attitude towards CAM, but desire further education to adequately address patient concerns [2,41]. In a national study of 648 pediatricians, less than one in five reported any formal training in CAM, and 84% of respondents desired a continuing medical education curriculum, exhibiting self-awareness of their low familiarity with the topic [3,41–43].

To meet the growing needs of patients and practitioners alike, representatives from eight institutions (including Stanford) met in Kalamazoo, Michigan in July 1999. The outcome of this conference was the creation of the Academic Consortium for Integrative Medicine and Health. The vision of this group was to support leaders in integrative medicine in their advocacy, expand familiarity with the field, and develop a scientific knowledge base and research opportunities. Most importantly, it aimed to establish a community of providers in this rapidly growing field of medicine. A survey in 2007 indicated that 16 of 143 North American medical schools had dedicated academic pediatric IM programs [44]. The growth of dedicated academic departments and training programs in IM highlight institutional interest and support for IM.

2. Pediatric Integrative Subspecialties in Academia

Academic medical centers are often the hub where education, research, and clinical care meet innovation to improve medical care. The field of pediatric integrative medicine thrives in this setting, which allows for collaboration across disciplines and the opportunity to treat medically complex patients across all socioeconomic and cultural backgrounds. Further, academic centers are conducive to the inception of novel scholarship and training initiatives.

The 2005 Institute of Medicine report recommended CAM education for all training levels in health professions schools [45]. From an educational standpoint, training in pediatric IM was spearheaded by the University of Arizona Center for Integrative Medicine. The 100-h online Pediatric Integrative Medicine in Residency (PIMR) program was designed to address the lack of IM training available to pediatric trainees [46]. The PIMR program teaches residents habits for their own personal wellness alongside an introduction to evidence-based IM principles. This program was adopted by five pediatric residency programs in 2012 as a pilot program. Inclusion of a curriculum on physician wellness in the PIMR program was intentional and necessary. Physician burnout and fatigue is associated with major medical errors and decreased productivity. Furthermore, it has been shown that healthy physicians are more likely to advise patients to follow healthy lifestyle habits and are more effective at motivating patients [47–54]. Embedding integrative medicine education in a pediatric academic setting has the additional advantage of increasing institution-wide exposure and comfort with IM modalities.

Pediatric IM is a much-needed subspecialty, emerging to meet the needs of today's children. From a research standpoint, rigorous studies evaluating the safety, efficacy, and cost effectiveness of IM approaches in pediatrics are needed to justify usage [3]. Research into the efficacy of a pediatric integrative care model is often conducted at academic medical centers where patient diversity and research support are available. Due, in part, to increased research, IM approaches are being integrated into the fields of pediatric gastroenterology, pain, neurology, oncology, and pulmonology, among others. Frequently, the multidisciplinary approach afforded by IM can effectively treat symptoms, decrease polypharmacy, and enhance overall wellness in pediatric illness.

2.1. Gastroenterology

Pediatric gastroenterology (GI) patients have a high frequency of CAM usage; studies estimate utilization to be between 36% and 72% [55,56]. Herbal medicines, dietary supplements, and special diets are the most prevalent therapies utilized [57]. The strongest predictor of CAM use was prior or feared side effects of conventional medicine [55].

Integrative approaches for inflammatory bowel disease (IBD) include dietary assessment to identify food intolerances, dietary and herbal supplements, and mind–body therapies (relaxation techniques, meditation, and aromatherapy) [58]. Some studies have suggested a modest effect of probiotics, curcumin, and acupuncture in promoting remission in patients with IBD [59–62]. Mind–body interventions also have a limited body of evidence showing benefit in adolescents with IBD. A 2010 study of 67 adolescents with IBD described frequent utilization of prayer (62%), relaxation (40%), and imagery (21%) for disease management [63,64].

In patients with irritable bowel syndrome (IBS), there exists increasing evidence for the bidirectional connection between the mind, body, and gut. Gut-directed hypnotherapy (both in-person and home-based exercises) is also showing promise for pediatric IBS symptom relief [65–67]. Small studies on enteric coated peppermint oil have also demonstrated improvement of pediatric IBS symptoms [68].

2.2. Pain/Perioperative

Complementary and alternative medicine therapies for pediatric pain management are becoming increasingly accessible. A 2005 survey of 43 pediatric anesthesia fellowship programs approved by the Accreditation Council for Graduate Medical Education (ACGME) showed that nearly 90% of institutions had CAM therapies available for pediatric pain management. Common available modalities included biofeedback (65%), guided imagery (49%), and hypnosis (44%) [69].

Children and adolescents experience both acute and chronic pain, and each requires a different clinical approach. Nearly 40% of children with chronic pain experience persistent or recurrent pain at least once weekly, with common diagnoses being headaches, abdominal pain, and musculoskeletal pain [70]. Chronic pain can negatively impact a patient's school functioning, sleep, and parent burden (e.g., financial obligations, missed work) [71]. Treating chronic pain requires a multidisciplinary approach. The complex interplay between the patient's effective coping skills, parental reinforcement of pain behavior, and patient's mood can all alter and affect patient functioning [71]. This patient demographic is, reassuringly, open to an integrative approach to their care. According to a study of 110 pediatric patients with chronic pain (headache, abdominal pain, and musculoskeletal pain) presenting at an academic integrative clinic, 100% of families were interested in additional counseling regarding diet, exercise, sleep, or stress management [70]. Further, evidence is emerging for non-pharmacologic treatments for pain. For instance, physical therapy (stretching, trigger point physiotherapy, massage) can relieve headaches, musculoskeletal pain, and chronic regional pain syndrome (CRPS) [72–74]. Cotton et al. found that after massage therapy, mean pain scores decreased in over 500 hospitalized children with chronic pain and anxiety [75]. Acupuncture and mindful meditation have been shown to be an effective treatment for chronic pain and can decrease opioid usage, but more robust randomized control trials (RCTs) are needed [29,76].

Acute pain in children can be experienced in acute illness, during procedures (including venipuncture or immunization), or post-operatively. Acute pain can also evolve into a chronic pain condition, requiring flexibility in diagnosis and management. Integrative modalities have been successfully used in the treatment of acute pain. For instance, acupuncture, clinical hypnosis, and breathing techniques have all been shown to improve pain scores in children with acute pain from illness or procedures [77–79]. Newer technologies, such as virtual reality devices, show significant promise in minimizing discomfort with vascular access and minor procedures [80,81].

2.3. Neurology/Neurodevelopmental Pediatrics

Pediatric patients with a wide variety of neurologic and neurodevelopmental conditions utilize CAM to alleviate symptoms and supplement conventional therapy. The use of CAM among pediatric neurology patients ranges from 24% to 78% [82,83]. In a survey of 327 pediatric neurology patients at the Mayo Clinic, over 40% used CAM, and melatonin for sleep disorders was the most commonly used therapy [84]. A 2014 survey of 206 pediatric neurology patients in a Canadian children's hospital diagnosed with epilepsy, headache, and cerebral palsy illustrated high use of multivitamins, massage, and chiropractic therapies (89.9%, 47.1%, and 36.8%, respectively); most practices were reported as helpful [85]. Among children with autism spectrum disorder (ASD), special diets are the most common form of CAM utilized according to eight independent studies [57,86].

In pediatric headache patients, headache frequency and intensity has been shown to improve with magnesium and riboflavin (vitamin B2) [87,88]. Furthermore, screening and treating comorbid sleep disorders such as sleep apnea, bruxism, insomnia, and restless leg syndrome can indirectly improve headache [89]. Neurofeedback has documented potential in treatment of epilepsy and headache [90,91]. Meditation, breath work, and relaxation activities have reduced school absences in patients with headaches, migraines, and seizures [83].

2.4. Pediatric Oncology

Between 1977 and 2011, 31 studies on the use of IM practices in pediatric oncology patients listed spirituality/prayer, positive mental imagery, and natural health products (multivitamins, megavitamins and herbals) as common interventions [57]. Mind–body therapies are readily accessible and low risk, with several trials showing decreased side effects of cancer therapy, increased patient self-confidence, and improved coping skills [92]. The largest study of pediatric oncology patients (1063 patients) found that 71% utilized IM modalities and only 4% reported adverse events [93]. The most common reasons cited by patients for using IM were to aid in treating cancer, symptomatic relief, support of conventional treatment, and management of side effects [94,95].

Integrative modalities may also play a role in long-term cancer risk reduction. Patient lifestyle factors such as stress, cigarette smoking, poor diet, alcohol consumption, and a sedentary lifestyle are revealed and discussed with greater frequency in the IM approach. Research has suggested numerous cancers to be primarily nutrition-responsive and preventable by dietary [96,97] and lifestyle changes [98,99]. The mechanism responsible may be by aliment-induced reversible epigenetic modification or the protective effects conferred by a diet high in fiber and antioxidants [20,100,101]. Establishing healthy habits in children to focus on healthy nutrition, mind–body interventions for stress reduction, quality sleep, and generous physical activity may be paramount in decreasing overall risk of some cancers (colon, lung, breast, and prostate) in later life [102].

2.5. Asthma and Allergy

Pediatric asthma is another area where an integrative approach may provide benefit. Elimination diets and those emphasizing core facets of the Mediterranean diet (high in fruits, vegetables, and legumes) have been shown to protect children from asthma and allergies [103–105]. A systematic review and meta-analysis by Cramer et al. in 2014 highlighted yoga as a supplementary intervention for asthma patients to improve symptoms and quality of life [106]. Breathing exercises and breath retraining techniques such as Buteyko breathing, yoga/pranayama, and physiotherapy have decreased bronchodilator usage [107,108]. Mark describes a multitude of integrative therapies as effective for pediatric asthma, including: (1) mind–body therapies to reduce anxiety and stress, lowering immune response and sympathetic activity; (2) proper prenatal and childhood nutrition that is high in fruits and vegetables; and (3) exercise and yoga to improve regimen adherence and decrease anxiety [109,110].

2.6. Other Subspecialties

There is a role for an integrative approach within many subspecialties. We know, for instance, that diet and exercise management can halt or reverse cardiovascular disease, diabetes, and obesity [10,13,23,111–113]. Integrative cardiology targets high body mass index (BMI) and poor nutrition using mind–body therapies to influence caloric consumption, sedentary or stressful lifestyles, and depression-associated symptoms [114]. Cognitive behavioral therapy has been used as an adjuvant in pediatric obesity management [115]. Mindfulness-based cognitive therapy has shown preliminary efficacy in youths with anxiety disorder and mindfulness based stress reduction programs in urban youth have improved psychological functioning and decreased negative effects of stress [33,116]. Furthermore, a recent study has proposed mechanistic pathways of action of acupuncture in alleviating cardiovascular disease [117–120].

As the evidence base to support the use of integrative approaches in each pediatric subspecialty grows, the use of CAM in pediatrics will increase. In light of this, clinical practices and academic centers are starting to integrate CAM modalities. Existing models of care can provide a foundation for future growth and utilization of integrative approaches for children.

3. Integrative Medicine at Stanford Children's Health

This section presents the historical development of Pediatric Integrative Medicine at Stanford Children's Health with the intent to afford inspiration and perspective for future programs in pediatric IM.

3.1. Program Background and History

Lucile Packard Children's Hospital and Stanford University School of Medicine are located in Palo Alto, California and serve the broader region of the San Francisco Bay area. The inpatient children's hospital houses 361 beds and outpatient clinics serve over 500,000 visits annually. Families travel from

50 states and 40 countries for care. Fifty-two percent of families have private insurance, while 45% have public health insurance.

The Pediatric Integrative Medicine (PIM) program was established at Stanford Children's Health in 2011 with support from the pediatric department leadership. The program was developed in recognition of the growing interests of patients and their families in the use, benefits, and potential complications of complementary therapies. The program's first activity was to survey all Stanford Children's Health medical providers (including nurse practitioners, residents, fellows, and attending physicians) and measure their knowledge of and interest in IM. The survey revealed that a majority of practitioners (over 75%) wished to learn more about IM. Reasons for wanting further education included: (1) a desire to learn more about different CAM therapies to better advise their patients and families about safety and efficacy of supplements and mind–body approaches (which they were already using); and (2) a need to knowledgably introduce evidence-based pediatric IM practices into patient care.

The PIM faculty prepared a business plan to ensure the new program's sustainability and improve access for families seeking expertise in these therapies. The business plan included: proposed faculty, support staff allocation (0.5 days per week), and projected revenue from clinical services. Rather than creating a separate PIM clinic, the four faculty members centered the integrative clinics within four established specialty clinics: pain, gastroenterology (GI), pulmonary, and rheumatology. This model aimed to decrease overhead cost (space, staff, supplies) and make PIM clinics easily accessible. This model was fiscally sustainable as it allowed continued financial support of the faculty for conventional work in their respective subspecialty in addition to the subspecialty PIM clinics. The anecdotal response to this model by patients, families, and institutional leadership was positive. Patients and families expressed satisfaction (e.g., >80% provider satisfaction scores on yearly Press Ganey reports) and gratitude for finding pediatric subspecialists that were knowledgeable in both mainstream treatments and integrative modalities. As the program grew, institutional leadership and division chiefs continued to support the program, allowing the IM faculty to shift more time toward integrative clinics. In addition, as pediatric providers in the community learned of the PIM faculty's expertise, they began referring families for consultation. Community providers were welcomed to educational sessions offered by the program leaders and began incorporating evidence-based IM practices into their own specialties. Figure 1 is a diagram of the program's accomplishments.

3.2. Clinical Work

The four subspecialty integrative clinics (staffed by four IM-trained faculties in the pulmonary, rheumatology, pain medicine, and gastroenterology fields), continue to grow. Clinical volume has increased significantly since inception in 2012. In 2016, there were 160 visits for integrative medicine, and by 2017 that number had nearly doubled to over 300 annual visits. The greatest growth was noted in integrative pain and gastroenterology clinics. Referrals have come from community alternative care providers (e.g., Chinese medicine practitioners and naturopathic practitioners), community pediatricians, providers within Stanford Children's Health, and self-referrals. Approximately 25% of encounters are new patient visits and the rest are follow-up visits.

Prior to an initial visit with a PIM provider, insurance authorization is obtained. If the visit is with an acupuncture provider, patients interested in acupuncture are given current procedure terminology (CPT) codes and instructed to determine insurance benefits and out-of-pocket costs. Many insurances in California do cover acupuncture services for certain indications. Authorization is also required for pain psychology services through the IM pain clinic. An insurance authorization team is available to assist in this process.

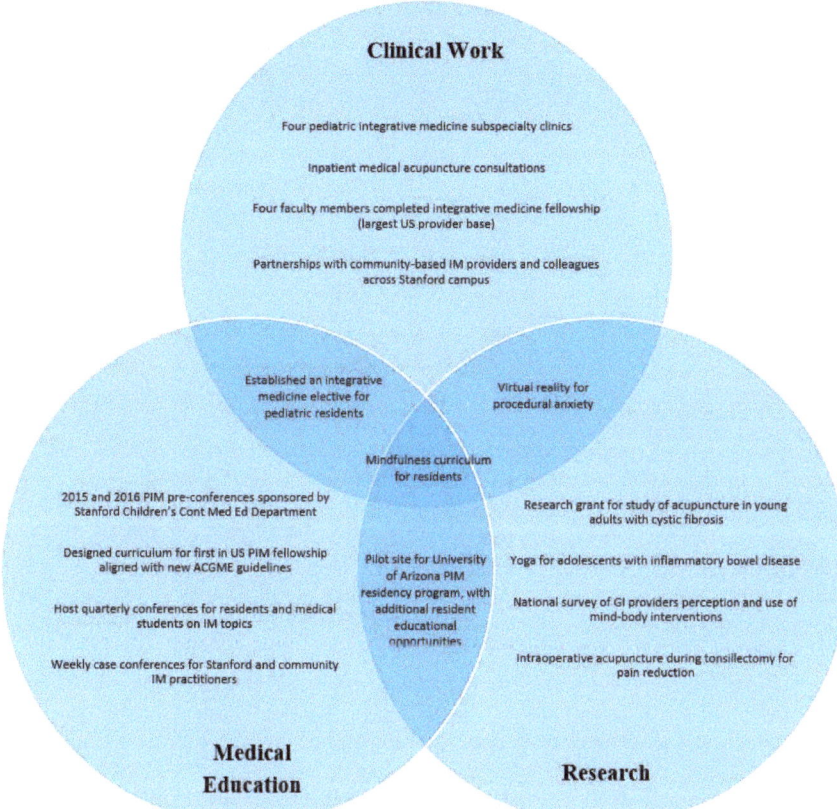

Figure 1. Program accomplishments. IM: integrative medicine; PIM: pediatric IM; GI: gastrointestinal; ACGME: Accreditation Council for Graduate Medical Education.

Each subspecialty clinic has a slightly different staffing structure. The integrative pain clinic includes a comprehensive initial pain evaluation for each new patient with the pain physician, nurse practitioner (NP), and pain psychologist. Depending on patient's needs, subsequent follow-up visits are with the pain medical doctor (MD)/NP and either the Stanford pain psychologist or community psychologist. Pain clinic NPs are also medical acupuncture-trained and therefore can continue treatment plans started by the acupuncture-trained physician. New patient visits in IM GI, pulmonary, and rheumatology clinics are for 90 min with an IM physician and follow-up visits are for 45 min. After a through intake evaluation, a comprehensive treatment plan is developed. The modalities offered depend largely on the individual training of the providers. The range of integrative treatment modalities include: nutrition recommendations, mind–body interventions, acupuncture, botanical or supplement review, and recommendations. The integrative GI clinic and integrative pulmonary clinic both have access to a registered dietician and social worker directly within the clinic. Pediatric IM providers will often refer to Stanford colleagues in the fields of nutrition, occupational therapy, psychiatry, child and pain psychology, and physical therapy. Frequency of referral to these services depends somewhat on the subspecialty, but the highest utilized services include psychology and occupational therapy for biofeedback. Further, the IM faculty will refer to community providers outside of the institution in acupuncture, massage, physical therapy, biofeedback, clinical hypnosis, mindfulness, and yoga. Community referrals are especially common when a patient lives a far distance from the Stanford campus and needs a particular therapy frequently (for example, weekly acupuncture for a patient who lives three hours away).

In the inpatient setting, a few IM modalities are available to inpatients through existing clinical departments. For example, the inpatient pain service provides acupressure and acupuncture. The child life department provides mind–body therapies, including guided imagery and virtual reality. The child psychology service provides clinical hypnosis as one of their treatment interventions. At this point there is not a dedicated PIM inpatient service but rather a meshwork of services offered by individual departments. For the future, an inpatient IM consultation service is a planned area for program expansion.

3.3. Research

Research for many integrative modalities is lacking, especially for pediatric patients. The Stanford faculties have produced a variety of publications including narrative reviews, book chapters, prospective pilot studies, retrospective studies of clinic outcomes, and position statements. Three faculty members are in the clinician educator track which does not afford protected research time. One faculty member is in the physician scientist track and has a dedicated 0.25 full time equivalent (FTE) of research time. Several generous foundation grants (Lawlor Foundation and Mayday Foundation) have allowed for support of the faculty and research assistants. Notable scholarly work includes faculty collaboration with PIM thought leaders to produce an Academy of Pediatrics (AAP) position statement on pediatric integrative medicine [3] and detailed results from the Pediatric Integrative Medicine in Residency (PIMR) pilot program [46,121]. A recent study found immersive virtual reality safe and effective for treating complex regional pain syndrome [80,122]. This has prompted further research on using virtual reality for other types of chronic, acute, and procedural pain. Intraoperative acupuncture for patients undergoing tonsillectomy and adenoidectomy was found to be feasible, decreased postoperative pain, and increased return of diet [77]. A pilot study on yoga for adolescents with inflammatory bowel disease found yoga to be widely acceptable, feasible, and safe [123]. For further details and a summary on research productivity and ongoing projects please see Table 1.

Challenges to studying the PIM program as a whole is that program providers often recommend a comprehensive treatment plan instead of a single intervention. This mirrors the wide array of interventions offered at other programs around the country (particularly for pain clinics) [69,124]. Therefore, developing research techniques to study multimodal interventions is needed to adequately study the integrative medicine approach as a whole [125]. This may include examining cost effectiveness and resource utilization (emergency visits, urgent care visits, and hospitalizations) in patients seen in a PIM program versus standard care.

Table 1. Summary of Published Scholarly Work on Integrative Medicine.

Category	Name of Study	Study Type	Findings	Funding
Pediatric integrative medicine	Pediatric Integrative Medicine [3]	Position Statement	Position Statement of Pediatric Integrative Medicine	N/A
Medical education	Pediatric Integrative Medicine in Residency (PIMR): Description of a New Online Educational Curriculum [46]	Retrospective review	Online curriculum targets integrative medicine (IM) knowledge gaps in pediatric residents	Funding received from foundation grants outside of Stanford
	Pediatric Integrative Medicine in Residency Program: Relationship between Lifestyle Behaviors and Burnout and Wellbeing Measures in First-Year Residents [121]	Retrospective review	Details burnout wellbeing in PIMR participants	Funding received from foundation grants outside of Stanford

Table 1. Cont.

Category	Name of Study	Study Type	Findings	Funding
Pediatric pulmonary	Complementary and Alternative Medicine in Pulmonology [126]	Literature review	Examines complementary and integrative medicine (CAM) use and effectiveness in children with pulmonary disorders	N/A
	Integrative Medicine in Asthma [127]	Literature review	Details integrative approach for children with asthma	N/A
	Nutrition in Pediatric Cystic Fibrosis [128]	Book chapter	Details evidence of nutritional therapies in children with cystic fibrosis	N/A
	Integrated Medicine and Asthma [129]	Book chapter	Details evidence of integrative approach to asthma	N/A
Pediatric gastroenterology	Yoga as adjunct therapy for adolescents with inflammatory bowel disease: A pilot clinical trial [127]	Prospective pilot	Yoga is acceptable, safe and feasible for adolescents with IBD	Tracie Lawlor Foundation, prAna
	Mind-Body Interventions for Pediatric Inflammatory Bowel Disease [130]	Literature review	Review of evidence on mind-body interventions for IBD	N/A
	Integrative Treatment of Reflux and Functional Dyspepsia in Children [130]	Case study and literature review	Describes integrative approach to children with reflux and functional dyspepsia	N/A
	Acupuncture and Integrative Medicine for Pediatric Gastroesophageal Reflux and Functional Dyspepsia [131]	Retrospective case series	Describes effect of acupuncture on children with GERD and functional dyspepsia	Stanford Medical Scholars Program
Pediatric neurology	Integrative Medicine in Child Neurology: what do providers think and what do they need to learn? [132]	National survey	Describes results of a national survey of IM modalities used in pediatric neurology	N/A
Pediatric pain	The Impact of Massage and Reading on Children's Pain and Anxiety After Cardiovascular Surgery: A Pilot Study [133]	Randomized prospective trial	Massage was safe and feasible for children undergoing cardiac surgery. Massage decreased anxiety scores and lowered exposure to benzodiazepines.	N/A
	Immersive Virtual Reality for Pediatric Pain [80]	Literature review	Review of evidence on using virtual reality for acute, chronic, and procedural pain	Mayday Foundation
	Two Virtual Reality Pilot Studies for the Treatment of Pediatric CRPS [122]	Prospective pilots	Virtual Reality feasible and effective for treating pediatric CRPS	Mayday Foundation
	Non-Pharmacological Techniques for Pain Management in Neonates [134]	Literature review	Details evidence of non-pharmacologic techniques to treat neonatal pain	N/A
Acupuncture	Acupuncture as an Anesthetic Adjuvant for Pediatric Orthopedic Patients: A Pilot Study and Protocol Description [79]	Prospective pilot	Acupuncture was associated with low pain scores and levels of nausea in patients undergoing orthopedic surgery	N/A
	Does Acupuncture Reduce Stress Over Time? A Clinical Heart Rate Variability Study in Hypertensive Patients [135]	Retrospective case study	Acupuncture increased heart rate variability after acupuncture treatment in adults undergoing treatment for hypertension	N/A
	Does Noninvasive Electrical Stimulation of Acupuncture Points Reduce Heelstick Pain in Neonates [136]	Randomized prospective trial	Noninvasive electrical stimulation at acupuncture points was not effective to decrease heelstick pain in neonates	Mayday Foundation
	Intraoperative acupuncture for post-tonsillectomy pain: a randomized, double-blind, placebo-controlled trial. [77]	Randomized prospective trial	Intraoperative acupuncture is feasible, well tolerated, and results in improved pain and earlier return of diet after tonsillectomy.	Stanford Medical Scholars Program, Howard Hughes Medical Institute Medical Fellows Program, Stanford Children's Health Research Institute Akiko Yamazaki and Jerry Yang Faculty Scholar

3.4. Medical Education

Stanford pediatric residents began participating in the University of Arizona's Pediatric Integrative Medicine Residency (PIMR) pilot online training curriculum in 2014. Trainee participation in this curriculum was a pivotal step towards formalizing PIM medical education efforts at Stanford Children's. In addition to providing a foundation in PIM knowledge, the curriculum enabled residents to improve their own lifestyle and wellness behaviors during the pilot [121]. To supplement the online curriculum offered by PIMR, the faculty developed a pediatric integrative medicine and wellness elective for pediatric residents who wanted in-depth exposure to integrative medicine in practice. The elective is currently offered as either a two-week or four-week in-person rotation. Residents taking the elective participate in the subspecialty PIM clinics (average four to five half-day clinic sessions per two-week rotation). Required readings and hands-on didactic sessions (average 4 h per two-week rotation) include lectures about plant-based nutrition and mind–body medicine. A field trip to a natural foods store provides the venue for a hands-on discussion of herbs and supplements. Residents are also asked to choose one integrative modality to experience for themselves to improve their own health. Meditation, massage, acupuncture, and yoga have been the most popular modalities that residents explore. Residents enrolled in the four-week elective are required to complete the 100-h PIMR online curriculum in addition to the above activities. The PIM elective at Stanford Children's has become one of the most popular electives, with approximately 20% of the 76 categorical pediatric residents participating annually.

At the fellow physician level, a new wellness curriculum has been developed by the Stanford Children's faculty, including the PIM faculty. The Fellowship WellBeing Program (FWP) focuses on fatigue mitigation, self-care, resiliency, and stress mitigation for over 100 pediatric fellows. This seven-hour curriculum emphasizes the use of breathing, movement, mindfulness and nutrition to help physician trainees find and maintain wellness.

In 2018, Stanford Children's launched the first one-year clinical fellowship in pediatric integrative medicine to formally train pediatricians in integrative medicine. The PIM fellowship includes partnership with the University of Arizona Fellowship in Integrative Medicine, a 1000-h, two-year distance learning program with three, week-long, hands-on training sessions. The fellow has a dedicated general pediatrics IM clinic precepted by the PIM faculty (average two half-day clinics per week) and also works alongside faculty members in their respective subspecialty PIM clinics (average two half-day clinics per week). Curriculum intensives—one to three-week mini courses—were developed by the PIM and adjunct faculty members to cover the important PIM topics of nutrition, mind–body medicine, botanical medicine, and inpatient consultation. The fellow may also work with non-Stanford affiliated community integrative medicine pediatric providers on an elective basis for niche skill development and clinical exposure. The fellow is also required to teach pediatric residents formally in several conferences per year and informally when residents are on the PIM elective. The fellowship curriculum includes weekly didactic and case conferences in the style of "Professor's Rounds" where a patient case is discussed with providers from various medical backgrounds and training expertise. The conferences are attended by community integrative medicine general pediatricians, PIM subspecialty providers (GI, pulmonary, pain, rheumatology), massage therapists, acupuncturists, psychologists, mind–body intervention providers, and nutritionists. After each case presentation, attendees offer their treatment recommendations (from their own unique perspectives), and these recommendations are provided to the patient at clinic follow-up.

Sample Case Presentation (Identifying Details Changed for Patient Privacy)

A 15-year-old girl presented to the outpatient pediatric integrative medicine clinic with chief complaint of abdominal pain for three years which had been diagnosed as abdominal migraines. A comprehensive history was taken regarding her pain including an evaluation of life stressors, a detailed diet history, and her extensive medication list.

Pertinent findings included a past medical history of anxiety and release of a tethered cord at nine months of age. Her prescription medications included duloxetine, cariprazine, amitriptyline, topiramate, polyethylene glycol, and a combined estrogen–progesterone oral contraceptive pill daily. She took clonazepam, ondansetron, sumatriptan, cyproheptadine, and simethicone on an as-needed basis for symptoms related to abdominal migraine. She did not find any of these as needed medications particularly helpful in treating her abdominal migraine episodes. Supplements included melatonin nightly and peppermint oil by mouth as needed for abdominal pain. She was an only child of her mother and father. She was starting the 10th grade and achieved good grades. Her bedtime was 22:00 h nightly and she fell asleep easily. She reported occasional overnight awakenings and feeling tired on waking at 06:00 h daily. She described herself as a worrier but also as willful and ambitious. Her favorite color was teal, and her favorite season was winter. She preferred salty foods. Both mom and patient readily offered that the patient's desire to please her teachers often led to high anxiety and tears if she felt like she was not working to her potential due to illness. Her self-reported personal strength was relating to other people, including classmates. She stated she was weak in mathematics. Her physical activity included biking to school or walking to the school bus stop. She was planning to join the school speech and debate team at the time of the visit.

On physical exam her weight was in the 73rd percentile and her height was in the 38th percentile. Her body mass index was 22. She was talkative and engaged. Abdominal exam was significant for hyperesthesia with light touch of all abdominal quadrants with significant epigastric tenderness. There was no palpable stool burden. The remainder of her physical exam was normal. Prior negative workup for her abdominal pain included infectious stool studies, *Helicobacter pylori*, fecal calprotectin, complete blood count with differential, and a comprehensive metabolic panel including liver function testing, amylase, lipase, sedimentation rate, lipids, tissue transglutaminase immunoglobulin A, ceruloplasmin, and thyroid stimulation hormone. The results of these studies were normal.

The patient's comprehensive treatment plan included mind–body, lifestyle, and diet recommendations. Mind–body therapies were discussed, and the patient elected to start attending a free yoga class at her primary medical center. She continued to see her outpatient psychiatrist for weekly psychotherapy including cognitive behavioral therapy. From a lifestyle perspective, she was recommended to increase physical activity and offered that she would start walking a few evenings per week with her mother. A therapy plan for acute abdominal discomfort was formulated, and, in addition to her current pharmaceutical regimen, included: acupressure massage, enteric coated peppermint oil, and aromatherapy.

At her first follow-up the patient reported acupressure massage helpful, and she and the family asked for further instruction on in-home use of acupressure massage. At the third visit, approximately six weeks later, the patient emphatically reported she had aborted two abdominal migraines using acupressure beads with massage—something she had never achieved before. She started receiving biweekly acupuncture. She continued yoga once per week. She also found benefit from using a mind–body application on her mobile phone for daily meditation to augment anxiety treatment. She weaned off amitriptyline and topiramate without incident and reserved only ondansetron and clonazepam on an as needed basis for acute discomfort. In the first three months of treatment the patient aborted abdominal migraines twice and experienced only two breakthrough episodes. Additionally, she missed fewer days of school due to abdominal pain. She continues to follow-up in the integrative medicine clinic every two–three weeks for acupuncture treatments.

4. Discussion

4.1. Pediatric Integrative Medicine in Academia

Pediatric Integrative Medicine is an emerging subspecialty that provides the foundation for whole-patient and whole-child preventative care and lifestyle medicine [44]. Within children's hospitals, patients are acutely sick, and in the outpatient setting, the incidence of children with complex and chronic medical problems has grown. According to a national survey performed by the Centers for Disease Control, in 2009, 15.1% of all children in the United States had special health care needs, up from 12.8% in 2001 [137]. These children often have multiple subspecialties involved in their care and their subsequent care coordination and communication between multiple consultants can be challenging. Specialists tend to focus on their organ system of interest, and the holistic approach to the care and healing of the child may be overlooked. Integrative medicine may help bring together all aspects of care since PIM is a blend of mainstream therapies with the other aspects of wellness. Further, our PIM faculty members are trained in both a pediatric subspecialty and integrative medicine. This affords a unique opportunity for specialized clinical care, education, and research in these integrative pediatric subspecialties.

4.2. Drivers for Success

A primary reason for our program's initial success was due to institutional support, strong leadership, and a financial model of embedding the integrative clinics within subspecialty divisions. Institutional leadership recognized that the PIM program is an attractive feature that is "uniquely Stanford" and serves the local San Francisco Bay Area community and beyond.

In addition, recruiting and collaborating with the well-respected existing faculty within the institution to provide consultations (rather than hiring or contracting with external providers) established trust, garnered respect for the program, and continued collegiality amongst providers. This mirrors an important key to success among other established non-pediatric integrative medicine centers around the world [44,138]. Given that integrative medicine at times can include treatment modalities that may not be well known to mainstream medicine, the faculty group also emphasizes evidence-informed treatment modalities to the extent available and emphasizes patient safety. Lifestyle recommendations that have minimal side effects such as good nutrition, sleep hygiene, physical activity, and mind–body modalities are often cornerstones of each treatment plan. When research on treatment efficacy in a pediatric population may not be available, providers extrapolate data from adult populations and utilize shared-decision making with families, and use the safety-effectiveness rubric to discuss and document efficacy [139]. Every effort is made to utilize available resources to ensure the safety of a treatment recommendation, especially in regard to botanicals or supplements. Further, pharmacy consultations are sometimes required in patients who have significant polypharmacy.

The medical education initiatives jumpstarted awareness of integrative medicine throughout the children's hospital faculty and leadership. The resident PIMR pilot and subsequent PIM elective required residency leadership approval of the residency curriculum change. The elective also increased resident exposure and engagement with the integrative medicine faculty, which led to several resident-initiated scholarly works [123,132]. The novel conception of the pediatric integrative medicine fellowship has additionally increased clinical services and education efforts. The weekly didactic conference (available in person and by webinar) had the unanticipated benefit of bringing together PIM providers within Stanford and the larger community. Continuing education courses for the pediatric community also stimulated community building and aided in patient referrals. As students, residents, and other community providers increase their exposure to and knowledge of integrative modalities, these treatment options become part of the norm, and then truly "integrated" into conventional care. Therefore, medical education and teaching are important keys to success.

Finally, the educational and research programs would not exist without generous philanthropic support—both in the form of private donations and research grants. These funds aided to establish funding for the program's research and have allowed the pediatric integrative medicine fellow to attend the Arizona Center for Integrative Medicine's distance learning fellowship.

4.3. Challenges and Financial Considerations

The program has faced several challenges. From a financial standpoint, integrative medicine bills using time-based evaluation and management codes, behavioral health codes, and acupuncture

CPT codes. Although we have not had significant challenges having physician billing codes covered, preventative services in the current fee-for-service model do not reimburse equally when more time is spent with the patient (compared to seeing several patients in the same time period). Currently, the PIM faculty members work in their respective pediatric subspecialties to offset some of the costs of the PIM clinic. A separate bill center was created to track financial progress and will add insight to this challenge. As newer models of care such as accountable care organizations (ACOs) are adopted in adult primary care fields [140], this will hopefully translate to novel prevention models for pediatrics.

While children from underserved populations are still able to be seen by PIM providers at our institution, additional services such as acupuncture, biofeedback, psychology, and nutrition may not be as readily covered. Further, these patients may not be able to afford additional supplements and suggested dietary changes. This continues to pose a significant challenge for our underserved population and deserves significant and sustained advocacy and philanthropy.

While the newly developed PIM fellowship currently has institutional and philanthropic support, the sustainability of this training program is uncertain. Given that it is a completely new fellowship program, accreditation by the ACGME is likely years away. Currently, a two-year pilot by the hospital and Pediatrics Department is currently funding the fellow salary, program director effort, and coordinator time; philanthropy is funding the educational programming for the fellow.

Lastly, the concept of an integrative approach is, at times, a difficult philosophical mindset for patients and families. Behavior, lifestyle, and diet changes are frequently more challenging to implement than taking medications. These changes also take time. Referring providers and patients may be looking for a "quick fix", which may not be feasible. While evidence on integrative modalities is emerging in pediatrics, colleagues often remain skeptical and have reservations on the value of integrative therapies.

4.4. Future Directions

The PIM program at Stanford hopes to increase clinical services, education efforts, and research productivity. Clinically, a pilot inpatient integrative medicine consultation service is planned for Spring 2019. Discussions are underway to integrate mind–body and acupuncture treatment modalities to perioperative and postoperative treatment protocols. The program also needs to formally survey patients and families on patient satisfaction of its current programs.

On a national level, the faculty aims to collaborate with national organizations such as the American Academy of Pediatrics and other pediatric subspecialty organizations to have a broader reach for educational efforts. Several faculties have participated in discussions about developing an integrative medicine core competency requirement for all pediatric residents. Additionally, our program leadership advocates for other academic centers to establish pediatric integrative medicine clinical training fellowships.

Continued research is needed to establish evidenced-based safety and efficacy data for integrative therapies in pediatrics. Specific ongoing projects at our center include examining acupuncture for patients undergoing craniotomy, mind–body interventions for pediatric inflammatory bowel disease, and utilizing virtual reality for procedural pain and anxiety. Our program would be open to collaborating with other centers to develop the recently proposed multi-center PIM research network [139]. Continued growth in these areas will require ongoing institutional support for faculty time, resource allocation, and financial support.

5. Conclusions

Evidence of safety and efficacy of pediatric integrative treatment modalities within pediatric subspecialties continues to grow. The establishment of a pediatric integrative medicine program within an academic setting is feasible. It requires sufficient institutional support, funding, and adequately trained physician faculty and staff. Important contributors to our program's success include medical education to drive provider and trainee education, an emphasis on patient safety and evidence-based medicine, and an incredible team of enthusiastic physician leaders.

Author Contributions: Conceptualization, A.Y., J.M. and B.G.; writing—original draft preparation, G.R., J.A. and A.Y.; writing—review and editing, G.R., J.A., A.Y., J.M., D.G. and B.G.; supervision, A.Y., B.G., D.G. and J.M.

Funding: This research received no external funding.

Acknowledgments: The authors would like to thank Kenneth Cox, Christy Sandborg, Daniel Murphy, and Mary Leonard for Stanford institutional leadership support. We acknowledge Leland Lei for assistance with pulling financial details for integrative clinics. We thank Ellen Gomes for technical editing, language editing, and proofreading. We would also like to thank Sudha K.V., the Weil Foundation, the Samuel Lawrence Foundation, and the Tracie Lawlor Foundation for philanthropic support.

Conflicts of Interest: The authors declare no conflict of interest.

References

1. Misra, S.M.; Guffey, D.; Roth, I.; Giardino, A.P. Complementary and Alternative Medicine Use in Uninsured Children in Texas. *Clin. Pediatr. (Phila.)* **2017**, *56*, 866–869. [CrossRef] [PubMed]
2. Kemper, K.J.; Vohra, S.; Walls, R. The Use of Complementary and Alternative Medicine in Pediatrics. *Pediatrics* **2008**, *122*, 1374–1386. [CrossRef] [PubMed]
3. McClafferty, H.; Vohra, S.; Bailey, M.; Brown, M.; Esparham, A.; Gerstbacher, D.; Golianu, B.; Niemi, A.-K.; Sibinga, E.; Weydert, J.; et al. Pediatric Integrative Medicine. *Pediatrics* **2017**, *140*, e20171961. [CrossRef]
4. Complementary, Alternative, or Integrative Health: What's In a Name? Available online: https://nccih.nih.gov/health/integrative-health (accessed on 20 July 2018).
5. Black, L.I.; Clarke, T.C.; Barnes, P.M.; Stussman, B.J.; Nahin, R.L. Use of Complementary Health Approaches Among Children Aged 4–17 Years in the United States: National Health Interview Survey, 2007–2012. *Natl. Health Stat. Rep.* **2015**, 1–19.
6. Clarke, T.C.; Black, L.I.; Stussman, B.J.; Barnes, P.M.; Nahin, R.L. Trends in the use of complementary health approaches among adults: United States, 2002–2012. *Natl. Health Stat. Rep.* **2015**, 1–16.
7. McCann, L.J.; Newell, S.J. Survey of paediatric complementary and alternative medicine use in health and chronic illness. *Arch. Dis. Child.* **2006**, *91*, 173–174. [CrossRef] [PubMed]
8. Eisenberg, D.M.; Davis, R.B.; Ettner, S.L.; Appel, S.; Wilkey, S.; Rompay, M.V.; Kessler, R.C. Trends in Alternative Medicine Use in the United States, 1990-1997: Results of a Follow-up National Survey. *JAMA* **1998**, *280*, 1569–1575. [CrossRef]
9. Taw, M.B. Integrative medicine, or not integrative medicine: That is the question. *J. Integr. Med.* **2015**, *13*, 350–352. [CrossRef]
10. Herman, P.M.; Poindexter, B.L.; Witt, C.M.; Eisenberg, D.M. Are complementary therapies and integrative care cost-effective? A systematic review of economic evaluations. *BMJ Open* **2012**, *2*, e001046. [CrossRef]
11. Ali, A.; Katz, D.L. Disease Prevention and Health Promotion: How Integrative Medicine Fits. *Am. J. Prev. Med.* **2015**, *49*, S230–S240. [CrossRef]
12. Vohra, S.; Schlegelmilch, M.; Jou, H.; Hartfield, D.; Mayan, M.; Ohinmaa, A.; Wilson, B.; Spavor, M.; Grundy, P. Comparative effectiveness of pediatric integrative medicine as an adjunct to usual care for pediatric inpatients of a North American tertiary care centre: A study protocol for a pragmatic cluster controlled trial. *Contemp. Clin. Trials Commun.* **2017**, *5*, 12–18. [CrossRef] [PubMed]
13. Cooney, G.; Dwan, K.; Mead, G. Exercise for Depression. *JAMA* **2014**, *311*, 2432–2433. [CrossRef] [PubMed]
14. Ornish, D.; Scherwitz, L.W.; Billings, J.H.; Gould, K.L.; Merritt, T.A.; Sparler, S.; Armstrong, W.T.; Ports, T.A.; Kirkeeide, R.L.; Hogeboom, C.; et al. Intensive Lifestyle Changes for Reversal of Coronary Heart Disease. *JAMA* **1998**, *280*, 2001–2007. [CrossRef] [PubMed]
15. Knowler, W.C.; Barrett-Connor, E.; Fowler, S.E.; Hamman, R.F.; Lachin, J.M.; Walker, E.A.; Nathan, D.M. Reduction in the Incidence of Type 2 Diabetes with Lifestyle Intervention or Metformin. *N. Engl. J. Med.* **2002**, *346*, 393–403.
16. Loef, M.; Walach, H. The combined effects of healthy lifestyle behaviors on all cause mortality: A systematic review and meta-analysis. *Prev. Med.* **2012**, *55*, 163–170. [CrossRef] [PubMed]

17. Ornish, D.; Lin, J.; Chan, J.M.; Epel, E.; Kemp, C.; Weidner, G.; Marlin, R.; Frenda, S.J.; Magbanua, M.J.M.; Daubenmier, J.; et al. Effect of comprehensive lifestyle changes on telomerase activity and telomere length in men with biopsy-proven low-risk prostate cancer: 5-year follow-up of a descriptive pilot study. *Lancet Oncol.* **2013**, *14*, 1112–1120. [CrossRef]
18. Ornish, D.; Magbanua, M.J.M.; Weidner, G.; Weinberg, V.; Kemp, C.; Green, C.; Mattie, M.D.; Marlin, R.; Simko, J.; Shinohara, K.; et al. Changes in prostate gene expression in men undergoing an intensive nutrition and lifestyle intervention. *Proc. Natl. Acad. Sci. USA* **2008**, *105*, 8369–8374. [CrossRef]
19. He, Z.-Y.; Shi, C.-B.; Wen, H.; Li, F.-L.; Wang, B.-L.; Wang, J. Upregulation of p53 Expression in Patients with Colorectal Cancer by Administration of Curcumin. *Cancer Investig.* **2011**, *29*, 208–213. [CrossRef]
20. Supic, G.; Jagodic, M.; Magic, Z. Epigenetics: A New Link Between Nutrition and Cancer. *Nutr. Cancer* **2013**, *65*, 781–792. [CrossRef]
21. Patel, V.H. Nutrition and prostate cancer: An overview. *Expert Rev. Anticancer Ther.* **2014**, *14*, 1295–1304. [CrossRef]
22. Riccio, P.; Rossano, R. Nutrition Facts in Multiple Sclerosis. *ASN Neuro* **2015**, *7*, 1759091414568185. [CrossRef] [PubMed]
23. Gustafson, D.R.; Clare Morris, M.; Scarmeas, N.; Shah, R.C.; Sijben, J.; Yaffe, K.; Zhu, X. New Perspectives on Alzheimer's Disease and Nutrition. *J. Alzheimer's Dis.* **2015**, *46*, 1111–1127. [CrossRef] [PubMed]
24. Kawicka, A.; Regulska-Ilow, B. How nutritional status, diet and dietary supplements can affect autism. A review. *Roczniki Państwowego Zakładu Higieny* **2013**, *64*, 1–12. [PubMed]
25. Eilat-Adar, S.; Sinai, T.; Yosefy, C.; Henkin, Y. Nutritional Recommendations for Cardiovascular Disease Prevention. *Nutrients* **2013**, *5*, 3646–3683. [CrossRef] [PubMed]
26. Rodriguez-Leyva, D.; Weighell, W.; Edel, A.L.; LaVallee, R.; Dibrov, E.; Pinneker, R.; Maddaford, T.G.; Ramjiawan, B.; Aliani, M.; Guzman, R.; et al. Potent Antihypertensive Action of Dietary Flaxseed in Hypertensive PatientsNovelty and Significance. *Hypertension* **2013**, *62*, 1081–1089. [CrossRef] [PubMed]
27. Chen, T.; Yan, F.; Qian, J.; Guo, M.; Zhang, H.; Tang, X.; Chen, F.; Stoner, G.D.; Wang, X. Randomized Phase II Trial of Lyophilized Strawberries in Patients with Dysplastic Precancerous Lesions of the Esophagus. *Cancer Prev. Res.* **2012**, *5*, 41–50. [CrossRef] [PubMed]
28. Zeidan, F.; Martucci, K.T.; Kraft, R.A.; Gordon, N.S.; McHaffie, J.G.; Coghill, R.C. Brain Mechanisms Supporting the Modulation of Pain by Mindfulness Meditation. *J. Neurosci.* **2011**, *31*, 5540–5548. [CrossRef]
29. Jacob, J.A. As Opioid Prescribing Guidelines Tighten, Mindfulness Meditation Holds Promise for Pain Relief. *JAMA* **2016**, *315*, 2385–2387. [CrossRef]
30. Cherkin, D.C.; Sherman, K.J.; Balderson, B.H.; Cook, A.J.; Anderson, M.L.; Hawkes, R.J.; Hansen, K.E.; Turner, J.A. Effect of Mindfulness-Based Stress Reduction vs Cognitive Behavioral Therapy or Usual Care on Back Pain and Functional Limitations in Adults With Chronic Low Back Pain: A Randomized Clinical Trial. *JAMA* **2016**, *315*, 1240–1249. [CrossRef]
31. Nidich, S.I.; Rainforth, M.V.; Haaga, D.A.F.; Hagelin, J.; Salerno, J.W.; Travis, F.; Tanner, M.; Gaylord-King, C.; Grosswald, S.; Schneider, R.H. A Randomized Controlled Trial on Effects of the Transcendental Meditation Program on Blood Pressure, Psychological Distress, and Coping in Young Adults. *Am. J. Hypertens.* **2009**, *22*, 1326–1331. [CrossRef]
32. Davidson, R.J.; Kabat-Zinn, J.; Schumacher, J.; Rosenkranz, M.; Muller, D.; Santorelli, S.F.; Urbanowski, F.; Harrington, A.; Bonus, K.; Sheridan, J.F. Alterations in Brain and Immune Function Produced by Mindfulness Meditation. *Psychosom. Med.* **2003**, *65*, 564. [CrossRef] [PubMed]
33. Cotton, S.; Luberto, C.M.; Sears, R.W.; Strawn, J.R.; Stahl, L.; Wasson, R.S.; Blom, T.J.; Delbello, M.P. Mindfulness-based cognitive therapy for youth with anxiety disorders at risk for bipolar disorder: A pilot trial. *Early Interv. Psychiatry* **2016**, *10*, 426–434. [CrossRef] [PubMed]
34. Spigelblatt, L.; Laîné-Ammara, G.; Pless, I.B.; Guyver, A. The Use of Alternative Medicine by Children. *Pediatrics* **1994**, *94*, 811–814. [PubMed]
35. Sawni-Sikand, A.; Schubiner, H.; Thomas, R.L. Use of Complementary/Alternative Therapies Among Children in Primary Care Pediatrics. *Ambul. Pediatr.* **2002**, *2*, 99–103. [CrossRef]
36. Sibinga, E.M.S.; Ottolini, M.C.; Duggan, A.K.; Wilson, M.H. Parent-Pediatrician Communication about Complementary and Alternative Medicine Use for Children. *Clin. Pediatr. (Phila.)* **2004**, *43*, 367–373. [CrossRef] [PubMed]

37. Pappas, S.; Perlman, A. Complementary and alternative medicine: The importance of doctor-patient communication. *Med. Clin. N. Am.* **2002**, *86*, 1–10. [CrossRef]
38. Eisenberg, D.M. Advising Patients Who Seek Alternative Medical Therapies. *Ann. Intern. Med.* **1997**, *127*, 61. [CrossRef]
39. Perlman, A.I.; Eisenberg, D.M.; Panush, R.S. Talking with Patients about Alternative and Complementary Medicine. *Rheum. Dis. Clin. N. Am.* **1999**, *25*, 815–822. [CrossRef]
40. Sugarman, J.; Burk, L. Physicians' Ethical Obligations Regarding Alternative Medicine. *JAMA* **1998**, *280*, 1623–1625. [CrossRef]
41. Kemper, K.J.; O'Connor, K.G. Pediatricians' Recommendations for Complementary and Alternative Medical (CAM) Therapies. *Ambul. Pediatr.* **2004**, *4*, 482–487. [CrossRef]
42. Sawni, A.; Thomas, R. Pediatricians' attitudes, experience and referral patterns regarding complementary/alternative medicine: A national survey. *BMC Complement. Altern. Med.* **2007**, *7*, 18. [CrossRef] [PubMed]
43. Winslow, L.C.; Shapiro, H. Physicians Want Education About Complementary and Alternative Medicine to Enhance Communication With Their Patients. *Arch. Intern. Med.* **2002**, *162*, 1176–1181. [CrossRef]
44. Vohra, S.; Surette, S.; Mittra, D.; Rosen, L.D.; Gardiner, P.; Kemper, K.J. Pediatric integrative medicine: Pediatrics' newest subspecialty? *BMC Pediatr.* **2012**, *12*, 123. [CrossRef]
45. Institute of Medicine (US) Committee on the Use of Complementary and Alternative Medicine by the American Public. *Complementary and Alternative Medicine in the United States*; The National Academies Collection: Reports funded by National Institutes of Health; National Academies Press (US): Washington, DC, USA, 2005; ISBN 978-0-309-09270-8.
46. McClafferty, H.; Dodds, S.; Brooks, A.J.; Brenner, M.G.; Brown, M.L.; Frazer, P.; Mark, J.D.; Weydert, J.A.; Wilcox, G.M.G.; Lebensohn, P.; et al. Pediatric Integrative Medicine in Residency (PIMR): Description of a New Online Educational Curriculum. *Children* **2015**, *2*, 98–107. [CrossRef] [PubMed]
47. Frank, E.; Breyan, J.; Elon, L. Physician disclosure of healthy personal behaviors improves credibility and ability to motivate. *Arch. Fam. Med.* **2000**, *9*, 287–290. [CrossRef] [PubMed]
48. McClafferty, H.; Brown, O.W.; Section on Integrative Medicine, Committee on Practice and Ambulatory Medicine. Physician Health and Wellness. *Pediatrics* **2014**, *134*, 830–835. [CrossRef] [PubMed]
49. Dewa, C.S.; Loong, D.; Bonato, S.; Thanh, N.X.; Jacobs, P. How does burnout affect physician productivity? A systematic literature review. *BMC Health Serv. Res.* **2014**, *14*, 325. [CrossRef]
50. Tawfik, D.S.; Profit, J.; Morgenthaler, T.I.; Satele, D.V.; Sinsky, C.A.; Dyrbye, L.N.; Tutty, M.A.; West, C.P.; Shanafelt, T.D. Physician Burnout, Well-being, and Work Unit Safety Grades in Relationship to Reported Medical Errors. *Mayo Clin. Proc.* **2018**, *93*, 1571–1580. [CrossRef]
51. Howe, A.; Smajdor, A.; Stöckl, A. Towards an understanding of resilience and its relevance to medical training. *Med. Educ.* **2012**, *46*, 349–356. [CrossRef]
52. Frank, E.; Rothenberg, R.; Lewis, C.; Belodoff, B.F. Correlates of physicians' prevention-related practices. Findings from the Women Physicians' Health Study. *Arch. Fam. Med.* **2000**, *9*, 359–367. [CrossRef]
53. Howe, M.; Leidel, A.; Krishnan, S.M.; Weber, A.; Rubenfire, M.; Jackson, E.A. Patient-Related Diet and Exercise Counseling: Do Providers' Own Lifestyle Habits Matter? *Prev. Cardiol.* **2010**, *13*, 180–185. [CrossRef] [PubMed]
54. Nguyen, C.T. Integrative Medicine as a Bridge to Physician Wellness. *Otolaryngol.-Head Neck Surg.* **2018**, *158*, 987–988. [CrossRef] [PubMed]
55. Vlieger, A.M.; Blink, M.; Tromp, E.; Benninga, M.A. Use of Complementary and Alternative Medicine by Pediatric Patients With Functional and Organic Gastrointestinal Diseases: Results From a Multicenter Survey. *Pediatrics* **2008**, *122*, e446–e451. [CrossRef] [PubMed]
56. Serpico, M.; Boyle, B.; Kemper, K.J.; Kim, S. Complementary and Alternative Medicine Use in Children with Inflammatory Bowel Diseases: A Single Center Survey. *J. Pediatr. Gastroenterol. Nutr.* **2016**, *63*, 651–657. [CrossRef] [PubMed]
57. Surette, S.; Vohra, S. Complementary, Holistic, and Integrative Medicine: Utilization Surveys of the Pediatric Literature. *Pediatr. Rev.* **2014**, *35*, 114–128. [CrossRef] [PubMed]
58. Misra, S.M. Integrative Therapies and Pediatric Inflammatory Bowel Disease: The Current Evidence. *Children* **2014**, *1*, 149–165. [CrossRef]

59. Miele, E.; Pascarella, F.; Giannetti, E.; Quaglietta, L.; Baldassano, R.N.; Staiano, A. Effect of a Probiotic Preparation (VSL#3) on Induction and Maintenance of Remission in Children With Ulcerative Colitis. *Am. J. Gastroenterol.* **2009**, *104*, 437–443.
60. Hanai, H.; Iida, T.; Takeuchi, K.; Watanabe, F.; Maruyama, Y.; Andoh, A.; Tsujikawa, T.; Fujiyama, Y.; Mitsuyama, K.; Sata, M.; et al. Curcumin Maintenance Therapy for Ulcerative Colitis: Randomized, Multicenter, Double-Blind, Placebo-Controlled Trial. *Clin. Gastroenterol. Hepatol.* **2006**, *4*, 1502–1506. [CrossRef]
61. Suskind, D.L.; Wahbeh, G.; Burpee, T.; Cohen, M.; Christie, D.; Weber, W. Tolerability of Curcumin in Pediatric Inflammatory Bowel Disease: A Forced-Dose Titration Study. *J. Pediatr. Gastroenterol. Nutr.* **2013**, *56*, 277. [CrossRef]
62. Ji, J.; Lu, Y.; Liu, H.; Feng, H.; Zhang, F.; Wu, L.; Cui, Y.; Wu, H. Acupuncture and Moxibustion for Inflammatory Bowel Diseases: A Systematic Review and Meta-Analysis of Randomized Controlled Trials. *J. Evid.-Based Complement. Altern. Med.* **2013**, *2013*, 158352. [CrossRef]
63. Timmer, A.; Preiss, J.C.; Motschall, E.; Rücker, G.; Jantschek, G.; Moser, G. Psychological interventions for treatment of inflammatory bowel disease. *Cochrane Database Syst. Rev.* **2011**. [CrossRef] [PubMed]
64. Cotton, S.; Roberts, Y.H.; Tsevat, J.; Britto, M.T.; Succop, P.; McGrady, M.E.; Yi, M.S. Mind-Body Complementary Alternative Medicine Use and Quality of Life in Adolescents with Inflammatory Bowel Disease. *Inflamm. Bowel Dis.* **2010**, *16*, 501–506. [CrossRef] [PubMed]
65. Mahler, T. Education and Hypnosis for Treatment of Functional Gastrointestinal Disorders (FGIDs) in Pediatrics. *Am. J. Clin. Hypn.* **2015**, *58*, 115–128. [CrossRef] [PubMed]
66. Mayer, E.A.; Tillisch, K. The brain-gut axis in abdominal pain syndromes. *Annu. Rev. Med.* **2011**, *62*, 381–396. [CrossRef] [PubMed]
67. Rutten, J.M.T.M.; Reitsma, J.B.; Vlieger, A.M.; Benninga, M.A. Gut-directed hypnotherapy for functional abdominal pain or irritable bowel syndrome in children: A systematic review. *Arch. Dis. Child.* **2013**, *98*, 252–257. [CrossRef] [PubMed]
68. Kline, R.M.; Kline, J.J.; Di Palma, J.; Barbero, G.J. Enteric-coated, pH-dependent peppermint oil capsules for the treatment of irritable bowel syndrome in children. *J. Pediatr.* **2001**, *138*, 125–128. [CrossRef] [PubMed]
69. Lin, Y.-C.; Lee, A.C.C.; Kemper, K.J.; Berde, C.B. Use of Complementary and Alternative Medicine in Pediatric Pain Management Service: A Survey. *Pain Med.* **2005**, *6*, 452–458. [CrossRef] [PubMed]
70. Young, L.; Kemper, K.J. Integrative care for pediatric patients with pain. *J. Altern. Complement. Med.* **2013**, *19*, 627–632. [CrossRef]
71. Palermo, T.M. Impact of recurrent and chronic pain on child and family daily functioning: A critical review of the literature. *J. Dev. Behav. Pediatr.* **2000**, *21*, 58–69. [CrossRef]
72. von Stülpnagel, C.; Reilich, P.; Straube, A.; Schäfer, J.; Blaschek, A.; Lee, S.-H.; Müller-Felber, W.; Henschel, V.; Mansmann, U.; Heinen, F. Myofascial trigger points in children with tension-type headache: A new diagnostic and therapeutic option. *J. Child Neurol.* **2009**, *24*, 406–409. [CrossRef]
73. Calvo-Muñoz, I.; Gómez-Conesa, A.; Sánchez-Meca, J. Physical therapy treatments for low back pain in children and adolescents: A meta-analysis. *BMC Musculoskelet. Disord.* **2013**, *14*, 55. [CrossRef] [PubMed]
74. Lee, B.H.; Scharff, L.; Sethna, N.F.; McCarthy, C.F.; Scott-Sutherland, J.; Shea, A.M.; Sullivan, P.; Meier, P.; Zurakowski, D.; Masek, B.J.; et al. Physical therapy and cognitive-behavioral treatment for complex regional pain syndromes. *J. Pediatr.* **2002**, *141*, 135–140. [CrossRef] [PubMed]
75. Cotton, S.; Luberto, C.M.; Bogenschutz, L.H.; Pelley, T.J.; Dusek, J. Integrative Care Therapies and Pain in Hospitalized Children and Adolescents: A Retrospective Database Review. *J. Altern. Complement. Med.* **2013**, *20*, 98–102. [CrossRef] [PubMed]
76. Lin, Y.-C.; Wan, L.; Jamison, R.N. Using Integrative Medicine in Pain Management: An Evaluation of Current Evidence. *Anesth. Analg.* **2017**, *125*, 2081.
77. Tsao, G.J.; Messner, A.H.; Seybold, J.; Sayyid, Z.N.; Cheng, A.G.; Golianu, B. Intraoperative acupuncture for posttonsillectomy pain: A randomized, double-blind, placebo-controlled trial. *Laryngoscope* **2015**, *125*, 1972–1978. [CrossRef] [PubMed]
78. Montgomery, G.H.; DuHamel, K.N.; Redd, W.H. A meta-analysis of hypnotically induced analgesia: How effective is hypnosis? *Int. J. Clin. Exp. Hypn.* **2000**, *48*, 138–153. [CrossRef] [PubMed]
79. Golianu, B.; Seybold, J.; D'Souza, G. Acupuncture as an Anesthetic Adjuvant for Pediatric Orthopedic Patients: A Pilot Study and Protocol Description. *Med. Acupunct.* **2015**, *27*, 475–480. [CrossRef]

80. Won, A.S.; Bailey, J.; Bailenson, J.; Tataru, C.; Yoon, I.A.; Golianu, B. Immersive Virtual Reality for Pediatric Pain. *Children* **2017**, *4*, 52. [CrossRef]
81. Yuan, J.C.; Rodriguez, S.; Caruso, T.J.; Tsui, J.H. Provider-controlled virtual reality experience may adjust for cognitive load during vascular access in pediatric patients. *Can. J. Anaesth.* **2017**, *64*, 1275–1276. [CrossRef]
82. Soo, I.; Mah, J.K.; Barlow, K.; Hamiwka, L.; Wirrell, E. Use of complementary and alternative medical therapies in a pediatric neurology clinic. *Can. J. Neurol. Sci.* **2005**, *32*, 524–528. [CrossRef]
83. Treat, L.; Liesinger, J.; Ziegenfuss, J.Y.; Humeniuk, K.; Prasad, K.; Tilburt, J.C. Patterns of Complementary and Alternative Medicine Use in Children with Common Neurological Conditions. *Glob. Adv. Health Med.* **2014**, *3*, 18–24. [CrossRef] [PubMed]
84. Kenney, D.; Jenkins, S.; Youssef, P.; Kotagal, S. Patient Use of Complementary and Alternative Medicines in an Outpatient Pediatric Neurology Clinic. *Pediatr. Neurol.* **2016**, *58*, 48–52.e7. [CrossRef] [PubMed]
85. Galicia-Connolly, E.; Adams, D.; Bateman, J.; Dagenais, S.; Clifford, T.; Baydala, L.; King, W.J.; Vohra, S. CAM Use in Pediatric Neurology: An Exploration of Concurrent Use with Conventional Medicine. *PLoS ONE* **2014**, *9*, e94078. [CrossRef] [PubMed]
86. Perrin, J.M.; Coury, D.L.; Hyman, S.L.; Cole, L.; Reynolds, A.M.; Clemons, T. Complementary and Alternative Medicine Use in a Large Pediatric Autism Sample. *Pediatrics* **2012**, *130*, S77–S82. [CrossRef] [PubMed]
87. Condò, M.; Posar, A.; Arbizzani, A.; Parmeggiani, A. Riboflavin prophylaxis in pediatric and adolescent migraine. *J. Headache Pain* **2009**, *10*, 361–365. [CrossRef] [PubMed]
88. Wang, F.; Van Den Eeden, S.K.; Ackerson, L.M.; Salk, S.E.; Reince, R.H.; Elin, R.J. Oral magnesium oxide prophylaxis of frequent migrainous headache in children: A randomized, double-blind, placebo-controlled trial. *Headache* **2003**, *43*, 601–610. [CrossRef] [PubMed]
89. Guidetti, V.; Dosi, C.; Bruni, O. The relationship between sleep and headache in children: Implications for treatment. *Cephalalgia* **2014**, *34*, 767–776. [CrossRef]
90. Legarda, S.B.; McMahon, D.; Othmer, S.; Othmer, S. Clinical Neurofeedback: Case Studies, Proposed Mechanism, and Implications for Pediatric Neurology Practice. *J. Child Neurol.* **2011**, *26*, 1045–1051. [CrossRef]
91. Tan, G.; Thornby, J.; Hammond, D.C.; Strehl, U.; Canady, B.; Arnemann, K.; Kaiser, D.A. Meta-Analysis of EEG Biofeedback in Treating Epilepsy. *Clin. Eeg. Neurosci.* **2009**, *40*, 173–179. [CrossRef]
92. Kanitz, J.L.; Camus, M.E.M.; Seifert, G. Keeping the balance—An overview of mind–body therapies in pediatric oncology. *Complement. Ther. Med.* **2013**, *21*, S20–S25. [CrossRef]
93. Laengler, A.; Spix, C.; Seifert, G.; Gottschling, S.; Graf, N.; Kaatsch, P. Complementary and alternative treatment methods in children with cancer: A population-based retrospective survey on the prevalence of use in Germany. *Eur. J. Cancer* **2008**, *44*, 2233–2240. [CrossRef] [PubMed]
94. Bishop, F.L.; Prescott, P.; Chan, Y.K.; Saville, J.; von Elm, E.; Lewith, G.T. Prevalence of Complementary Medicine Use in Pediatric Cancer: A Systematic Review. *Pediatrics* **2010**, *125*, 768–776. [CrossRef] [PubMed]
95. Jacobs, S.S. Integrative Therapy Use for Management of Side Effects and Toxicities Experienced by Pediatric Oncology Patients. *Children* **2014**, *1*, 424–440. [CrossRef] [PubMed]
96. Campbell, T.C. Cancer Prevention and Treatment by Wholistic Nutrition. *J. Nat. Sci.* **2017**, *3*.
97. Campbell, T.C. Nutrition and Cancer: An Historical Perspective—The Past, Present, and Future of Nutrition and Cancer. Part 2. Misunderstanding and Ignoring Nutrition. *Nutr. Cancer* **2017**, *69*, 962–968. [CrossRef] [PubMed]
98. Harvie, M.; Howell, A.; Evans, D.G. Can diet and lifestyle prevent breast cancer: What is the evidence? *Am. Soc. Clin. Oncol. Educ. Book* **2015**, e66-73. [CrossRef]
99. Lee, J.; Jeon, J.Y.; Meyerhardt, J.A. Diet and Lifestyle in Survivors of Colorectal Cancer. *Hematol. Oncol. Clin. N. Am.* **2015**, *29*, 1–27. [CrossRef] [PubMed]
100. Correa, P. Human Gastric Carcinogenesis: A Multistep and Multifactorial Process—First American Cancer Society Award Lecture on Cancer Epidemiology and Prevention. *Cancer Res.* **1992**, *52*, 6735–6740.
101. Vance, T.M.; Su, J.; Fontham, E.T.H.; Koo, S.I.; Chun, O.K. Dietary Antioxidants and Prostate Cancer: A Review. *Nutr. Cancer* **2013**, *65*, 793–801. [CrossRef]
102. Anand, P.; Kunnumakara, A.B.; Sundaram, C.; Harikumar, K.B.; Tharakan, S.T.; Lai, O.S.; Sung, B.; Aggarwal, B.B. Cancer is a Preventable Disease that Requires Major Lifestyle Changes. *Pharm. Res.* **2008**, *25*, 2097–2116. [CrossRef]

103. Chatzi, L.; Apostolaki, G.; Bibakis, I.; Skypala, I.; Bibaki-Liakou, V.; Tzanakis, N.; Kogevinas, M.; Cullinan, P. Protective effect of fruits, vegetables and the Mediterranean diet on asthma and allergies among children in Crete. *Thorax* **2007**, *62*, 677–683. [CrossRef] [PubMed]
104. Lozinsky, A.C.; Meyer, R.; Koker, C.D.; Dziubak, R.; Godwin, H.; Reeve, K.; Ortega, G.D.; Shah, N. Time to symptom improvement using elimination diets in non-IgE-mediated gastrointestinal food allergies. *Pediatr. Allergy Immunol.* **2015**, *26*, 403–408. [CrossRef] [PubMed]
105. Castro-Rodriguez, J.A.; Ramirez-Hernandez, M.; Padilla, O.; Pacheco-Gonzalez, R.M.; Pérez-Fernández, V.; Garcia-Marcos, L. Effect of foods and Mediterranean diet during pregnancy and first years of life on wheezing, rhinitis and dermatitis in preschoolers. *Allergol. Immunopathol. (Madrid)* **2016**, *44*, 400–409. [CrossRef] [PubMed]
106. Cramer, H.; Posadzki, P.; Dobos, G.; Langhorst, J. Yoga for asthma: A systematic review and meta-analysis. *Ann. Allergy Asthma Immunol.* **2014**, *112*, 503–510.e5.
107. Sankar, J.; Das, R.R. Asthma—A Disease of How We Breathe: Role of Breathing Exercises and Pranayam. *Indian J. Pediatr.* **2018**, *85*, 905–910. [CrossRef] [PubMed]
108. Burgess, J.; Ekanayake, B.; Lowe, A.; Dunt, D.; Thien, F.; Dharmage, S.C. Systematic review of the effectiveness of breathing retraining in asthma management. *Expert Rev. Respir. Med.* **2011**, *5*, 789–807. [CrossRef] [PubMed]
109. Mark, J.D. Pediatric Asthma. *Nutr. Clin. Pract.* **2009**, *24*, 578–588. [CrossRef]
110. Misra, S.M. The Current Evidence of Integrative Approaches to Pediatric Asthma. *Curr. Probl. Pediatr. Adolesc. Health Care* **2016**, *46*, 190–194. [CrossRef]
111. Guardamagna, O.; Abello, F.; Cagliero, P.; Lughetti, L. Impact of nutrition since early life on cardiovascular prevention. *Ital. J. Pediatr.* **2012**, *38*, 73. [CrossRef]
112. Kaikkonen, J.E.; Mikkilä, V.; Raitakari, O.T. Role of Childhood Food Patterns on Adult Cardiovascular Disease Risk. *Curr. Atheroscler. Rep.* **2014**, *16*, 443. [CrossRef]
113. Kavey, R.-E.W.; Allada, V.; Daniels, S.R.; Hayman, L.L.; McCrindle, B.W.; Newburger, J.W.; Parekh, R.S.; Steinberger, J. Cardiovascular Risk Reduction in High-Risk Pediatric Patients*: A Scientific Statement From the American Heart Association Expert Panel on Population and Prevention Science; the Councils on Cardiovascular Disease in the Young, Epidemiology and Prevention, Nutrition, Physical Activity and Metabolism, High Blood Pressure Research, Cardiovascular Nursing, and the Kidney in Heart Disease; and the Interdisciplinary Working Group on Quality of Care and Outcomes Research Endorsed by the American Academy of Pediatrics. *J. Cardiovasc. Nurs.* **2007**, *22*, 218–253. [PubMed]
114. Guarneri, M.; Mercado, N.; Suhar, C. Integrative Approaches for Cardiovascular Disease. *Nutr. Clin. Pract.* **2009**, *24*, 701–708. [CrossRef] [PubMed]
115. Boisvert, J.A.; Harrell, W.A. Integrative Treatment of Pediatric Obesity: Psychological and Spiritual Considerations. *Integr. Med. (Encinitas)* **2015**, *14*, 40–47. [PubMed]
116. Sibinga, E.M.S.; Webb, L.; Ghazarian, S.R.; Ellen, J.M. School-Based Mindfulness Instruction: An RCT. *Pediatrics* **2016**, *137*, e20152532. [CrossRef] [PubMed]
117. Nesvold, A.; Fagerland, M.W.; Davanger, S.; Ellingsen, Ø.; Solberg, E.E.; Holen, A.; Sevre, K.; Atar, D. Increased heart rate variability during nondirective meditation. *Eur. J. Prev. Cardiol.* **2012**, *19*, 773–780. [CrossRef] [PubMed]
118. Nijjar, P.S.; Puppala, V.K.; Dickinson, O.; Duval, S.; Duprez, D.; Kreitzer, M.J.; Benditt, D.G. Modulation of the autonomic nervous system assessed through heart rate variability by a mindfulness based stress reduction program. *Int. J. Cardiol.* **2014**, *177*, 557–559. [CrossRef] [PubMed]
119. Olex, S.; Newberg, A.; Figueredo, V.M. Meditation: Should a cardiologist care? *Int. J. Cardiol.* **2013**, *168*, 1805–1810. [CrossRef]
120. Painovich, J.; Longhurst, J. Integrating acupuncture into the cardiology clinic: Can it play a role? *Sheng Li Xue Bao* **2015**, *67*, 19–31.
121. McClafferty, H.; Brooks, A.J.; Chen, M.-K.; Brenner, M.; Brown, M.; Esparham, A.; Gerstbacher, D.; Golianu, B.; Mark, J.; Weydert, J.; et al. Pediatric Integrative Medicine in Residency Program: Relationship between Lifestyle Behaviors and Burnout and Wellbeing Measures in First-Year Residents. *Children* **2018**, *5*, 54. [CrossRef]
122. Won, A.S.; Tataru, C.A.; Cojocaru, C.M.; Krane, E.J.; Bailenson, J.N.; Niswonger, S.; Golianu, B. Two Virtual Reality Pilot Studies for the Treatment of Pediatric CRPS. *Pain Med.* **2015**, *16*, 1644–1647. [CrossRef]

123. Arruda, J.M.; Bogetz, A.L.; Vellanki, S.; Wren, A.; Yeh, A.M. Yoga as adjunct therapy for adolescents with inflammatory bowel disease: A pilot clinical trial. *Complement. Ther. Med.* **2018**, *41*, 99–104. [CrossRef] [PubMed]
124. Bodner, K.; D'Amico, S.; Luo, M.; Sommers, E.; Goldstein, L.; Neri, C.; Gardiner, P. A cross-sectional review of the prevalence of integrative medicine in pediatric pain clinics across the United States. *Complement. Ther. Med.* **2018**, *38*, 79–84. [CrossRef] [PubMed]
125. Kemper, K.J. Integrative medicine is becoming mainstream: Research on multimodal interventions needs to catch up. *Complement. Ther. Med.* **2018**, *39*, A1. [CrossRef] [PubMed]
126. Mark, J.D.; Chung, Y. Complementary and alternative medicine in pulmonology. *Curr. Opin. Pediatr.* **2015**, *27*, 334–340. [CrossRef]
127. Mark, J.D. Integrative medicine and asthma. *Pediatr. Clin. N. Am.* **2007**, *54*, 1007–1023. [CrossRef]
128. Coates, A.C.; Mark, J.D. Nutrition in Cystic Fibrosis. In *Nutrition in Pediatric Pulmonary Disease*; Dumont, R., Chung, Y., Eds.; Nutrition and Health; Springer: New York, NY, USA, 2014; pp. 81–97, ISBN 978-1-4614-8474-5.
129. Mark, J.D. Chapter 29—Asthma. In *Integrative Medicine (Fourth Edition)*; Rakel, D., Ed.; Elsevier: Amsterdam, The Netherlands, 2018; pp. 288–299.e2, ISBN 978-0-323-35868-2.
130. Yeh, A.M.; Wren, A.; Golianu, B. Mind-Body Interventions for Pediatric Inflammatory Bowel Disease. *Children* **2017**, *4*, 22. [CrossRef] [PubMed]
131. Kanak, M.; Park, K.T.; Yeh, A.M. Acupuncture and Integrative Medicine for Pediatric Gastroesophageal Reflux and Functional Dyspepsia. *Med. Acupunct.* **2015**, *27*, 467–474. [CrossRef]
132. Karamian, A.S.; Yeh, A.M.; Wusthoff, C. Integrative Medicine in Child Neurology: What do providers think and what do they need to learn? In Proceedings of the Annual Meeting of American Academy of Neurology, Los Angeles, CA, USA, 21 April 2018.
133. Staveski, S.L.; Boulanger, K.; Erman, L.; Lin, L.; Almgren, C.; Journel, C.; Roth, S.J.; Golianu, B. The Impact of Massage and Reading on Children's Pain and Anxiety After Cardiovascular Surgery: A Pilot Study. *Pediatr. Crit. Care Med.* **2018**, *19*, 725–732. [CrossRef]
134. Golianu, B.; Krane, E.; Seybold, J.; Almgren, C.; Anand, K.J.S. Non-pharmacological techniques for pain management in neonates. *Semin. Perinatol.* **2007**, *31*, 318–322. [CrossRef]
135. Sparrow, K.; Golianu, B. Does Acupuncture Reduce Stress Over Time? A Clinical Heart Rate Variability Study in Hypertensive Patients. *Med. Acupunct.* **2014**, *26*, 286–294. [CrossRef]
136. Mitchell, A.J.; Hall, R.W.; Golianu, B.; Yates, C.; Williams, D.K.; Chang, J.; Anand, K.J.S. Does noninvasive electrical stimulation of acupuncture points reduce heelstick pain in neonates? *Acta Paediatr.* **2016**, *105*, 1434–1439. [CrossRef] [PubMed]
137. NS-CSHCN Compare All Years: How Many Children/Youth Have Special Health Care Needs? Nationwide. Available online: http://childhealthdata.org/browse/survey/results?q=1792&r=1&t=1&ta=116 (accessed on 27 November 2018).
138. Eckert, M.; Amarell, C.; Anheyer, D.; Cramer, H.; Dobos, G. Integrative Pediatrics: Successful Implementation of Integrative Medicine in a German Hospital Setting-Concept and Realization. *Children* **2018**, *5*, 122. [CrossRef] [PubMed]
139. Esparham, A.; Misra, S.; Sibinga, E.; Culbert, T.; Kemper, K.; McClafferty, H.; Vohra, S.; Rosen, L. Pediatric Integrative Medicine: Vision for the Future. *Children* **2018**, *5*, 111. [CrossRef] [PubMed]
140. Bell, I.R.; Caspi, O.; Schwartz, G.E.R.; Grant, K.L.; Gaudet, T.W.; Rychener, D.; Maizes, V.; Weil, A. Integrative medicine and systemic outcomes research: Issues in the emergence of a new model for primary health care. *Arch. Intern. Med.* **2002**, *162*, 133–140. [CrossRef] [PubMed]

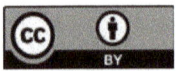

© 2018 by the authors. Licensee MDPI, Basel, Switzerland. This article is an open access article distributed under the terms and conditions of the Creative Commons Attribution (CC BY) license (http://creativecommons.org/licenses/by/4.0/).

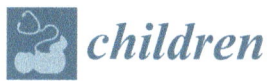

Article

Integrative Pediatrics: Successful Implementation of Integrative Medicine in a German Hospital Setting—Concept and Realization

Marion Eckert [1,*], Catharina Amarell [1], Dennis Anheyer [2], Holger Cramer [2] and Gustav Dobos [2]

1. Kinderkrankenhaus St. Marien, Grillparzerstr. 9, 84036 Landshut, Germany; catharina.amarell@st-marien-la.de
2. Department of Internal and Integrative Medicine, Kliniken Essen-Mitte, Faculty of Medicine, University of Duisburg-Essen, Am Deimelsberg 34a, 45276 Essen, Germany; D.Anheyer@kliniken-essen-mitte.de (D.A.); H.Cramer@kliniken-essen-mitte.de (H.C.); g.dobos@kliniken-essen-mitte.de (G.D.)
* Correspondence: dr-eckert@t-online.de; Tel.: +49-171-178-6524

Received: 26 July 2018; Accepted: 28 August 2018; Published: 4 September 2018

Abstract: Complementary and Alternative Medicine (CAM) has not been systematically institutionalized in pediatric hospital care in Germany so far. For the responsible implementation and systematic evaluation of CAM in pediatric care, a model project was initialized in three different pediatric hospitals in Germany, one of them being the "Kinderkrankenhaus St. Marien" in Landshut, Germany. During this project, a concept of the implementation process was developed based on clinical care, teaching, and scientific evaluation. A project group was formed in St. Marien, which included leaders of the hospital, physicians, nurses, and physiotherapists. Over a period of three years, pediatric treatment modalities of the CAM-spectrum were systematically integrated into routine pediatric care and a new integrative medicine department was established. CAM is now being applied in an inpatient as well as outpatient setting, in addition to conventional medical treatments. The modalities now applied include Traditional Chinese Medicine (TCM), relaxation, hypnosis, reflexology, wraps and poultices, aromatherapy, homeopathy, yoga, and herbal medicine. Studies were initiated in some areas. The process and concept leading up to this successful implementation will be described in this article. We show that with motivated team players and structured proceedings, implementation of integrative medicine in a children's hospital can be successful.

Keywords: integrative medicine; pediatrics; clinical practice

1. Introduction

Integrative Medicine (IM) is an emerging field, even if the increasingly wide use of Complementary and Alternative Medicine (CAM) and its incorporation into conventional medicine has been described in numerous publications [1–3]. IM incorporates the use of methods of the CAM spectrum into conventional medicine in an evidence-based way and integrates the whole person and the environment that person lives in into the treatment of adults as well as children. The Academic Consortium of Integrative Medicine & Health (ACIMH) states that "Integrative Medicine is the practice of medicine that reaffirms the importance of the relationship between practitioner and patient, focuses on the whole person, is informed by evidence, and makes use of all appropriate therapeutic approaches, healthcare professionals and disciplines to achieve optimal health and healing" [4].

Many authors have described the substantial increase in the use of CAM, not only in adults, but also in children [3,5–11], as well as the lack of information the treating physicians receive about the methods used and the possible side-effects that some of these treatments may have [12–14]. A variety of treatment modalities are nowadays applied in integrative medicine in the field of pediatrics [2]. Teaching programs for physicians and residents have been developed to increase their knowledge about and widen their spectrum of CAM treatments [15–17]. Many institutions have implemented integrative medicine in various models, even in hospitals [1,18–20]. Some of them have identified important factors and strategies that are vital for successful implementation [18,19]. Yet, CAM has not been widely systematically institutionalized in pediatric care in Germany so far—in hospitals or private practice.

Our intent was to implement integrative medicine in a pediatric hospital, by building a concept upon our and other's experiences that can be applicable and useful for different hospitals that strive to develop such programs. We also aimed at contributing to scientific insights on the modalities used. Therefore, at the very start of the project, an overview regarding the scientific situation of CAM in pediatrics was compiled and possible indications for CAM in children identified in a multidisciplinary meeting.

2. The Hospital Setting of St. Marien

The Children's Hospital "Kinderkrankenhaus St. Marien" in Landshut, Germany, is an academic teaching hospital of the LMU (Ludwig-Maximilians-University) München. It is equipped with 120 beds. An average of 6500 children are treated annually on the wards and about 16,000 children in the specialized outpatient departments. Seventeen thousand children are seen in the pediatric emergency department annually. A social pediatric center, which takes care of about 5200 patients per year, is affiliated with the hospital.

St. Marien Hospital has always been dedicated to promoting integrative approaches for the medical treatment of children. Besides conventional medicine, additional certifications of attending physicians allowed for naturopathic and homeopathic treatments, even in the years before our project started. For the past 10 years for example, a pediatrician with certification in homeopathy has been employed in the hospital treating inpatients as well as children in the outpatient department. A pediatrician certified in naturopathic medicine had also established policies for the application of naturopathic treatments for pertinent indications like upper airway infections or certain pain conditions.

3. Preparation

Whenever an institution takes a new direction, it is important that its leaders make decisions on the new course of action to be taken from then on. This needs to be communicated and future expectations made clear to the rest of the organization. This also applies to establishing an integrative medical care model within a hospital. Only then does the body of the organization know that a new corporate strategy is being pursued and employees are expected to act upon it in certain ways. In addition, a decision needs to be made on the areas in which CAM is supposed to be integrated in the hospital. The areas can be clinical, teaching, or research [19], depending on the structure of the hospital and interests of the organization. Not every institution will want to or be able to serve all three areas and this is not necessary. Various models, from e.g., focusing on pain management, research orientation, or offering a wide variety of integrative care modalities to patients, can work [19]. Furthermore, there are different approaches that can be taken in order to execute the new strategy. One is a model from "inside" the institution; the other would be a more external approach in which new staff with new skills is employed to start a new venture. We chose the model from inside, in which we built upon the skills and motivation of staff members. This offers the advantage of using existing resources and preventing resistance from staff members on new treatment methods. This has been described as one of the cornerstones of a successful implementation [19].

4. First Steps

First, a project group with members of different disciplines of the hospital with one coordinating leader was formed. This group met once a month to determine next steps to be taken and goals to accomplish.

It was beneficial to have the executive director of the hospital as a part of the group, amongst attending physicians of different disciplines, nursing management, nurses, physiotherapists, and psychologists in order to reach staff members from different disciplines and to build integrative medicine from inside the organization. A new sense of a common comprehensive project led to the necessary enthusiasm in all participants. It was important for the coordinating leader to be an experienced senior pediatrician, also trained in a broad field of complementary medicine, and someone who was accepted by all members of the project group. This leader was responsible for coordinating activities, establishment of contacts, development of next steps, creating questionnaires, communication with other facilities and researchers, networking, and motivation. Leaders from other pediatric integrative medicine programs were contacted and literature was reviewed for advice and ideas on how to successfully establish integrative medicine within a hospital [18,19,21].

The second step involved the determination of resources existing within the hospital. Hospital staff—be it nurses, doctors or physiotherapists—have a variety of additional qualifications in the area of complementary medicine, which they would readily apply in their work. To determine the existing resources, a questionnaire was designed, as other centers had done before in a similar way [22]. The questionnaire included questions about additional qualifications, overall interest in CAM being introduced in the hospital, and interest to use those qualifications in the treatment of children. We found that there was an immense variety of knowledge and skills already present in St. Marien (Table 1), similar to modalities applied in other centers in the US [2]. It was these resources that we utilized to build upon in the process of implementing IM in our institution.

Table 1. Existing staff expertise within St. Marien revealed through questionnaires.

Aromatherapy	Foot Reflexology	Massage
Art therapy	Homeopathy	Music therapy
Biofeedback	Naturopathy	Therapeutic riding
Craniosacral therapy	Nutritional counseling	Yoga

Thirdly we were interested in the assessment of desires of parents. Many studies showed that CAM methods are readily applied in children and that parents also desire the use of CAM in the treatment of their children [3,23]. There are regional differences though, so we wanted to know about the wishes of the parents in the local area as well as their past experiences with CAM and willingness to make additional payments for the integration of CAM in the treatment of their child. Therefore, another questionnaire was created and given to the parents arriving at the hospital. The majority of parents were very approving of CAM treatments for their children. These data will be published in a separate article and therefore will not be further described.

The fourth step was to start educating the nurses, physicians and other staff on different kinds of CAM methods. It is an advantage if there is a culture of regular teaching schedules (like lunch symposia or in-house trainings) already established within the institution. In St. Marien, CAM trainings were included in the in-house trainings taking place regularly. Teachings about aromatherapy, foot reflexology, wraps and poultices, homeopathy, hypnosis, and naturopathic treatment options were given by experts (physicians and nurses) this way. Instructions on the application of acupuncture needles, acupressure, aromatherapy, and homeopathy were also given to smaller groups on the wards. In addition, the staff gained practical experience and training in guided imagery and hypnosis as well as in naturopathic treatments over weekends and in half-day courses. This way, the staff learned about new treatment options and how and when to apply them. Knowledge was disseminated this way and new competencies were acquired (e.g., hypnosis for pain management, acupressure, etc.) and applied by nurses and physicians. Regular refresher teachings, including practical exercises to ensure quality of care, are being given.

In the process, it turned out to be essential to have one responsible, qualified physician, with additional qualifications in naturopathy and Traditional Chinese Medicine (TCM), who was able to anchor CAM deeper on the wards by making sure the new ways of treatment were being applied and by staff were being given repeated teachings. An outpatient clinic for CAM also was established. This is also according to the experience of other medical centers that emphasized on the advantage of having one protagonist leading the initiative in the hospital [19].

In order to publicize our institution's new corporate strategy and promote its presence, different paths were taken, within and outside the hospital. Flyers and posters were designed and displayed in the building, and the hospital website now provides specific details of the CAM services offered and the new department now in operation. A consult service was established and in-house teachings were held regularly. Medical discharge reports now include CAM treatments applied on children, in a bid to inform primary care physicians and make a public statement about the new corporate policy. In addition, articles in magazines and journals were published and interviews videotaped (available online [24,25]). All these efforts help in communicating the significance and new philosophy of the hospital to its staff and the public.

Another important step was creating structures within the hospital. Wards were specialized in different areas like aromatherapy or homeopathy according to interests and competencies of the nurses assigned to the wards. For example, nurses are responsible for keeping a track of stocks of homeopathic remedies or aroma oils, teachings on other wards, etc. CAM was made part of every ward conference meeting held by these nurses. Furthermore, policies for specific treatments were established and were made readily available on the intranet for physicians and nurses to refer to and download. CAM consult services were established across the hospital, as well as a CAM clinic. A curriculum has also been compiled, which every staff member—new and old—is required to go through (it takes approximately 8 h).

5. Financing

The challenge of financing CAM services has been addressed as an issue in most institutions [19,21]. It is absolutely necessary to have enough philanthropic support or available funds at least in the early stages, as financial resources are often scarce and money is needed for salaries, education of staff, and to generate research projects. In our case, this turned out to be the biggest cost factor at the beginning, diminishing over time though, as most staff was trained and the new treatment methods became routine. Trained staff members can now partly assume the teaching of colleagues and therefore diminish the need of external, costly teachers. The clinical care component was self-supporting and not too expensive. In the US as well as in Germany, CAM services are mostly not covered by health insurances. Endowment funding therefore is essential to support sustainability. All of the biggest centers that offer CAM services in the US (e.g., Osher Centers at Harvard and Penny George Institute for Health and Healing) have several million dollars of endowment funding for support. In Germany, foundations can provide substantial monetary inputs. In addition, it turned out beneficial to negotiate special deals with insurance companies that at least many families now profit from. Cost effectiveness of integrative care over time has been demonstrated on numerous occasions [26–28].

6. Results of Our Project

Starting in 2015, complementary medicine was introduced step by step in the routine care of children and an integrative approach was established, which led to the foundation of an integrative medicine department with an attending physician in 2017. One of the first steps we took was identifying the resources present in the hospital, which we could draw upon. A questionnaire for the staff was designed and handed out to all staff members. Questions included the overall interest in the introduction of CAM treatments in the hospital as well as additional certifications of staff members. Seventy-seven percent of those who had answered the questionnaire reported having an interest in CAM methods. While most of them were nursing staff members (58%), 31% were physicians. Areas that garnered most interest were acupuncture, osteopathy, aromatherapy, and naturopathy. As these results will be published in a separate article, they will not be described in detail here.

In the feedback part of the questionnaire, interest in the research topic was evident through several remarks like:

- "I think it is wonderful that our hospital belongs to the more progressive ones. I support CAM treatments 100%."
- "I am VERY happy, that CAM is now being established in our hospital and I hope that nursing staff can participate in trainings and teachings."
- "I think this area is really interesting and important, I would love to receive additional training and participate."

CAM Services Now Offered at St. Marien

Apart from homeopathy, which has a long history at St. Marien, many other treatment modalities were integrated in the everyday care of the children at St. Marien, within three years of our project:

1. Aromatherapy is now being used regularly on hospitalized patients as roll-on sticks and in form of wraps and poultices. One nurse successfully completed her certification as an aromatherapist.
2. Acupuncture points have been taught to nurses and physicians and are now being applied in the form of pyonex press needles inserted in the acupuncture point P6 (pericard 6) to almost all children under anesthesia to prevent post-operative nausea and vomiting. Several studies have shown that P6 can be as effective as antiemetic drugs in preventing post-operative nausea and vomiting [29]. Nurses and doctors have been trained to insert the needles and regular refresher teachings take place.
3. Acupressure points are being taught to children and parents for cough, anxiety, abdominal pain, and nausea.
4. Another treatment modality is foot reflexology according to Hanne Marquardt [30]. Two indications were chosen—abdominal and lung conditions—and their treatment methods were taught to staff and parents. It is now being used regularly. A study was initiated and started in September 2016 to determine the effect of reflexology on children with these conditions.
5. Yoga is being offered in the hospital now and a study was initiated and completed by our research partner in Essen, Germany, about the effect of yoga for headaches in children.
6. Basic hypnotherapy methods (like "the magic glove") were taught to physicians and nurses over the course of two weekends and are now being applied regularly.
7. Wraps and poultices are used in combination with aroma oils in the Newborn Intensive Care Unit (NICU) and the pediatric wards on patients with rheumatic diseases, anxiety, fever, joint pain, sleep problems, abdominal pain, and cough, among others.
8. Two doctors are now consulting on the wards on request for integrative treatment options for a variety of conditions. One of them is a certified homeopath, the other one is certified in naturopathy and TCM.
9. A "handling" course for parents has been held a few times since September 2016 to enable them to touch and move their babies in a more supportive and physiologic way to help their developmental process.
10. Herbal remedies are being applied and medical reference cards (detailing indications and dosage) have been designed for physicians.
11. A multidisciplinary pain management team now applies CAM Methods for treating pain in children.
12. Relaxation techniques of mind-body medicine are applied in the psychosomatic unit and social pediatric center.

7. Discussion

Integrating CAM methods into routine care for children within a hospital to create a real "integrative care" can be challenging. However, through our program, we demonstrated that CAM can successfully be integrated into a pediatric hospital in a relatively short time. The cornerstones that were essential to our process are summarized here and overlap some of which have been described as important components of other successful programs [18,19] as well as learned through personal communications (Kemper 2015).

1. The institution in which methods of the CAM spectrum require establishment has to make a clear decision on the path that should be taken.
2. Institutional support from the executive leader and medical director of the institution is essential. They represent the hospital and determine the overall concept of the institution. In our case, the leaders communicated well with each other about the new business concept, relayed this to their staff and put plans in place for it to be introduced by them. This enabled efficient evolution of the project and offered the prospect of sustainability.
3. It is important to have back-up support within the organization, as leaders can change over time. The project becomes vulnerable if the primary protagonist leaves. At least one well-respected person, preferably a qualified physician, should take the lead in the beginning. This person does not have to be an expert in all offered CAM modalities, but must be willing to cooperate with other CAM experts so that all team members can learn from each other. In St. Marien, two physicians led the project—one in the coordinating role and the other as an integrative physician present and active in the hospital.
4. It is crucial to have philanthropic support or available funds. Financial resources are often scarce and money is required for salaries, education of staff, and to generate research projects.
5. To minimize resistance, it is advisable to build on the prevalent interest of the institution. Depending on the organization, it could be research or clinical applications, or education, or a combination of both. It is easier to first follow that path and strengthen it before starting new ventures. In our case, clinical applications and education of staff were where the most interest was found, followed by research. We followed that interest, used existing resources, and tapped on motivation of the staff members (identified through a questionnaire) and subsequently built the new concept from inside out to keep staff members motivated.
6. It is essential to have motivated, creative colleagues working together, who can solve problems and find solutions one person can't see.
7. Networking with like-minded colleagues and institutions creates motivation and inspiration. Sharing ideas and experiences can help expand the project. In our project, three hospitals were involved and common projects were created and ideas exchanged in regular meetings with all participants. Networking with international colleagues also created inspiration and offered new ideas.
8. It is important to not implement several modalities at once. To have a clear and simple treatment plan in which the patient can develop a relationship with the therapist is better that an overwhelming and expensive plan. In addition, too many new modalities can lead to an overload of the staff and therefore lead to resistance, which is not good for the project. We selected our modalities by identifying evidence-based knowledge and experience present within the hospital. Although there is a lack of evidence in the treatment of children, in accordance with other centers, we did not exclude modalities that had inadequate evidence [19]; instead, we evaluated efficacy by performing meta-analyses and reviews on various topics [31–34].
9. Multidisciplinary meetings can help broaden one's spectrum of knowledge and experiences within the institution.

10. Research programs can be important in some institutions. Academic centers mostly want and need to add research to the project. Again, it is essential to follow the interest of the staff members and collaborate with other disciplines.
11. Education is an important aspect of any facility, be it in the form of lectures for students, training and rotations for staff members, or workshops.
12. Financing is a challenge in all centers. Financial plans have to be made, fundings organized, and payments by patients considered.
13. Cooperation and communication with colleagues in other hospitals as well as in private practices have to be established, in order to ensure complete integration into the field. In Germany, resistance can be quite high if the hospital offers treatments that colleagues in private practices don't. This can hinder the success of the project. A qualified physician or well-respected person has to represent the project in order to raise acceptance and reputation of the institution.

Pediatric Integrative Medicine programs are found in several US medical centers and a few in Europe [18,19,35]. In 2009, nine US medical centers that played an important pioneer role in integrative medicine were interviewed on the critical factors leading to success or failure of the establishment of IM in hospitals in the fields of research, education, and clinical application [19]. Many of the factors discussed are consistent with our findings, and therefore can be considered essential in the process of implementing an integrative medicine program in any institution.

8. Conclusions

Integrative medicine can be established in a pediatric hospital, if there is support from leaders, has a motivated, multidisciplinary team with a qualified leader, and enough philanthropic or institutional initial funding. Regular team meetings to identify and pursue goals, communication of these within the institution, and repeated teaching modules that meet the interest of the staff are essential strategies to ensure motivation and sustainability. Also, the addition of CAM treatments into the curriculum of residents and nurses will allow for an even-deeper anchoring of integrative medicine into the institution. As a next step, new treatment standards and policies encompassing CAM treatments for various conditions can be defined, so they become a natural part of routine care of the hospital. Parental desire for CAM treatments is strong and a variety of indications are suitable for their application.

Author Contributions: M.E. was primarily responsible for the coordination of the project as well as the conception and design of this article. C.A. is the leading physician for integrative medicine at St. Marien and was responsible for the implementation of the new treatment concepts and critically revised the manuscript. D.A. and H.C. were responsible for the scientific supervision of the project, participated in conception and design of the project, and critically revised the manuscript. G.D. initiated and designed the whole project and critically revised the manuscript. All authors approved the final manuscript.

Funding: The project was supported by a grant from the Karl and Veronica-Carstens Foundation. Further funds were received from the Weil Foundation.

Acknowledgments: We thank Hilary McClafferty and Kathi Kemper for all the support provided during and for the finalization of this project. We also thank Bernhard Brand for the support and encouragement in the realization of new pathways at St. Marien. We also thank Anita Eder, without whom our success would not have been possible.

Conflicts of Interest: On behalf of all authors, the corresponding author states that there is no conflict of interest.

References

1. Horrigan, B.; Lewis, S.; Abrams, D.I.; Pechura, C. *How Integrative Medicine Is Being Practiced in Clinical Centers across the United States*; The Bravewell Collaborative: Minneapolis, MN, USA, 2012. Available online: http://www.bravewell.org/current_projects/mapping_field/ (accessed on 20 May 2018).
2. Vohra, S.; Surette, S.; Mittra, D.; Rosen, L.D.; Gardiner, P.; Kemper, K.J. Pediatric integrative medicine: Pediatrics' newest subspecialty? *BMC Pediatr.* **2012**, *12*, 123. [CrossRef] [PubMed]

3. Zuzak, T.J.; Boňková, J.; Careddu, D.; Garami, M.; Hadjipanayis, A.; Jazbec, J.; Merrick, J.; Miller, J.; Ozturk, C.; Persson, I.A.; et al. Use of complementary and alternative medicine by children in Europe: Published data and expert perspectives. *Complement. Ther. Med.* **2013**, *21* (Suppl. 1), S34–S47. [CrossRef] [PubMed]
4. Academic Consortium of Integrative Medicine and Health (ACIMH). Definition of Integrative Medicine and Health. Available online: https://www.imconsortium.org/about/about-us.cfm (accessed on 5 June 2018).
5. Du, Y.; Wolf, I.K.; Zhuang, W.; Bodemann, S.; Knöss, W.; Knopf, H. Use of herbal medicinal products among children and adolescents in Germany. *BMC Complement. Altern. Med.* **2014**, *14*, 218. [CrossRef] [PubMed]
6. Du, Y.; Knopf, H. Paediatric homoeopathy in Germany: Results of the German Health Interview and Examination Survey for Children and Adolescents (KiGGS). *Pharmacoepidemiol. Drug Saf.* **2009**, *18*, 370–379. [CrossRef] [PubMed]
7. Du, Y.; Knopf, H. Self-medication among children and adolescents in Germany: Results of the National Health Survey for Children and Adolescents (KiGGS). *Br. J. Clin. Pharmacol.* **2009**, *68*, 599–608. [CrossRef] [PubMed]
8. Italia, S.; Wolfenstetter, S.B.; Teuner, C.M. Patterns of complementary and alternative medicine (CAM) use in children: A systematic review. *Eur. J. Pediatr.* **2014**, *173*, 1413–1428. [CrossRef] [PubMed]
9. Kemper, K.J.; Vohra, S.; Walls, R. American Academy of Pediatrics. The use of complementary and alternative medicine in pediatrics. *Pediatrics* **2008**, *122*, 1374–1386. [CrossRef] [PubMed]
10. Lin, Y.C.; Lee, A.C.; Kemper, K.J.; Berde, C.B. Use of complementary and alternative medicine in pediatric pain management service: A survey. *Pain Med.* **2005**, *6*, 452–458. [CrossRef] [PubMed]
11. Groenewald, C.B.; Beals-Erickson, S.E.; Ralston-Wilson, J.; Rabbitts, J.A.; Palermo, T.M. Complementary and Alternative Medicine Use by Children With Pain in the United States. *Acad. Pediatr.* **2017**, *17*, 785–793. [CrossRef] [PubMed]
12. Sidora-Arcoleo, K.; Yoos, H.L.; Kitzman, H.; McMullen, A.; Anson, E. Don't ask, don't tell: Parental nondisclosure of complementary and alternative medicine and over-the-counter medication use in children's asthma management. *J. Pediatr. Health Care* **2008**, *22*, 221–229. [CrossRef] [PubMed]
13. Lindly, O.; Thorburn, S.; Zuckerman, K. Use and Nondisclosure of Complementary Health Approaches Among US Children with Developmental Disabilities. *J. Dev. Behav. Pediatr.* **2018**, *39*, 217–227. [CrossRef] [PubMed]
14. Sibinga, E.M.; Ottolini, M.C.; Duggan, A.K.; Wilson, M.H. Parent-pediatrician communication about complementary and alternative medicine use for children. *Clin. Pediatr.* **2004**, *43*, 367–373. [CrossRef] [PubMed]
15. McClafferty, H.; Dodds, S.; Brooks, A.J.; Brenner, M.G.; Brown, M.L.; Frazer, P.; Mark, J.D.; Weydert, J.A.; Wilcox, G.M.; Lebensohn, P.; et al. Pediatric Integrative Medicine in Residency (PIMR): Description of a New Online Educational Curriculum. *Children* **2015**, *2*, 98–107. [CrossRef] [PubMed]
16. Lebensohn, P.; Kligler, B.; Brooks, A.J.; Teets, R.; Birch, M.; Cook, P.; Maizes, V. Integrative Medicine in Residency: Feasibility and Effectiveness of an Online Program. *Fam. Med.* **2017**, *49*, 514–521. [PubMed]
17. Academy of Integrative Health & Medicine (AIHM). Available online: https://www.aihm.org (accessed on 20 July 2018).
18. Von Rosenstiel, I.A.; Schats, W.; Bongers, K.; Jong, M.C. Integrative paediatrics: A Dutch experience. *Focus Altern. Complement. Ther.* **2011**, *16*, 22–27. [CrossRef]
19. Vohra, S.; Feldman, K.; Johnston, B.; Waters, K.; Boon, H. Integrating complementary and alternative medicine into academic medical centers: Experience and perceptions of nine leading centers in North America. *BMC Health Serv. Res.* **2005**, *5*, 78. [CrossRef] [PubMed]
20. Highfield, E.S.; McLellan, M.C.; Kemper, K.J.; Risko, W.; Woolf, A.D. Integration of complementary and alternative medicine in a major pediatric teaching hospital: An initial overview. *J. Altern. Complement. Med.* **2005**, *11*, 373–380. [CrossRef] [PubMed]
21. Eisenberg, D.M.; Kaptchuk, T.; Post, D.E.; Hrbek, A.L.; O'connor, B.B.; Osypiuk, K.; Wayne, P.M.; Buring, J.E.; Levy, D.B. Establishing an Integrative Medicine Program within an Academic Health Center: Essential Considerations. *Acad. Med.* **2016**, *91*, 1223–1230. [CrossRef] [PubMed]
22. Kemper, K.J.; Dirkse, D.; Eadie, D.; Pennington, M. What do clinicians want? Interest in integrative health services at a North Carolina academic medical center. *BMC Complement. Altern. Med.* **2007**, *7*, 5. [CrossRef] [PubMed]

23. Sencer, S.F.; Kelly, K.M. Complementary and alternative therapies in pediatric oncology. *Pediatr. Clin. N. Am.* **2007**, *54*, 1043–1060. [CrossRef] [PubMed]
24. Carstens Stiftung. Available online: https://www.carstens-stiftung.de/paediatrie.html (accessed on 20 July 2018).
25. Carstens Stiftung. Available online: https://www.youtube.com/results?search_query=integrative+pädiatrie (accessed on 20 July 2018).
26. Herman, P.M.; Poindexter, B.L.; Witt, C.M.; Eisenberg, D.M. Are complementary therapies and integrative care cost-effective? A systematic review of economic evaluations. *BMJ Open* **2012**, *2*, e001046. [CrossRef] [PubMed]
27. Baars, E.W.; Kooreman, P. A 6-year comparative economic evaluation of healthcare costs and mortality rates of Dutch patients from conventional and CAM GPs. *BMJ Open* **2014**, *4*, e005332. [CrossRef] [PubMed]
28. Deng, G.; Cassileth, B.R. Integrative oncology: Complementary therapies for pain, anxiety, and mood disturbance. *CA Cancer J. Clin.* **2005**, *55*, 109–116. [CrossRef] [PubMed]
29. Lee, A.; Chan, S.K.; Fan, L.T. Stimulation of the wrist acupuncture point PC6 for preventing postoperative nausea and vomiting. *Cochrane Database Syst. Rev.* **2015**, *11*, CD003281. [CrossRef] [PubMed]
30. Lett, A. The scope and limitations of treatment. An interview with Ann Lett, Principle, British School—Reflex Zone Therapy of the Feet. *Complement. Ther. Nurs. Midwifery* **2001**, *7*, 146–149. [CrossRef] [PubMed]
31. Anheyer, D.; Dobos, G.; Cramer, H. Evidenzlage pflanzlicher Präparate in der Anwendung bei Kindern und Jugendlichen. [Herbal medicines in children and adolescents—A narrative overview]. *Zeitschrift für Phytotherapie* **2016**, *6*, 236–241.
32. Anheyer, D.; Lauche, R.; Schumann, D.; Dobos, G.; Cramer, H. Herbal medicines in children with attention deficit hyperactivity disorder: A systematic review. *Complement. Ther. Med.* **2017**, *30*, 14–23. [CrossRef] [PubMed]
33. Anheyer, D.; Frawley, J.; Koch, A.K.; Lauche, R.; Langhorst, J.; Dobos, G.; Cramer, H. Herbal medicines for gastrointestinal disorders in children and adolescents: A systematic review. *Pediatrics* **2017**, *139*, e20170062. [CrossRef] [PubMed]
34. Anheyer, D.; Cramer, H.; Lauche, R.; Saha, F.J.; Dobos, G. Herbal medicine in children with respiratory tract infection: Systematic review and meta-analysis. *Acad. Pediatr.* **2018**, *18*, 8–19. [CrossRef] [PubMed]
35. Winther, C.; Von Rosenstiel, I.; Robinson, N.; Lee, R.; Shah, P.; Bukutu, C.; Koolen, R.; Vlieger, A.; Bongers, K.; Eckert, M.; et al. It'a small world—Pediatric CAM initiatives in the EU. *Focus Altern. Complement. Ther.* **2008**, *13*, 90–94. [CrossRef]

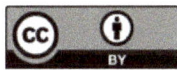

© 2018 by the authors. Licensee MDPI, Basel, Switzerland. This article is an open access article distributed under the terms and conditions of the Creative Commons Attribution (CC BY) license (http://creativecommons.org/licenses/by/4.0/).

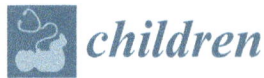

Article

Applied Pediatric Integrative Medicine: What We Can Learn from the Ancient Teachings of Sebastian Kneipp in a Kindergarten Setting

Marion Eckert [1,*] and Melanie Anheyer [2]

1. Kinderkrankenhaus St. Marien, 84036 Landshut, Germany
2. Elisabeth Krankenhaus, 45138 Essen, Germany; m.anheyer@contilia.de
* Correspondence: dr-eckert@t-online.de; Tel.: +49-171-178-6524

Received: 13 June 2018; Accepted: 24 July 2018; Published: 26 July 2018

Abstract: Pediatric integrative medicine focuses on the whole child and the environment in which the child grows up during the treatment of a child's illness. Nowadays, many different treatment modalities are applied even in children, and doctors need to know about them and, ideally, be able to apply different approaches in the process of treating a child themselves. The program Pediatric Integrative Medicine in Residency (PIMR) already provides residents with several tools to provide this kind of service for the child. In our PIMR pilot program in Germany, we chose to diversify our knowledge about treatment and prevention options by visiting a Kneipp-certified kindergarten in Germany. The philosophy of Sebastian Kneipp focuses on five pillars of health, which incorporate aspects of prevention, self-awareness, self-responsibility, and consciousness of health by means of hydrotherapy, herbal medicine, exercise, nutrition, and lifestyle-medicine. These are being taught to the children during the early years they spend in kindergarten, and represent integral parts of integrative medicine. Integration of Kneipp-based health programs within a kindergarten setting can work well and provides an effective means of early prevention education in childhood.

Keywords: Kneipp; kindergarten; PIMR

---

1. Introduction

In Germany, there has been a long tradition of naturopathic medicine. Hildegard von Bingen (1098–1179), a Benedictine abbess, is considered the founder of natural history and her work still greatly influences modern naturopathic medicine movements. One of the more recent forefathers of the naturopathic movement was the priest, Sebastian Kneipp (1821–1897), who is most commonly associated with hydrotherapy and the "Kneipp-Cure", which he claimed had therapeutic or healing effects. But, it was not only hydrotherapy that he based his principles of achieving and maintaining health on. In fact, he proposed an entire system of healing, which rested on five pillars: Hydrotherapy, herbal medicine, exercise, nutrition, and lifestyle-medicine (order and balance) [1]. Even nowadays, his teachings and philosophy are a part of many naturopathic teachings in Germany, being represented in national and regional Kneipp-associations who certify a wide variety of qualified facilities with the "Kneipp certificate", such as schools and kindergartens as well as health resorts and spas, campgrounds, and guest houses, who must fulfill certain requirements according to the Kneipp philosophy. As Kneipp's principles form the basis for European traditional naturopathic medicine, they are an essential part of the curriculum offered for physicians in Germany who want to become legally certified naturopathic doctors. The pillars of Kneipp can also be found in modern and international integrative and naturopathic medicine and teaching curriculums [2,3], which makes them an essential part of knowledge for the integrative physician.

Integrative medicine in pediatrics focuses on the whole child and the environment in which the child grows up. Currently, obesity in children and allergies as well as stress related disorders are on the rise. An immediate reward principle, with everything readily available and a focus outside of oneself, is an increasing phenomenon. Therefore, prevention aspects, as well as self-awareness and mindfulness in life and health, have become important aspects of modern medicine. Especially, children need tools to grow up healthy in this kind of environment. Nowadays, many treatment modalities are being applied in integrative medicine and in the field of pediatrics [2]. The teaching program, "Pediatric Integrative Medicine in Residency (PIMR)" [3], provides residents with the knowledge about a wide variety of complementary healing approaches. In Germany, the PIMR program was used as a pilot program at three different childrens' hospitals. To deepen and diversify their knowledge about integrative medicine approaches, the group explored the principles of a Kneipp-certified kindergarten in Germany as an extracurricular activity. As described above, the philosophy of Sebastian Kneipp focuses on five pillars of health, which incorporate prevention, self-awareness, self-responsibility, and consciousness of health. These principles are being taught to the children during the years they spend in kindergarten.

2. Visit of the Kneipp Kindergarten

2.1. General Information

The kindergarten, St. Stephanus, in Essen, Germany, is one of 400 Kneipp-certified child daycare facilities in Germany. Certification by the Kneipp-Bund requires the offer of a multitude of self-awareness and self-experience opportunities that lie within the Kneipp principles to attain the ability of prevention in everyday life. In the case of a kindergarten, at least 50% of the teachers are required to attend an advanced 30-h training in health concepts according to Kneipp, and must attend yearly refresher courses. For implementation in daily life, a set of guidelines has been laid out, which must be fulfilled by the kindergarten to be certified [4]. These guidelines incorporate adequate outdoor and physical activity spaces, integration of parents, balance of life (e.g., daily routine, time for sleep and rest), offer of physical activities in- and outdoors, healthy nutrition, use of herbs, and, finally, daily water treatments according to Kneipp. After 18 months of gaining experience, certification of the facility ensues.

In the facility of St. Stephanus, the children are divided into three groups, with a total of 54 children. Two of the groups have children aged 3–6 years and one group is for children aged 0.3 months–3 years of age. The children can stay in the kindergarten either 35 h (7:00 a.m. through 2:00 p.m.) or 45 h (7:00 a.m. through 4:30 p.m.) per week. Still, there are many intergroup activities so children experience a greater variety of experiences and decision processes. There is a total of six teachers, one pediatric nurse, one childcare assistant, and the director of the facility. Children have two group rooms, two side rooms, a big common room, two wash rooms, a sleep room, one activity room, and a wide outdoor area at their disposal. They can play in all weather conditions, as the facility considers itself an all-weather kindergarten.

This kindergarten is closely associated with the local catholic community. Religious work is characterized by the appreciation of others and their beliefs, so acceptance and tolerance of different religions is actively lived. St. Stephanus is under the administration union of the "KiTa Zweckverband", a union of child daycare facilities in the Bishopric of Essen, and is financed partly by the union, the parents, and the city of Essen.

St. Stephanus is situated amidst one of the most densely populated parts of the city of Essen, namely Essen Holsterhausen, with close to 27,000 inhabitants. This part of Essen is characterized by a mixed population of all social classes where many single parents are in need of long hours of care for their child. The kindergarten is well accessible by car, bus, and is in walking distance of the surrounding residential areas.

2.2. Conceptual Design

Life in the kindergarten, St. Stephanus, has been lived according to the principles of Sebastian Kneipp since April 2013, when the kindergarten was officially certified by the "Kneipp-Bund".

As soon as you enter the facility the spirit of Kneipp's principles becomes evident: Binders in different colours and decorated stones representing the five pillars welcome the visitor. Throughout the kindergarten, it is obvious how deeply the Kneipp concept is integrated into everyday life. The following examples show how each of the five pillars of hydrotherapy, phytotherapy, physical activity, nutrition, and lifestyle-medicine is lived and applied by the children and their teachers.

Hydrotherapy is applied in many ways: The children learn through the effects of cold- or warm water washings or brushings how to calm themselves down or energize themselves. Every child has their own washcloth or brush and learns how to use it. There are tubs for arm-baths and foot-baths. In winter, children with warm feet go for a short walk in the snow, and, in spring and summer, the dew on the lawn is used for the "dew cure". This is one of the more than 120 forms of hydrotherapies of Kneipp, where a barefoot walk with initially warm feet in the fresh morning grass is performed for 2–5 min to boost the circulation, and strengthen the immune system and foot muscles. Water basins with cold water are used for water treading, the most well-known water application of Sebastian Kneipp. Always, the individual child, its health condition, body temperature etc. is considered so the child learns to listen to signs of their own body to determine what is good for them and what can be potentially harmful. Therefore, a self-determined and responsible care for their own health and body condition is taught to the children.

Herbs also play a central role in the kindergarten. An outdoor herb garden is used for planting and identifying herbs with the children. They pick and dry them and use them for making herb sachets and herbal teas as well as reference books. Also, aroma-oil diffusions are done in the group rooms, and herbal inhalations in a tent under supervision of a teacher. This way the children learn about the properties of the herbs and how they can be applied. Herbs used are common traditional European medicinal plants, for example chamomile, fennel, peppermint, anise, and lavender. Throughout the kindergarten, herbs and information sheets on how to use them are displayed for parents. This provides the families and children with respect and knowledge about nature as well as with tools for their own health.

Physical activity is also an important module in the kindergarten as well as promoting feeling and sensing the own body. Hence, there is a movement room in which children can move freely, climb, and be wild. To promote sensation, all is done barefoot. Also, the large outdoor area of the kindergarten gives the children the opportunity to move around outdoors in all weather conditions. With a feeling parcours, on which they also walk barefoot, children learn the different feeling of grass, asphalt, rocks, snow etc. in a mindful way. Thus, the children's innate joy of movement can be considered. The aim is to promote this in a sustainable way, which also shapes the social and emotional development of the children.

In early childhood, the foundations for a consciousness of healthy nutrition and way of eating can be built and shaped. Nutrition in the kindergarten is according to the recommendations of the Germany society for nutrition, incorporating seasonal and regional foods as well as whole grain products. A healthy diet is promoted through a daily changing breakfast buffet from which children can choose, serve themselves, and thereby determine what it is they want to eat. The lunch menu is selected each week by a different group of children. This way the children learn to listen to their body's needs while being able to choose from a healthy buffet.

The principle of order and balance is taught by the rules of Papilio for children as well as through daily and seasonal rituals, which promote a feeling of safety and assurance for the children. Balance between sleep and activity during the day, and a regulated day with fixed meal and play times is as important as lunch rituals, sleep rituals, birthday rituals, etc. Papilio is a program for the primary prevention of behavioral problems and for supporting the socio-emotional competencies of children. It has been designed for three different age groups and aims for the prevention of addictions and violence. The program is based on scientific studies and the effects have been proven by a controlled longitudinal study [5]. The kindergarten uses the program designed for children aged 3–6 years. According to the principles of Papilio, children learn how to interact with themselves and others in a respectful way, how to contribute their own matters, and how to be considerate of others.

The first principle is: Learn how to play with others and how to make yourself happy without the use of specific toys. Therefore, one day per week there is a "toys are on vacation day" where children only work with natural materials or must come up with own interactive ideas for playing.

The second principle is learning social rules and awareness of others in a playful way. Daily rules are made up together with the children, and one child always makes sure the rules are kept. For example, "I let others finish their sentence", "I listen to what others are saying", and "I put toys away after I'm finished playing with them".

The third principle is about teaching the children about emotions, so that they learn to recognize these in themselves and others, and, this way, learn how to deal with them. Puppets, in the form of emotion-goblins, displaying the major emotions of anger, happiness, sadness, and fear are applied in various ways. The happiness-goblin always smiles and cannot understand that anyone could feel different, the anger-goblin could explode upon every opportunity, the crying-goblin is always sad, and the fright-goblin is always afraid because something bad could happen at any time. The children learn how to recognize their own feelings as well as the feelings of others, and develop an understanding for the feelings of someone else. This is an important task in the development of a personality.

3. Discussion

In the kindergarten of St. Stephanus, the children live the principles of Kneipp in everyday life. In a playful way, they learn the basics for a healthy lifestyle, not only about "what can make me sick", but, even more so, "what keeps me healthy". Health-conscious behaviors and attitudes are being learned and practiced so that they become natural to the child and can provide the basis for a better consciousness of health and a healthier lifestyle later in life.

Despite health problems being a rising phenomenon in children, health education is usually not a teaching subject in schools and kindergartens. Different concepts of education can be found in kindergartens in Germany, yet, a concept based on physical and mental health education is unique to a Kneipp kindergarten.

The principle of order and balance forms the basis for the other four pillars according to the principles of Kneipp. It helps and supports children in implementing health-promoting attitudes into their daily life. In the kindergarten, this is achieved by the rules according to Papilio, as well as rituals, so that children can orient themselves and have a sense of stability. Thus, they can acquire skills that help them to find the balance between resources and everyday requirements.

There are no studies that have been performed specifically on Kneipp kindergarten children. However, studies done on children in various ages and adults show that water treatments lead to active training of blood vessels. Cold and warm water treatments increase blood flow and result in the training of blood vessels, which leads to a stabilization of the immune system [6]. A variety of benefits have been described, including a lowering of the frequency of coughing in respiratory tract infections and various immunological modulations [7–11]. As most children love water, washings, arm- and foot-baths, and walking in dew, snow, and water are perfect ways to playfully help in the prevention of common colds [7]. By directly experiencing their bodily reactions to the water-stimuli, they can learn to develop a better awareness of their own body.

Herbs, which the children grow in their own herb garden, are an essential component of complementary medicine as well as an integral part of the Kneipp philosophy. The direct contact with nature teaches the children respect and lays the foundation of an understanding of the benefits and damages of nature. The child recognizes the involvement of the human being in its environment. The sense of responsibility towards the environment and one's own body is supported and promoted.

Physical activity is a fundamental need and an integral part in the mental and physical development and well-being of children. In the kindergarten of St. Stephanus, the children are allowed to follow their daily urge to move. The focus is on elementary forms of movement and combines movement with positive experiences. This can prevent physical inactivity, which is associated with various diseases, such as metabolic syndrome and back pain.

Sebastian Kneipp recognized that many diseases occur due to the wrong type of nutrition. Therefore, he promoted a simple, natural diet with enough calories to support the functions of the organs and the body. Nutrition has also gained importance in conventional medicine, as the influence of malnutrition and over-nutrition on the development of civilization diseases is widely recognized nowadays. In St. Stephanus, the children receive a healthy, balanced diet, which is as natural and seasonal as possible. This can help establish a healthy eating pattern in the children. As parents are integrated into the activities of the kindergarten, this is also transported into the homes and families of the children.

Many publications show that despite huge medical advances, many children suffer from lifestyle (obesity, stress related disorders), chronic, and severe diseases [12–15]. Therefore, the promotion of health and wellness in childhood is essential. Kneipp had already recognized, in the 19th century, that the relationship between the body, mind, and soul plays a pivotal role in health and disease. Accordingly, he placed the whole human being, with its physical, psychological, and social needs, in the center of his prevention and therapy system, just like modern integrative medicine is dedicated to. He demanded responsibility for one's own health, including an active participation in one's own lifestyle and social relationships. Apart from a certain way and order of life, he claimed that physical activity, nutrition, and the use of herbs can be used to prevent and treat sickness. Those aspects are an integral part of modern integrative and complementary medicine, and are also represented in the curriculum of the PIMR [3].

The fact that this can already effectively be applied to children makes the Kneipp concept an ideal target for kindergartens and early priming for a healthy lifestyle. Most children are open and curious and love to learn [16,17]. This provides an excellent ground for laying new and lasting foundations regarding their own health. Teaching them Kneipp's prevention and treatment tools in a fun way at an early age provides an effective way to make those principles a palpable experience for children and allows for a holistic childhood education.

The limitation of applying some of Kneipp's principles in a kindergarten lies in the fact that treatments of sick children cannot be performed by teachers or nurses due to legal issues. Therefore, the use of Kneipp is limited to prevention aspects in this setting.

In Germany, no curriculum for a certification in naturopathic or integrative pediatrics exists. To obtain the certification of a naturopathic physician, only doctors can go through a curriculum designed for adult patients. In this curriculum, the principles according to Kneipp are an essential part and even a specific certification as a Kneipp physician exists. Visiting a Kneipp certified kindergarten helps pediatric residents and physicians to directly gain knowledge about the application of those principles to children so that they can use that knowledge in their care of children and transfer theory into practice. In this way, they can advise parents or educate kindergartens and schools in the application of Kneipp's principles and, therefore, support the inclusion of health promoting activities (both physical and social-emotional) in educational settings. Also, certain modalities, like hydrotherapy, can be introduced by adept doctors into pediatric hospitals interested in holistic healthcare approaches.

4. Conclusions

It has been shown that even in early childhood basic attitudes and patterns regarding one's own health and healing can be developed. Kneipp's system of healing, with its pillars of hydrotherapy, phytotherapy, exercise, and nutrition as well as order and balance, can be well integrated within a kindergarten setting and are perfectly suitable for teaching children about responsibility and connectedness towards self, others, and nature. In this way, the Kneipp principles can provide holistic support for the development of personality and health-conscious behaviors of the child. An awareness of individual health resources and avoidance of risk factors are promoted, as well as the development of a natural feeling for physical and emotional health, respect for others and the environment, mindfulness towards one's own resources, self-empowerment, and self-responsibility for health and emotional competencies.

A significant proportion of children worldwide suffer from health problems and with an increasing age the risk of civilizational diseases rises. A healthy lifestyle can prevent diseases or diminish their progression. Child day care facilities offer an ideal setting to introduce children to a health-promoting and health-conscious way of living: For one, children are curious, and their behavioral patterns can still be shaped. Secondly, kindergarten is a universal area of life for pre-school children, which makes it possible to reach children and parents from all social backgrounds. Even though there are currently no studies existing that give evidence about the advantages of a Kneipp based education in kindergarten, the principles of Kneipp are integral parts of modern integrative and naturopathic medicine. Kneipp based educational systems for children provide a good opportunity for physicians to observe and promote self-care strategies applied in children.

Author Contributions: M.E. is primarily responsible for the conception and design of this article. M.E. and M.A. drafted the text. Both authors provided evaluation and revision of the manuscript and have given final approval of the manuscript.

Funding: This research was funded by the Weil Foundation.

Acknowledgments: The authors thank Gustav Dobos, without whom this project and article would not exist. We thank the Weil Foundation for their funding of the pilot program PIMR in Germany and Birgit Drückler for the visit in the Kindergarten and her support regarding this publication. Thank you, Dennis Anheyer, for your input during the writing of this article and Mr. Brand for his overall support of our project.

Conflicts of Interest: The authors declare no conflict of interest. The funders had no role in the writing of the manuscript, and in the decision to publish the results.

References

1. Locher, C.; Pforr, C. The legacy of Sebastian Kneipp: Linking wellness, naturopathic, and allopathic medicine. *J. Altern. Complement. Med.* **2014**, *20*, 521–526. [CrossRef] [PubMed]
2. Vohra, S.; Surette, S.; Mittra, D.; Rosen, L.D.; Gardiner, P.; Kemper, K.J. Pediatric integrative medicine: Pediatrics' newest subspecialty? *BMC Pediatr.* **2012**, *12*, 123. [CrossRef] [PubMed]
3. McClafferty, H.; Dodds, S.; Brooks, A.J.; Brenner, M.G.; Brown, M.L.; Frazer, P.; Mark, J.D.; Weydert, J.A.; Wilcox, G.M.G.; Lebensohn, P.; et al. Pediatric Integrative Medicine in Residency (PIMR): Description of a New Online Educational Curriculum. *Children* **2015**, *2*, 98–107. [CrossRef] [PubMed]
4. Kneipp-Bund e.V. Available online: https://www.kneippbund.de/fileadmin/user_upload/kneipp-bund/dokumente/guetesiegel_zertifizierung/Richtlinien_2014/Richtlinien_Kitas_2014.pdf (accessed on 8 June 2018).
5. Scheithauer, H.; Bondü, R.; Niebank, K.; Mayer, H. Prävention von Verhaltensproblemen und Förderung prosozialen Verhaltens bei Hoch-und Niedrig-Risikokindern im Kindergarten: Erste Ergebnisse der Augsburger Längsschnittstudie zur Evaluation des Programms Papilio®(ALEPP). *Praxis der Rechtspsychologie* **2007**, *17*, 376–391.
6. Mooventhan, A.; Nivethitha, L. Scientific evidence-based effects of hydrotherapy on various systems of the body. *N. Am. J. Med. Sci.* **2014**, *6*, 199–209. [CrossRef] [PubMed]
7. Goedsche, K.; Förster, M.; Kroegel, C.; Uhlemann, C. Repeated cold water stimulations (hydrotherapy according to Kneipp) in patients with COPD. *Forsch. Komplementmed.* **2007**, *14*, 158–166. [PubMed]
8. Ring, J.; Teichmann, W. Immunological changes during hydrotherapy. *Dtsch. Med. Wochenschr.* **1977**, *102*, 1625–1630. [CrossRef] [PubMed]
9. Grüber, C.; Riesberg, A.; Mansmann, U.; Knipschild, P.; Wahn, U.; Bühring, M. The effect of hydrotherapy on the incidence of common cold episodes in children: A randomised clinical trial. *Eur. J. Pediatr.* **2003**, *162*, 168–176. [CrossRef] [PubMed]

10. Pilch, W.; Pokora, I.; Szyguła, Z.; Pałka, T.; Pilch, P.; Cisoń, T.; Malik, L.; Wiecha, S. Effect of a single finnish sauna session on white blood cell profile and cortisol levels in athletes and non-athletes. *J. Hum. Kinet* **2013**, *39*, 127–135. [CrossRef] [PubMed]
11. Werner, G.T.; Drinovac, V.; Penz, M.G. Immunologic testing on the effects of hydrotherapy according to Kneipp. *Münch. Med. Wochenschr.* **1998**, *140*, 566–569.
12. Miller, G.F.; Coffield, E.; Leroy, Z.; Wallin, R. Prevalence and Costs of Five Chronic Conditions in Children. *J. Sch. Nurs.* **2016**, *32*, 357–364. [CrossRef] [PubMed]
13. Burns, K.H.; Casey, P.H.; Lyle, R.E.; Bird, T.M.; Fussell, J.J.; Robbins, J.M. Increasing prevalence of medically complex children in US hospitals. *Pediatrics* **2010**, *126*, 638–646. [CrossRef] [PubMed]
14. Juonala, M.; Magnussen, C.G.; Berenson, G.S.; Venn, A.; Burns, T.L.; Sabin, M.A.; Srinivasan, S.R.; Daniels, S.R.; Davis, P.H.; Chen, W.; et al. Childhood adiposity, adult adiposity, and cardiovascular risk factors. *N. Engl. J. Med.* **2011**, *365*, 1876–1885. [CrossRef] [PubMed]
15. Messerli-Burgy, N.; Kakebeeke, T.H.; Arhab, A.; Stülb, K.; Zysset, A.E.; Leeger-Aschmann, C.S.; Schmutz, E.A.; Fares, F.; Meyer, A.H.; Munsch, S.; et al. The Swiss Preschoolers' health study (SPLASHY): Objectives and design of a prospective multi-site cohort study assessing psychological and physiological health in young children. *BMC Pediatr.* **2016**, *16*, 85. [CrossRef] [PubMed]
16. Perry, B.D. Why Young Children Are Curious. Available online: https://www.scholastic.com/teachers/articles/teaching-content/why-young-children-are-curious/ (accessed on 8 June 2018).
17. Kiser, B. Early child development: Body of knowledge. *Nature* **2015**, *523*, 286–289. [PubMed]

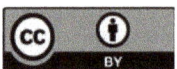

© 2018 by the authors. Licensee MDPI, Basel, Switzerland. This article is an open access article distributed under the terms and conditions of the Creative Commons Attribution (CC BY) license (http://creativecommons.org/licenses/by/4.0/).

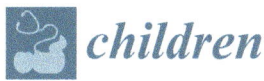

Article

Family-Based Mindful Eating Intervention in Adolescents with Obesity: A Pilot Randomized Clinical Trial

Seema Kumar [1,*], Ivana T. Croghan [2], Bridget K. Biggs [3], Katrina Croghan [4], Rose Prissel [5], Debbie Fuehrer [6], Bonnie Donelan-Dunlap [2] and Amit Sood [6]

1. Division of Pediatric Endocrinology, Department of Pediatric and Adolescent Medicine, Mayo Clinic, Rochester, MN 55905, USA
2. Primary Care Internal Medicine, Mayo Clinic, Rochester, MN 55905, USA; croghan.ivana@mayo.edu (I.T.C.); DonelanDunlap.bonnie@mayo.edu (B.D.-D.)
3. Department of Psychiatry and Psychology, Mayo Clinic, Rochester, MN 55905, USA; biggs.bridget@mayo.edu
4. Cancer Center, Mayo Clinic, Rochester, MN 55905, USA; croghan.katrina@mayo.edu
5. Endocrinology/Nutrition, Mayo Clinic, Rochester, MN 55905, USA; prissel.rose@mayo.edu
6. General Internal Medicine, Mayo Clinic, Rochester, MN 55905, USA; fuehrer.debbie@mayo.edu (D.F.); sood.amit@mayo.edu (A.S.)
* Correspondence: kumar.seema@mayo.edu; Tel.: +1-507-284-3300; Fax: +1-507-284-0727

Received: 23 May 2018; Accepted: 3 July 2018; Published: 6 July 2018

Abstract: Mindfulness has gained attention in the treatment of obesity. However, there is a paucity of data on family-based training in mindful eating in children. The objective of this pilot randomized clinical trial was to evaluate the feasibility and acceptability of a family-based mindful eating intervention (MEI) in adolescents with obesity, and to compare the efficacy of the MEI versus standard dietary counseling (SDC) for decreasing weight and improving cardiometabolic risk markers. Twenty-two adolescents (age 14.5–17.9 years) and parent pairs were randomized to the MEI or SDC. The MEI was administered in four 90-min sessions over 10 weeks and SDC was provided at baseline, 12 weeks, and 24 weeks. Despite the requirement of more frequent visits with the MEI, adolescents and parents attended 100% of the sessions and there were no dropouts in that group. High density lipoprotein (HDL) cholesterol increased in the SDC group, but not in the MEI group. Adolescents receiving the MEI demonstrated an increase in awareness at 24 weeks ($p = 0.01$) and a decrease in distraction during eating at 12 weeks ($p = 0.04$), when compared with the SDC group. The family-based MEI showed feasibility and acceptability in adolescents with obesity. Future studies with more intense therapy and larger sample sizes are warranted to examine the role of mindful eating in treating pediatric obesity.

Keywords: mindful eating; obesity; adolescents

1. Background

The problem of childhood obesity has reached epidemic proportions [1]. Currently, 18.5% of children in the United States have obesity and 6% have severe obesity [1]. Childhood obesity is associated with several adverse health consequences, including type 2 diabetes, dyslipidemia, and hypertension [2–4]. If established by adolescence, obesity, and its associated health problems, is likely to persist into adulthood [2]. While lifestyle modification is considered the cornerstone of pediatric obesity treatment, the efficacy of behavioral modification programs to address obesity through the promotion of healthier eating and an active lifestyle is modest and is limited by dropout rates of 27–73% [5–9]. Additionally, there is limited evidence for the long-term sustainability of weight loss in children with obesity [10–12]. Therefore, additional strategies are warranted to enhance the efficacy and sustainability of lifestyle modifications, including dietary habits, in the management of childhood obesity.

Mindfulness is defined as "the awareness that arises from paying attention on purpose, in the present moment and non-judgmentally" [13]. Eating behaviors play an important role in excess weight gain. Mindfulness has gained attention as an avenue for the treatment of obesity through modification of problematic eating behaviors, such as excess caloric intake in response to external cues (e.g., portion size) [14–17]. Studies investigating the effects of mindfulness on obesity-related eating behaviors have focused almost exclusively on adult samples, with only two including late-adolescent/young adult participants [15]. Several studies have demonstrated the benefits of mindfulness-based weight loss intervention for adults [18,19]. Mindfulness-based interventions have demonstrated effectiveness in improving binge eating, emotional eating, and external eating behaviors [15], as well as improving self-control [20]. Mindfulness techniques have been adapted for use with adolescents and children as young as preschool age, with at least 15 reported studies supporting their feasibility and acceptability when taught to children or to children and parents together [21,22]. The limited research suggests mindfulness can improve adolescents' self-regulation, particularly in response to stress [23]. However, there is a paucity of data on the effect of family-based mindful eating interventions (MEI) in the management of pediatric obesity or in young people's eating behaviors [24].

The objectives of this pilot randomized clinical trial were to (i) evaluate the feasibility and acceptability of a family-based MEI in adolescents with obesity and (ii) compare the efficacy of a family-based MEI versus standard dietary counseling (SDC) for decreasing weight and improving cardiometabolic risk markers in adolescents with obesity.

2. Subjects and Methods

2.1. Design Overview

This was a two-arm, parallel-group, pilot, randomized, blinded (outcome assessor and statistician), dietary counseling group controlled clinical trial in adolescents with obesity. The trial was registered on ClinicalTrials.gov (NCT01764113), and was approved by the Mayo Clinic Institutional Review Board (12-006349).

2.2. Setting and Participants

Adolescents between the ages of 14–17 years were considered eligible if their body mass index (BMI) was at or above the 95th percentile for age and gender. Age and gender-specific BMI percentiles and z-scores were calculated using the standards recommended by the Centers for Disease Control and Prevention [25].

Exclusion criteria included: (i) currently attending a supervised weight loss program; (ii) underlying genetic or endocrine cause for weight gain; (iii) type 1 or type 2 diabetes mellitus; (iv) ongoing treatment with receiving insulin, metformin, or oral hypoglycemic medications; (v) use of oral glucocorticoids in the previous two months; (vi) current cancer; (vii) established diagnosis of psychiatric illness in the previous six months; (viii) inability of the participant or parent to provide informed assent/consent or inability of the same parent to attend all of the intervention sessions and (ix) study visits along with their adolescent.

Participants were recruited from primary care practices (general pediatrics and family medicine) and pediatric specialties at the Mayo Clinic, Rochester, MN, USA.

2.3. Randomization and Interventions

Participants and one parent were randomized in a 1:1 ratio to the MEI group or SDC. Randomization was performed using a computer-generated randomization schedule. The same parent was required to attend the intervention sessions, as well as the study visits, in either group throughout the duration of the study.

Informed assent was obtained from the adolescents and informed consent was obtained from the parent who had enrolled in the study. Interventions for both the arms were group based (3–4 adolescent and parent pairs per group). The sessions in both the MEI and SDC treatment arms were conducted in an outpatient clinic setting on a weekday between 6 p.m. and 7:30 p.m. A healthy meal consisting of a sub sandwich with low fat meats and veggies with fruit, baked chips, and zero calorie lemonade was served before the meetings at 5:30 p.m.

The mindful eating program was administered over four 90-min sessions (baseline, 1 week, 6 weeks, and 10 weeks) by a team comprised of a physician and a trained mind-body therapist.

The adolescents and parents in the MEI arm attended concurrent sessions (one for adolescents and the other one for parents only) held in different rooms and met each other at the end of the session only. The program had two components: an approach toward mindfulness, and an application of the mindfulness principles to eating. The first session emphasized mindfulness and stress management strategies, including brief practices to improve attention and bring greater gratitude and compassion in life. In the next three sessions, participants learned mindful eating principles, including learning to be more cognizant of what one is eating, attuning with one's body to assess hunger and appropriate size of serving, cultivating gratitude for food and its preparers, relaxing for a moment prior to eating, paying purposeful attention to the color and aroma of food, eating slowly in small bites, enjoying each bite fully, and paying attention to the sensation of fullness from the stomach. Participants were also taught skills to avoid automatic eating, develop better self-control when offered appetitive calorie dense foods, and shopping with better awareness of the calorie density and nutritive value of foods. Each session offered a combination of a scientific perspective combined with stories and specific skills in mindfulness and mindful eating.

Adolescent/parent pairs in the SDC arm received three 90-min sessions of dietary counseling (parents and adolescents together) by a registered pediatric dietician at baseline, 12 weeks, and 24 weeks. The dietary counseling in the SDC group focused on portion control, decreasing intakes of calorie dense fast food/convenience store foods, and substituting with healthier foods consistent with routine care for youth with obesity. Throughout each session, the focus was on further educating teens and their caregiver through discussion and utilization of educational tools, such as using the provided meal to discuss portion control, satiety, energy density, and the nutrients provided in the food. In addition, using meaningful food labels, food models, and various plate, cup, and bowl sizes to engage thought provoking discussion were used along with the didactic means of educating teens and their care provider.

2.4. Outcomes and Follow Up

Participants were evaluated by study staff at baseline, 12 weeks, and 24 weeks. The primary outcomes measures were change in weight, BMI, and BMI z-score. The secondary outcomes measures were change in fasting glucose, insulin, lipids, high sensitivity C-reactive protein (hs-CRP), and domains in the mindful eating questionnaire (MEQ) and weight-efficacy lifestyle questionnaire (WEL).

Weight, height, and blood pressure were obtained at baseline, 12 weeks, and 24 weeks, and were collected by trained research assistants using standardized instruments. Blood glucose, insulin, total cholesterol, high density lipoprotein (HDL) cholesterol, triglycerides, and hs-CRP were obtained after a 10–12 h overnight fast at baseline and at 24 weeks. Plasma glucose was measured by hexokinase enzymatic assay, and serum insulin was measured using commercial electrochemiluminescence immunoassay kits. Total cholesterol, HDL cholesterol, and triglyceride levels were measured by an enzymatic calorimetric assay. Non-HDL cholesterol was calculated as total cholesterol minus HDL cholesterol. Low density lipoprotein (LDL) cholesterol was calculated using the equation: LDL = total cholesterol − HDL cholesterol − (triglycerides/5). Measurement of hs-CRP was performed using particle-enhanced immunonephelometry (Siemens Healthcare Diagnostics, Deerfield, IL, USA).

The MEQ [26] and WEL [27] were administered at baseline, 12, and 24 weeks. The MEQ is a 28-item scale designed to assess non-judgmental awareness of physical and emotional cues associated with eating. For each item, respondents rate the frequency of the listed behavior and items are scored 1–4, with 4 indicating higher mindfulness. Resulting scores include a summary score and five subscales: disinhibition, awareness, external cues, emotional response, and distraction. The WEL is a 20-item eating self-efficacy scale consisting of a total score and five situational factors: negative emotions, availability, social pressure, physical discomfort, and positive activities. For each item, respondents rate their level of confidence in their ability to resist eating in the given situation on a 10-point scale, from 0—"not confident", to 9—"very confident".

2.5. Sample Size Calculation and Statistical Analysis

A priori power analysis conducted using G*Power 3 [28] indicated that a sample size of 40 participants (20 for each arm) would be required to detect the medium to large effect sizes observed in similar previous research assuming 0.80 power with a two-tailed test and α set at 0.05. Since the trial was of a pilot nature and the primary aim was to examine the feasibility and acceptability of the MEI, recruitment was discontinued at the end of the trial despite a total enrollment of only 22 participants.

Continuous variables were summarized with mean ± standard deviation (SD), or median and interquartile range (IQR), as appropriate. Categorical variables were summarized as a frequency and percentage. Differences between time points were assessed within each study group with Wilcoxon signed-rank tests, and the paired differences were compared between study groups with Wilcoxon rank-sum tests. p-Values less than 0.05 were considered statistically significant. All analyses were performed using SAS version 9.3 (SAS Institute Inc., Cary, NC, USA) [29]. Subgroup analyses were not performed due to the small sample size.

3. Results

A total of 22 adolescents (age range 14.5–17.9 years) were enrolled in the study (Figure 1). Out of 45 adolescents that were called in and prescreened for the study, 31 passed the phone screen and 14 did not meet the study criteria (Figure 1). Twenty-nine adolescents consented to the study and two declined. Seven out of the 29 consented adolescents withdrew consent and; therefore, 22 adolescents were randomized to either of the study arms (11 in each group). The study was conducted between 7 December 2012 and 19 December 2013. The interventions were conducted at two different times of the year due to the convenience in the recruitment timing. The first group of 14 participants (8 males, 6 females) began intervention in winter (February 2013) and these were equally divided between the MEI and SDC (7 in each group). The remaining 8 patients (4 males, 4 females) began receiving the intervention in June 2013 and these were also equally split between the two intervention groups (4 in each group).

Anthropometric and laboratory characteristics of the participants are detailed in Table 1.

Age, gender, and race were not different between the two groups ($p > 0.05$). The median age (quartile, Q1, Q3) was 15.6 (15.2, 16.8) years in the SDC group and 17.1 (15.5, 17.4) years in the MEI group. There were 12 male and 10 female participants, with 7/11 (63.6%) participants in the SDC group (63.6%) and 5/11 (45.5%) participants in the MEI group were male. Nineteen out of 22 participants were white and three were non-white (one in the SDC group and two in the MEI group).

Baseline BMI was not significantly different between the two groups (median (Q1, Q3): 32.9 (30.9, 36.2) kg/m^2 and 34.9 (32, 36.6) kg/m^2 in the SDC and MEI group, respectively; $p > 0.05$). Baseline BMI z-score also was not different between the two groups (median (Q1, Q3): 2.4 (1.9, 3.2) and 2.5 (2.3, 3.0) in the SDC and MEI group, respectively; $p > 0.05$). There were no differences in the laboratory parameters between the two groups ($p > 0.05$, Table 1).

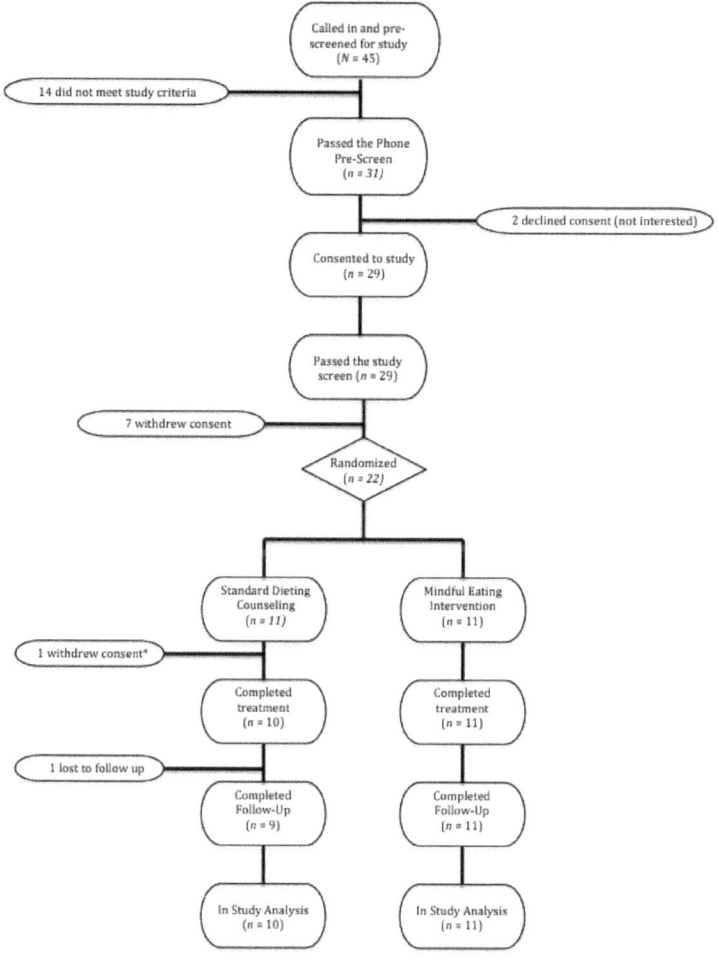

Figure 1. Study flow.

Table 1. Anthropometric and laboratory characteristics of study participants.

	Standard Dietary Counseling (n = 11)		Mindful Eating Intervention (n = 11)		Difference between the Two Arms
	Median	Q1, Q3	Median	Q1, Q3	p-Value
Age (years)	15.6	15.2, 16.8	17.1	15.5, 17.4	NS
Weight (kg)	103.7	87, 123	98.7	95.9, 106.4	NS
BMI (kg/m^2)	32.9	30.9, 36.2	34.9	32, 36.6	NS
BMI z-score	2.4	1.9, 3.2	2.5	2.3, 3.0	NS
Glucose (mg/dL)	88	81, 96	92	88, 99	NS
Insulin (mcIU/mL)	21.8	17.7, 24.5	29.3	15.6, 35.1	NS
Total cholesterol (mg/dL)	176	133, 183	144	124, 180	NS
HDL cholesterol (mg/dL)	41	33, 53	35	31, 48	NS
LDL cholesterol (mg/dL)	101	69, 106	81	77, 112	NS
Non-HDL cholesterol (mg/dL)	126	91, 146	108	93, 132	NS
Triglycerides (mg/dL)	174	81, 219	104	80, 134	NS
hs-CRP (mg/L)	1.7	0.5, 4.3	3.2	0.4, 5.7	NS

NS, $p > 0.05$. BMI, body mass index; HDL, high density lipoprotein; LDL, low density lipoprotein; hs-CRP, high sensitivity C-reactive protein; Q, quartile.

All 11 adolescent and parents in the MEI group attended all four intervention sessions, as well as the study visits, at 12 weeks and 24 weeks. Therefore, there were no drop outs in the MEI group. One participant in the SDC group dropped out after the first session and did not return for the 12-week or 24-week visit. Data from 10 participants in the SDC group and from 11 participants in the MEI group were included in the analysis.

Body mass index and BMI z-score in the MEI group were higher at 12 weeks and 24 weeks ($p < 0.05$) relative to baseline (Table 2). Body mass index and BMI z-scores in the SDC group were higher ($p < 0.05$) at 24 weeks compared to baseline (Table 2). However, there were no significant differences in the change in weight, BMI, and BMI z-score from baseline to 12-week or 24-week time points between the two groups ($p > 0.05$ for all, Table 2).

Table 2. Change in anthropometric and laboratory measures during follow up.

Parameter	Time	Standard Dietary Counseling (n = 10)		Mindful Eating Intervention (n = 11)		Difference between the Two Groups
		Median	Q1, Q3	Median	Q1, Q3	p-Value
Weight (kg)	Week 12	−0.1	−1.4, 1.2	2.3	−0.7, 3.2	NS
	Week 24	2.5	1.5, 3.3	4.0	−0.2, 5.2	NS
BMI (kg/m²)	Week 12	−0.3	−0.9, −0.1	0.6	−0.2, 1.2	NS
	Week 24	1	0.4, 1.1	0.9	0.2, 2.3	NS
BMI z-score	Week 12	−0.1	−0.2, 0	0.1	0, 0.2	NS
	Week 24	0.2	0.1, 0.2	0.2	0, 0.4	NS
Glucose (mg/dL)	Week 24	2	−3, 6	−4	−8, 6	NS
Insulin (mcIU/mL)	Week 24	3.5	1.4, 6.6	0.3	−4.5, 4.8	NS
Total cholesterol (mg/dL)	Week 24	14	4, 24	3	−11, 28	NS
LDL cholesterol (mg/dL)	Week 24	1	−7, 12	8	−11, 20	NS
HDL cholesterol (mg/dL)	Week 24	7	2, 10	−1	−2, 3	0.0245
Triglycerides (mg/dL)	Week 24	9	2, 27	7	−8, 24	NS
hs-CRP (mg/L)	Week 24	0.3	0.2, 0.4	0.2	−1.4, 1.2	NS

NS, $p > 0.05$.

There was a statistically significant difference in the δ HDL cholesterol between the SDC and MEI groups, with HDL cholesterol increasing in the SDC group (median (Q1, Q3): 7 (2, 10) mg/dL), but not in the MEI group ((−1 (−2, 3) mg/dL); $p = 0.0245$). There was no difference in changes in other laboratory measures between the two groups.

No adverse side effects were reported by study participants in either of the groups.

Adolescents in the MEI group demonstrated an increase in awareness at 24 weeks and a decrease in distraction during eating at 12 weeks relative to the SDC group ($p = 0.01$ and $p = 0.04$, respectively, Table 3).

Table 3. Changes in mindful eating questionnaire (MEQ) and weight-efficiency lifestyle questionnaire (WEL) domains.

	Standard Dietary Counseling (SDC) (n = 10)			Mindless Eating Intervention (MEI) (n = 11)		
	Baseline [a]	Week 12 [a]	Week 24 [a]	Baseline [a]	Week 12 [a]	Week 24 [a]
Mindful eating questionnaire						
Awareness	2.5 (0.6)	2.5 (0.7)	2.4 (0.7)	2.1 (0.5)	2.4 (0.4)	2.5 (0.5) *
Disinhibition	2.7 (0.7)	2.7 (0.6)	2.6 (0.8)	3.0 (0.4)	2.9 (0.3)	2.9 (0.4)
Distraction	3.7 (0.3)	3.6 (0.3)	3.7 (0.5)	3.8 (0.2)	3.4 (0.4) **	3.6 (0.4)
Emotional	2.6 (0.3)	3.1 (0.4)	2.9 (0.3)	2.9 (0.4)	2.8 (0.5)	2.9 (0.3)
Weight efficacy lifestyle questionnaire						
Total score	6.2 (2.0)	6.5 (1.9)	6.5 (2.0)	7.0 (1.2)	6.5 (1.2)	7.0 (1.1)
Negative emotions	6.5 (2.5)	6.4 (2.8)	6.9 (2.4)	6.8 (2.2)	6.7 (1.7)	7.0 (1.6)
Availability	5.2 (2.2)	5.7 (2.3)	5.6 (2.2)	5.9 (1.5)	5.4 (1.9)	6.1 (1.4)
Social pressure	5.8 (2.7)	6.3 (2.4)	5.7 (2.0)	7.0 (1.2)	6.2 (1.7)	6.8 (1.5)
Physical discomfort	6.9 (1.8)	7.3 (1.6)	7.4 (1.9)	7.7 (1.2)	7.3 (1.3)	7.7 (1.4)
Positive activities	6.7 (1.8)	7.0 (1.7)	6.8 (2.1)	7.4 (1.1)	7.0 (0.8)	(0.9)

[a] Data are presented as mean ± SD (standard deviation); difference between MEI and SDC groups with regards to change from baseline: * MEQ awareness (week 24-baseline difference), $p = 0.01$; ** MEQ distraction (week 12-baseline difference), $p = 0.04$.

4. Discussion

We demonstrate the feasibility and acceptability of a family-based mindful eating intervention in adolescents with obesity. To our knowledge, this is the first randomized clinical trial to test the feasibility, acceptability, and short term weight loss efficacy of a family-based mindful eating intervention in adolescents with obesity.

Despite the need for four 90-min sessions for adolescents and their parents over a period of 10 weeks, we noted 100% attendance in the four training sessions by adolescents and their parents. In addition, all participants in the MEI group returned for assessments at 12 weeks and 24 weeks. This level of attendance in the intervention sessions and retention over the 24-week period is remarkable given reported dropout rates in behavioral treatments for pediatric obesity [9], and the scant data on the feasibility and acceptability of a mindful eating-based intervention in children and adolescents with obesity [30]. In contrast to our findings, Daly and colleagues reported only 57% retention in a randomized feasibility study aimed at weight loss in adolescent Latino females [30]. The mindful eating intervention in that study was administered to adolescents recruited in a public high school in southwestern United States and was not delivered to parents. The differences in retention rates may be related to differences in the ethnicity and gender distribution of participants as the majority of our study participants were white, and males comprised more than half of our study population. Additionally, there were several differences in the specifics of the mindful eating intervention, such as the frequency of the intervention sessions (90-min session every week for six weeks in the study by Daly versus four 90-min sessions over a period of 10 weeks in our study), time of the day (afterschool setting versus evening time in our study), and setting (classroom versus outpatient clinic in our study). The mindful eating intervention in our study, on the other hand, was conducted in the late evening with an evening meal provided to all participants and their parents. Finally, involvement of the family, as was required in our study, could have also contributed to a greater retention. Our finding of a higher retention in the MEI group is all the more remarkable in view of the longer follow up period in our study (24 weeks versus 10 weeks in the study by Daly and colleagues [30]).

The MEI was not efficacious in decreasing BMI or BMI z-score at 12 weeks or 24 weeks in our study. Participants in both groups had an increase in BMI and BMI z-scores at 24 weeks. These findings are not surprising given the modest efficacy of behavior modifications on severity of adiposity [31]. Similar to our study, overweight/obese adolescent females in another study by Shomaker and colleagues also exhibited an increase in BMI despite receiving mindfulness-based group intervention [32]. In contrast, a 1.4 kg/m^2 decrease in BMI was noted at 10 weeks in Latino adolescent females receiving MEI, but no subsequent BMI measurements were available at 24 weeks in their study [30]. The greater frequency of MEI in the study in Latino adolescent females (six weekly 90-min sessions) compared to our study (four 90-min sessions over a period of 10 weeks) may partly account for differences in the effects on BMI. Mindful eating-based interventions have been shown to result in weight loss among children with Prader-Willi syndrome [33–35]. Several studies in adults have also demonstrated modest benefits in adults [18,19,36], with a mean weight loss of 4 kg and a mean decrease in BMI of 1.3 kg/m^2 in one study [19]. The lack of improvement in weight or BMI in the participants in our MEI or SDS groups may be due to the low intensity of the intervention, with only 6 h of contact over a period of six months, despite the most recent The United States Preventive Task Force guidelines recommending >26 h "over a period of 2–12 months" [37]. It remains unknown if an addition of a greater number of hours of mindfulness-based intervention would lead to an improvement in outcomes of adolescents with obesity.

We noted improvements in awareness and in reduced distraction during eating among the adolescents receiving the mindful eating intervention. No differences in mindfulness awareness were noted in adolescent Latino females receiving a mindful eating intervention [30]. Unfortunately, changes in these domains did not result in an improved weight status during the study period. The inclusion of dietary assessments in future studies would further the understanding of whether changes in these mindful eating domains translate into changes in dietary quality or caloric intake that could, over time, lead to changes in weight status.

The strengths of our study include the randomized clinical trial design with the presence of a control group receiving standard dietary counseling on a low fat, portion controlled dietary plan. We had excellent retention with follow up on all but one out of the 22 participants at six months from the time of enrollment.

The most significant limitation of our study is its pilot nature and small sample size. The study was underpowered to determine the efficacy of the MEI on weight and cardiometabolic risk factors in adolescents with obesity. Another limitation was the low intensity of the intervention, with the total number of hours of contact of 6 h being significantly below the >26 h "over a period of 2–12 months" recently recommended by national experts [37]. The duration of follow up was short and, therefore, outcomes beyond six months could not be assessed. Other important limitations were the lack of information regarding pubertal staging and body composition, and lack of data on disordered eating patterns, such as binge eating and emotional eating, as well as on quality/quantity of dietary intake and physical activity. Finally, the study findings cannot be generalized due to a lack of ethnic and racial diversity among the participants.

5. Conclusions

A family-based mindful eating intervention was found to be feasible and acceptable in adolescents with obesity. No beneficial changes in weight, BMI, or any of the cardiometabolic risk factors were observed. Further studies with a greater intensity of interventions and larger sample size are warranted to examine the role of mindful eating interventions in the treatment of childhood obesity.

Author Contributions: Conceptualization, S.K. and A.S.; Methodology, S.K., A.S., I.T.C., B.K.B., R.P. and A.S.; Validation, S.K., I.T.C. and A.S.; Formal Analysis, S.K., A.S. and I.T.C.; Investigation, S.K., K.C., and A.S.; Resources, I.T.C., A.S. and S.K.; Writing-Original Draft Preparation, S.K.; Writing-Review & Editing, S.K., I.T.C., B.K.B., A.S., K.C., D.F., B.D.-D. and R.P.; Supervision, I.T.C. and A.S.; Project Administration, I.T.C., K.C., R.P., D.F., B.D.-D.; Funding Acquisition, S.K. and A.S.

Funding: The funding for the study was provided by the Sanford T. Denny Sanford Pediatric Collaborative Research Fund.

Conflicts of Interest: Amit Sood is the owner of Global Center for Resiliency and Wellbeing. None of the other authors have any conflict of interest to disclose.

References

1. Skinner, A.C.; Ravanbakht, S.N.; Skelton, J.A.; Perrin, E.M.; Armstrong, S.C. Prevalence of obesity and severe obesity in us children, 1999–2016. *Pediatrics* **2018**. [CrossRef] [PubMed]
2. Kelly, A.S.; Barlow, S.E.; Rao, G.; Inge, T.H.; Hayman, L.L.; Steinberger, J.; Urbina, E.M.; Ewing, L.J.; Daniels, S.R. Severe obesity in children and adolescents: Identification, associated health risks, and treatment approaches: A scientific statement from the american heart association. *Circulation* **2013**, *128*, 1689–1712. [CrossRef] [PubMed]
3. Weiss, R.; Dziura, J.; Burgert, T.S.; Tamborlane, W.V.; Taksali, S.E.; Yeckel, C.W.; Allen, K.; Lopes, M.; Savoye, M.; Morrison, J.; et al. Obesity and the metabolic syndrome in children and adolescents. *N. Engl. J. Med.* **2004**, *350*, 2362–2374. [CrossRef] [PubMed]
4. Skinner, A.C.; Perrin, E.M.; Moss, L.A.; Skelton, J.A. Cardiometabolic risks and severity of obesity in children and young adults. *N. Engl. J. Med.* **2015**, *373*, 1307–1317. [CrossRef] [PubMed]
5. Barlow, S.E. Expert committee recommendations regarding the prevention, assessment, and treatment of child and adolescent overweight and obesity: Summary report. *Pediatrics* **2007**, *120*, S164–S192. [CrossRef] [PubMed]
6. Epstein, L.H.; Valoski, A.M.; Vara, L.S.; McCurley, J.; Wisniewski, L.; Kalarchian, M.A.; Klein, K.R.; Shrager, L.R. Effects of decreasing sedentary behavior and increasing activity on weight change in obese children. *Health Psychol.* **1995**, *14*, 109–115. [CrossRef] [PubMed]

7. Whitlock, E.P.; O'Connor, E.A.; Williams, S.B.; Beil, T.L.; Lutz, K.W. Effectiveness of weight management interventions in children: A targeted systematic review for the uspstf. *Pediatrics* **2010**, *125*, e396–e418. [CrossRef] [PubMed]
8. Ho, M.; Garnett, S.P.; Baur, L.; Burrows, T.; Stewart, L.; Neve, M.; Collins, C. Effectiveness of lifestyle interventions in child obesity: Systematic review with meta-analysis. *Pediatrics* **2012**, *130*, e1647–e1671. [CrossRef] [PubMed]
9. Skelton, J.A.; Beech, B.M. Attrition in paediatric weight management: A review of the literature and new directions. *Obes. Rev.* **2011**, *12*, e273–e281. [CrossRef] [PubMed]
10. Butryn, M.L.; Wadden, T.A.; Rukstalis, M.R.; Bishop-Gilyard, C.; Xanthopoulos, M.S.; Louden, D.; Berkowitz, R.I. Maintenance of weight loss in adolescents: Current status and future directions. *J. Obes.* **2010**, *2010*, 789280. [CrossRef] [PubMed]
11. Nguyen, B.; Shrewsbury, V.A.; O'Connor, J.; Steinbeck, K.S.; Lee, A.; Hill, A.J.; Shah, S.; Kohn, M.R.; Torvaldsen, S.; Baur, L.A. Twelve-month outcomes of the loozit randomized controlled trial: A community-based healthy lifestyle program for overweight and obese adolescents. *Arch. Pediatr. Adolesc. Med.* **2012**, *166*, 170–177. [CrossRef] [PubMed]
12. Mameli, C.; Krakauer, J.C.; Krakauer, N.Y.; Bosetti, A.; Ferrari, C.M.; Schneider, L.; Borsani, B.; Arrigoni, S.; Pendezza, E.; Zuccotti, G.V. Effects of a multidisciplinary weight loss intervention in overweight and obese children and adolescents: 11 years of experience. *PLoS ONE* **2017**, *12*, e0181095. [CrossRef] [PubMed]
13. Paulson, S.; Davidson, R.; Jha, A.; Kabat-Zinn, J. Becoming conscious: The science of mindfulness. *Ann. N. Y. Acad. Sci.* **2013**, *1303*, 87–104. [CrossRef] [PubMed]
14. Godsey, J. The role of mindfulness-based interventions in the treatment of obesity and eating disorders: An integrative review. *Complement. Ther. Med.* **2013**, *21*, 430–439. [CrossRef] [PubMed]
15. O'Reilly, G.A.; Cook, L.; Spruijt-Metz, D.; Black, D.S. Mindfulness-based interventions for obesity-related eating behaviours: A literature review. *Obes. Rev.* **2014**, *15*, 453–461. [CrossRef] [PubMed]
16. Sojcher, R.; Gould Fogerite, S.; Perlman, A. Evidence and potential mechanisms for mindfulness practices and energy psychology for obesity and binge-eating disorder. *Explore* **2012**, *8*, 271–276. [CrossRef] [PubMed]
17. Dunn, C.; Haubenreiser, M.; Johnson, M.; Nordby, K.; Aggarwal, S.; Myer, S.; Thomas, C. Mindfulness approaches and weight loss, weight maintenance, and weight regain. *Curr. Obes. Rep.* **2018**, *7*, 37–49. [CrossRef] [PubMed]
18. Tapper, K.; Shaw, C.; Ilsley, J.; Hill, A.J.; Bond, F.W.; Moore, L. Exploratory randomised controlled trial of a mindfulness-based weight loss intervention for women. *Appetite* **2009**, *52*, 396–404. [CrossRef] [PubMed]
19. Dalen, J.; Smith, B.W.; Shelley, B.M.; Sloan, A.L.; Leahigh, L.; Begay, D. Pilot study: Mindful eating and living (meal): Weight, eating behavior, and psychological outcomes associated with a mindfulness-based intervention for people with obesity. *Complement. Ther. Med.* **2010**, *18*, 260–264. [CrossRef] [PubMed]
20. Hendrickson, K.L.; Rasmussen, E.B. Effects of mindful eating training on delay and probability discounting for food and money in obese and healthy-weight individuals. *Behav. Res. Ther.* **2013**, *51*, 399–409. [CrossRef] [PubMed]
21. Black, D.S.; Fernando, R. Mindfulness training and classroom behavior among lower-income and ethnic minority elementary school children. *J. Child Fam. Stud.* **2014**, *23*, 1242–1246. [CrossRef] [PubMed]
22. Black, D.S.; Milam, J.; Sussman, S. Sitting-meditation interventions among youth: A review of treatment efficacy. *Pediatrics* **2009**, *124*, e532–e541. [CrossRef] [PubMed]
23. Adams, C.E.; McVay, M.A.; Kinsaul, J.; Benitez, L.; Vinci, C.; Stewart, D.W.; Copeland, A.L. Unique relationships between facets of mindfulness and eating pathology among female smokers. *Eat* **2012**, *13*, 390–393. [CrossRef] [PubMed]
24. Dalen, J.; Brody, J.L.; Staples, J.K.; Sedillo, D. A conceptual framework for the expansion of behavioral interventions for youth obesity: A family-based mindful eating approach. *Child. Obes.* **2015**, *11*, 577–584. [CrossRef] [PubMed]
25. Kuczmarski, R.J.; Ogden, C.L.; Guo, S.S.; Grummer-Strawn, L.M.; Flegal, K.M.; Mei, Z.; Wei, R.; Curtin, L.R.; Roche, A.F.; Johnson, C.L. 2000 CDC growth charts for the united states: Methods and development. *Vital Health Stat.* **2002**, *11*, 1–190.
26. Framson, C.; Kristal, A.R.; Schenk, J.M.; Littman, A.J.; Zeliadt, S.; Benitez, D. Development and validation of the mindful eating questionnaire. *J. Am. Diet. Assoc.* **2009**, *109*, 1439–1444. [CrossRef] [PubMed]

27. Clark, M.M.; Abrams, D.B.; Niaura, R.S.; Eaton, C.A.; Rossi, J.S. Self-efficacy in weight management. *J. Consult. Clin. Psychol.* **1991**, *59*, 739–744. [CrossRef] [PubMed]
28. Faul, F.; Erdfelder, E.; Lang, A.-G.; Buchner, A. G*Power 3: A flexible statistical power analysis program for the social, behavioral, and biomedical sciences. *Behav. Res. Methods* **2007**, *39*, 175–191. [CrossRef] [PubMed]
29. SAS Institute Inc. *Sas/Stat User's Guide—Version 9.4*; SAS Institute: Cary, NC, USA, 2017.
30. Daly, P.; Pace, T.; Berg, J.; Menon, U.; Szalacha, L.A. A mindful eating intervention: A theory-guided randomized anti-obesity feasibility study with adolescent latino females. *Complement. Ther. Med.* **2016**, *28*, 22–28. [CrossRef] [PubMed]
31. McGovern, L.; Johnson, J.N.; Paulo, R.; Hettinger, A.; Singhal, V.; Kamath, C.; Erwin, P.J.; Montori, V.M. Clinical review: Treatment of pediatric obesity: A systematic review and meta-analysis of randomized trials. *J. Clin. Endocrinol. Metab.* **2008**, *93*, 4600–4605. [CrossRef] [PubMed]
32. Shomaker, L.B.; Bruggink, S.; Pivarunas, B.; Skoranski, A.; Foss, J.; Chaffin, E.; Dalager, S.; Annameier, S.; Quaglia, J.; Brown, K.W.; et al. Pilot randomized controlled trial of a mindfulness-based group intervention in adolescent girls at risk for type 2 diabetes with depressive symptoms. *Complement. Ther. Med.* **2017**, *32*, 66–74. [CrossRef] [PubMed]
33. Singh, N.N.; Lancioni, G.E.; Singh, A.N.; Winton, A.S.; Singh, A.D.; Singh, J. A mindfulness-based health wellness program for individuals with Prader-Willi syndrome. *J. Ment. Health Res. Intellect. Disabil.* **2011**, *4*, 90–106. [CrossRef]
34. Singh, N.N.; Lancioni, G.E.; Singh, A.N.; Winton, A.S.; Singh, J.; McAleavey, K.M.; Adkins, A.D. A mindfulness-based health wellness program for an adolescent with Prader-Willi syndrome. *Behav. Modif.* **2008**, *32*, 167–181. [CrossRef] [PubMed]
35. Singh, N.N.; Lancioni, G.E.; Singh, A.N.; Winton, A.S.; Singh, J.; McAleavey, K.M.; Adkins, A.D.; Joy, S.D. A mindfulness-based health wellness program for managing morbid obesity. *Clin. Case Stud.* **2008**, *7*, 327–339. [CrossRef]
36. Lillis, J.; Hayes, S.C.; Bunting, K.; Masuda, A. Teaching acceptance and mindfulness to improve the lives of the obese: A preliminary test of a theoretical model. *Ann. Behav. Med.* **2009**, *37*, 58–69. [CrossRef] [PubMed]
37. Force, U.S.P.S.T.; Grossman, D.C.; Bibbins-Domingo, K.; Curry, S.J.; Barry, M.J.; Davidson, K.W.; Doubeni, C.A.; Epling, J.W., Jr.; Kemper, A.R.; Krist, A.H.; et al. Screening for obesity in children and adolescents: US preventive services task force recommendation statement. *JAMA* **2017**, *317*, 2417–2426.

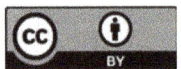

© 2018 by the authors. Licensee MDPI, Basel, Switzerland. This article is an open access article distributed under the terms and conditions of the Creative Commons Attribution (CC BY) license (http://creativecommons.org/licenses/by/4.0/).

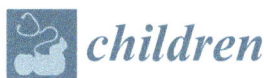

Article

Can the Mindful Awareness and Resilience Skills for Adolescents (MARS-A) Program Be Provided Online? Voices from the Youth

Nicholas Chadi [1,*], Elli Weisbaum [2], Catherine Malboeuf-Hurtubise [3], Sara Ahola Kohut [4], Christine Viner [5], Miriam Kaufman [6], Jake Locke [7] and Dzung X. Vo [8]

1. Department of Pediatrics, Boston Children's Hospital, Harvard Medical School, 300 Longwood Avenue, Boston, MA 02115, USA
2. Institute of Medical Sciences, University of Toronto, 1 King's College Circle, Room 2374, Toronto, ON M5S 1A8, Canada; elliweisbaum@gmail.com
3. Department of Psychology, Bishop's University, 2600 College Street, Sherbrooke, QC J1M 1Z7, Canada; catherine.malboeuf.hurtubise@gmail.com
4. Department of Psychiatry, Hospital for Sick Children, University of Toronto, 555 University Avenue, Toronto, ON M5G 1X8, Canada; sara.aholakohut@sickkids.ca
5. Department of Pediatrics, Downstate Medical Center, State University of New York, 450 Clarkson Ave, Brooklyn, NY 11203, USA; christine.viner@gmail.com
6. Division of Adolescent Medicine, Department of Pediatrics, Hospital for Sick Children, University of Toronto, 555 University Avenue, Toronto, ON M5G 1X8, Canada; meejum1@icloud.com
7. Department of Child and Adolescent Psychiatry, British Columbia Children's Hospital, University of British Columbia, Vancouver, BCV6H 3N1, Canada; jlocke@cw.bc.ca
8. Division of Adolescent Health and Medicine, Department of Pediatrics, BC Children's Hospital, University of British Columbia, 4480 Oak St, Vancouver, BC V6H 3N1, Canada; dvo@cw.bc.ca
* Correspondence: nicholas.chadi@childrens.harvard.edu; Tel.: +1-617-919-6367

Received: 27 July 2018; Accepted: 23 August 2018; Published: 28 August 2018

Abstract: Mindfulness-based interventions (MBIs) have been shown to improve health and well-being in adolescents with chronic illnesses. Because they are most often delivered in person in a group setting, there are several barriers that limit access to MBIs for youth with limited mobility or who cannot access in-person MBIs in their communities. The objective of this study was to determine if eHealth is a viable platform to increase accessibility to MBIs for teens with chronic illnesses. This study reports the qualitative results of a mixed method randomized trial describing the experience of the Mindful Awareness and Resilience Skills for Adolescents (MARS-A) program, an eight-week MBI, delivered either in person or via eHealth. Participants were adolescents between the ages of 13 and 18 with a chronic illness recruited at a tertiary pediatric hospital in Toronto, Canada. Individual semi-structured post-participation audio-video interviews were conducted by a research assistant. A multiple-pass inductive process was used to review interview transcripts and interpret emergent themes from the participants' lived experiences. Fifteen participants (8 online and 7 in person) completed post-participation interviews. Four distinct themes emerged from participants in both groups: Creation of a safe space, fostering peer support and connection, integration of mindfulness skills into daily life, and improved well-being through the application of mindfulness. Direct quotations representative of those four themes are reported. Results from this study suggest that eHealth delivery of an adapted MBI for adolescents with chronic illnesses may be an acceptable and feasible mode of delivery for MBIs in this population. EHealth should be considered in future studies of MBIs for adolescents with chronic illnesses as a promising avenue to increase access to MBIs for youth who might not be able to access in-person programs.

Keywords: qualitative; mindfulness; meditation; chronic illness; adolescents; eHealth

1. Introduction

Adolescents with chronic illnesses face unique challenges that can have significant impacts on their development and well-being [1]. Adolescence is a period that typically involves the acquisition of independence and of a personal and social identity [2]. Managing a chronic illness and its associated appointments, procedures, and medications can disrupt this process [3]. Chronic health conditions (whether visible or not) can also cause emotional challenges and significant coping difficulties [4].

Mindfulness has been defined as "paying attention in a particular way: On purpose, in the present moment, and nonjudgmentally" [5]. Historically rooted in Eastern Buddhist and other contemplative traditions, mindfulness has recently gained popularity in both education and healthcare settings to promote health and well-being among adolescent populations [6]. In addition, mindfulness-based interventions (MBIs) for adolescents have been shown to have benefits on mood, stress, sleep, pain control, and concentration among many others in both clinical and non-clinical samples [7,8]. Emerging research has looked specifically at the feasibility and effectiveness of adapted MBIs for adolescents with chronic illnesses [9]. A randomized study conducted in 72 youth HIV-infected youth aged 14–22 who received an MBI or an active control intervention showed that mindfulness improved life satisfaction and cognitive accuracy in the context of negative emotion stimuli [10]. Another study conducted in 18 adolescents with functional somatic syndromes showed the high feasibility of an MBI and significant improvements in anxiety symptoms and level of functioning [11]. Finally, a number of small studies have shown that MBIs are well-received by adolescents with cancer and chronic pain conditions [12–16].

Despite these promising results, researchers have identified multiple barriers to implementation and dissemination of MBIs with adolescents with chronic illnesses. One barrier is that MBIs have traditionally been delivered in person in group settings [9]. This can pose a challenge for adolescents with mobility limitations, living in remote areas, or with limited access to transportation. Research conducted in adults has shown promise in the eHealth delivery of MBIs via online apps, web-based platforms, or hybrid modes of delivery [17–20]. To our knowledge, in-person and eHealth real-time group moderated MBIs have not been compared head-to-head in teens with chronic illnesses. Demonstrating the effectiveness of this new mode of delivery could have important implications to increase access to MBIs and potentially save costs of delivering this type of programming.

Studies conducted with adolescents have described the experience of participating in an MBI adapted for youth [21,22]. Qualitative data have revealed a number of benefits, including reduction of daily stressors and transformational shifts in life orientation and well-being [23]. It has been suggested that the incorporation of mindfulness practice in daily life demonstrates effective transmission of mindfulness skills to adolescents [24]. In this paper, we aim to describe the experience of adolescents with chronic illnesses receiving an MBI either in person or online. The overarching research question for this study was to determine if eHealth is a viable platform for teens with chronic illnesses. We hypothesized that eHealth would be an acceptable and feasible modality for the delivery of an adapted MBI in this population.

2. Materials and Methods

This paper will focus on the qualitative portion of a randomized mixed methods trial comparing the in-person and eHealth delivery of an adapted MBI for adolescents with chronic illnesses. All participants were included in both qualitative and quantitative analyses. Quantitative analyses sought to compare the acquisition of mindfulness skills and changes in mental health scores using standardized research questionnaires, changes in pre- and post-mindfulness salivary cortisol levels, and tracking of individual home practice between groups. The full description of the study protocol, including both qualitative and quantitative methods, has been published previously [25], and quantitative data will be reported separately. This study was a registered trial (ClinicalTrials.org: NCT03067207). All subjects gave their informed consent for inclusion before they participated in the study. The study was conducted in accordance with the Declaration of Helsinki, and the protocol was approved by the Ethics Committee of the Hospital for Sick Children in Toronto (project identification number: 1000053600).

Given our study's mixed methods design and to allow more flexibility in interpretation of the data, we decided to use a generic qualitative approach, combining elements of qualitative description [26] and interpretive description [27], rather than being guided by an explicit set of philosophical assumptions from an established qualitative methodology [28,29]. For our analysis of the in-depth interviews, we were guided by an interpretive lens, allowing concepts to emerge from the lived experiences of the participants, rather than from our own preconceived notions [30].

Participants were adolescents aged between 13 and 18 recruited from different subspecialty clinics in a tertiary pediatric hospital in Toronto, Canada. Participants were eligible to participate if they lived close enough to attend weekly in-person sessions. They needed to have a diagnosis of a medical or mental health condition requiring ongoing medical care, which included at least one physical symptom, such as chronic pain or headaches. Potential participants were referred by one of their health providers and later contacted by a research assistant (CV) who invited them to a recruitment meeting where the details of the study were explained and written informed consent was obtained from the teen and parent/guardian. Interested participants were then randomized and allocated to an in-person or eHealth group. In total, 58 participants were assessed for eligibility, 40 were excluded for not meeting inclusion criteria, for declining to participate, or for other reasons, including living too far and only being interested in the eHealth arm of the study. Eighteen participants were randomized (9 per group) and 14 (7 in each group) completed the MBI and post-participation interview. Two participants who had not completed the MBI, but had attended at least two mindfulness sessions (both in the eHealth group), were invited to participate in a post-participation interview, and one of them accepted.

Both groups received an eight-week evidence-informed MBI, the Mindful Awareness and Resilience Skills for Adolescents [31] (MARS-A) program, delivered either via eHealth, through a secure online platform allowing audio-visual group interactions in real time (Zoom Video Conferencing—Zoom Video Communications Inc., San Jose, CA, USA), or in person at the hospital. MARS-A sessions are 90 min in length, and the curriculum and facilitation are adapted for adolescents from eight-week evidence-based adult MBI's, including Mindfulness-Based Stress Reduction [32,33] and Mindfulness-Based Cognitive Therapy [34,35]. Each week, a different theme is explored, including introduction to mindfulness, informal mindfulness practice and gratitude, handling difficult emotions, and how best to take care of oneself. A more detailed thematic overview of the program can be found elsewhere [25,36]. Adaptations from adult MBIs include shorter sessions (90 min instead of 150 min), discussions focused on the challenges of coping with mental and physical illness in adolescence, and shorter group and home mindfulness practices. In-session activities included interactive group discussions related to weekly themes, mindfulness practices (i.e., sitting/breathing meditation, mindful movement, body scan, mindful eating, mindful listening), and review/inquiry of individual home practice. In-person and online groups were facilitated by co-authors, NC and EW, who both had extensive experience in MBIs for youth, were formally trained in teaching MARS-A, and had a long-standing personal mindfulness practice.

All participants took part in individual post-participation interviews through the same password-protected video conferencing platform used for the delivery of the MBI to the participants of the eHealth group. The video conferencing platform was chosen over phone or in-person interviews, since all participants, even participants in the in-person group, had been introduced to the platform at the time of enrollment. It was felt that this platform would allow a deeper connection with the interviewer than a phone interview and avoided the need for transportation for participants in the eHealth group. Interviews (average length 14 min, range 10–28 min) were conducted by a female research assistant with a medical degree (co-author, CV) who had received prior training in conducting semi-structured interviews and had met with participants at the moment of enrollment in the study. The interview template utilized was inspired by previous qualitative work with adolescents by co-authors, SAK [37] and NC [12]. Open-ended and semi-structured questions followed by specific probes were used to foster personal reflections about participants' lived experience of the MARS-A program (see Appendix A). The interviews were approached as an opportunity for data to be co-created, with space given for participants to elaborate on each question. Participants completed the interviews from a quiet room at home and were made aware that all interviews were audio-recorded and de-identified prior to transcription and analysis.

Data was analyzed manually through a multiple-pass inductive process [38]. In a first pass, co-authors, CV, NC, and EW, independently read through all the transcripts and coded them to identify emergent themes. Codes were generated using participants' own words whenever possible to minimize subjectivity. Co-authors, CV, NC, and EW, then met in person with the co-author, CMH, a child psychologist with extensive mindfulness facilitation experience who had reviewed the video-recordings of the MARS-A sessions to ensure facilitator quality and uniformity, and to review the themes that had been identified from the participants' semi-structured interviews. From this analysis, four key themes emerged, and a common coding scheme was developed. In a second pass, transcripts were recoded by NC and EW using the common coding scheme. In a third pass, codes were compared by EW and placed into corresponding theme categories. A final review of the transcripts was conducted by NC and EW to discuss classification until consensus was reached and to ensure that the language of participants, and not that of the investigators, guided the theme names and descriptions.

3. Results

The average number of sessions attended among participants who completed the MBI was 6.7 in the in-person group and 7 in the eHealth group. The average participant age was 15.3 years. There were two male participants in each group and all four of them completed post-participation interviews. Participants who did not complete the intervention mentioned lack of time (online group) and difficulty with transportation (in-person group) as reasons for non-completion. Table 1 details participant characteristics at baseline.

Four prominent themes emerged from the interview data: (1) Creating a safe space; (2) fostering peer support and connection; (3) integration of mindfulness skills into daily life; and (4) improved well-being through the application of mindfulness. These themes were similar, with only subtle differences between the in-person and eHealth groups and reflected the lived experience of the MARS-A participants. For brevity and clarity, we have used ellipses, (...), to indicate pauses and square brackets, ([...]), to indicate edits/omitted material when reporting supporting excerpts from interviews [39].

3.1. Creating a Safe Space

During their interviews, participants in both groups used the word, "safe", to describe their experience or environment. The use of the word, "safe", or concept of "safe space" arose most frequently in relation to the question, "What did you like the most about the program?" For both in-person and eHealth participants, the non-judgmental attitude of other group members who were experiencing similar challenges related to their chronic health condition allowed them to feel at ease during the MBI.

- In-person participant (IPP): [...] *it felt like a really safe space. Like it felt like you could really say whatever was on your mind.*
- IPP: [...] *you could say what you need to say, so like, afterwards if you're like stressed out about something then no one will like, judge you or make a comment ...*
- EHealth participant (EHP): *I felt like it was a very safe environment ... I felt like they were very welcoming, and it was comforting.*
- EHP: [...] *they made you feel like whatever you were feeling was like OK [...] Like, anytime I thought of something, I shared.*

Table 1. Participant characteristics at baseline.

Parameters	In-Person Group (n = 9)	Online Group (n = 9)
Average age (range)	15.2 (13–17)	15.4 (13–18)
Gender (%)		
Female	78	78
Male	22	22
Ethnicity (%)		
White/Caucasian	67	78
Asian	22	11
African-American	11	11
Primary diagnosis (%)		
Epilepsy	22	11
Anxiety	22	11
Somatic symptom disorder	11	11
Anorexia nervosa	11	11
Thalassemia	11	11
Diabetes	0	11
Obsessive-compulsive disorder	11	0
Juvenile idiopathic arthritis	0	11
Lupus	11	0
Cystic fibrosis	0	11
Asthma	0	11
Chronic pain (%)	44	44
Sleep difficulties (%)	67	78
Mental health (%)		
Any mental health diagnosis	89	78
Anxiety	78	67
Mood disorder	56	44
History of suicidal ideation	33	33
Other mental health diagnosis	33	22
Currently taking medication (%)	67	89
Substance use (past month) (%)		
Smoking/vaping (last month)	0	11
Alcohol (last month)	0	33
Other drugs	0	11
Past yoga/tai chi experience (%)	78	67
Previous meditation/mindfulness experience	44	44

3.2. Fostering Peer Support and Connection

Peer support and connection was reported in participants from both the in-person and online groups, with a focus on interaction with others either in person or through the audio-visual platform. These interactions were described as useful and allowed participants to compare their own challenges to those faced by their peers.

- IPP: [...] *you get to see like, other teens—what they're going through and stuff [...] I thought it was really useful.*
- IPP: [...] *then we started to get to know each other and like before the sessions started, or like when it ended we would talk to each other afterwards.*
- EHP: [...] *it was really interesting to hear the other kids and what they were saying [...] because I could relate to it, and I just didn't expect other people to be going through the same thing as me ...*
- EHP: *I liked how I was able to interact with other people ... other people who are in similar situations as me*

3.3. Integration of Mindfulness Skills into Daily Life

Implementing mindfulness practices outside of the formal sessions was a theme that emerged from both groups. Participants in both groups reported several concrete examples of how they were able to use the skills learned during the MBI to help them in their everyday life.

- IPP: *I liked how we could always learn new practices every week. And I feel like being able to try the practices out at school really helped.*
- IPP: *I liked the eating [practice] one too, because I could fit that into my daily life.*
- EHP: *I'm working and in the process of forgiving a bunch of people in my life, [...] so I definitely think that's going to be a helpful thing.*
- EHP: *I liked the techniques that I learned, the different kind of mindfulness things we went through because I use them throughout the day all the time.*

3.4. Improved Well-Being through the Application of Mindfulness

Reports from participants in the in-person and online groups suggested a positive impact of the intervention on well-being. Some of the benefits mentioned included: A reduction of anxiety and mood symptoms, an improvement in sleep, and the acquisition of new coping skills.

- IPP: *I feel like I'm less anxious about stuff and I feel a little bit happier about stuff now.*
- IPP: *I know that a couple times my stress level was a little bit lower which was helpful [...] like my sleeping patterns were consistent.*
- EHP: *I think the most useful part was how the program helps you cope with a lot of different things [...] it just helps you cope all around.*
- EHP: *I don't know what it is with the body scan, but it helps me go to sleep.*

4. Discussion

This article presents the qualitative results of a randomized study of an MBI for adolescents with chronic illnesses delivered in-person or via eHealth. The parallel emergence of four key themes—the creation of a safe space, the fostering of peer support and connections, the integration of mindfulness skills into daily life, and improved well-being through the application of mindfulness—in both the in-person and online groups suggests that an eHealth platform could present a viable alternative for the delivery of MBIs in this population.

Creating a safe space for learning, listening, and inquiry in which each participant feels comfortable and relaxed is an integral component of the MARS-A program and other eight-week mindfulness programs for adolescents [7,40]. This concept of creation of a safe space has been described in previous studies of adolescent MBIs [41] and was reported on several occasions by participants in both groups, yet, interestingly, was not included in any of the interview questions. Participants from the in-person group suggested that the lived experience of safe space allowed them to feel comfortable sharing their thoughts and emotions with the rest of the group. EHealth group participants' reflections mirrored the experience of safe space described by the in-person group, also describing an ease to share with others. An important question that remains unanswered is whether the creation of a safe space was the result of a non-specific group effect (unrelated to the mindfulness intervention) or, rather, was related to the facilitators' embodied mindfulness, which is considered to be integral to the pedagogy of mindfulness [42,43].

Although online participants' interactions, unlike in-person participants, were limited to viewing one another on screen during the formal session, with no designated time for informal social interactions before, after, or during sessions, the theme of fostering peer support and connection was reported in both groups. There was a slight difference in the nature of the connection described by each group, with the word, "friendship", used only by the in-person group and descriptors, like "similar", used more frequently by the online group. Nevertheless, both groups reported benefiting from meeting others with whom they had a shared lived experience, which is frequently reported in in-person studies of MBIs in pediatric populations [11,16].

A primary research question was whether the feeling of support and mutual learning could be fostered within the confines of online interaction. Online facilitation comes with its own novel set of challenges [44]. One of these challenges is having less physical cues to the emotional state of participants. During in-person sessions, facilitators have the chance to observe participants in informal interactions before and after the session and during the break. These informal interactions are removed in the online setting, which did not appear to limit participants' reports of group connectedness or the effectiveness of the intervention, as described in adult studies of MBIs delivered remotely [45].

One particularly striking finding regarding the group dynamic was seen in the reflection, "I got the sense that I wasn't alone", which was voiced by several participants. For individuals in the online group to feel this level of connection to their peers described in qualitative studies of in-person MBIs [15] speaks strongly to the viability of eHealth as a delivery platform for MBIs with adolescent populations. It also shows that a sense of community was fostered amongst participants, even though their description of their relationship to their peers—"friendship" vs. "support"—had a different quality between the in-person and online groups.

The question of whether the reported peer connectedness was attributed to the mindfulness intervention itself, or to a non-specific group effect, is challenging to answer without the presence of an active control group (e.g., non-mindfulness group therapy) [46,47]. It is worth noting that the intention of MBIs is usually not focused on fostering friendships per se, but rather on creating a sense of mindful peer connection and support [48], which was clearly reported by both groups. One could add that participants were part of a generation that has been exposed to technology and social media from an early age, which might have facilitated peer connection through the online platform [49].

Studies have indicated that pediatric participants in eight-week MBIs acquire the skillsets needed to apply mindfulness practices in their daily lives [11,15]. This integration of mindfulness skills can be assessed in different ways, including patient report and validated measurement scales [50], and is often used as a proxy to measure the effectiveness of MBIs [12,51]. In our study, participants were able to identify several real-life situations where the acquisition of new mindfulness skills would be useful for them (e.g., when eating, increased forgiveness). Both groups' willingness and ability to apply diverse mindful practices outside of the sessions suggests a successful adoption of the practices via in-person and online modalities.

Pediatric in-person studies have shown that the application of mindfulness can improve participants' well-being, specifically in relation to anxiety, pain, and sleep [14,16]. Both the in-person and online groups reported positive impacts in these three areas. In addition, participants explained that mindfulness had benefits on their happiness, body awareness, and reactions to difficult situations. On multiple occasions, participants went beyond simply describing foundational practices, such as sitting meditation, and were able to share high-level concepts, such as insight that their pain is connected to stress. This specific association has been described in previous in-person MBI studies, and is considered an indicator of increased mindfulness [16].

Qualitative data from post-participation interviews were meant to complement quantitative data from validated scales, logging of individual home practice, and measures of salivary cortisol levels also gathered during this study [52]. In brief, quantitative analyses from measurement scales and saliva samples were limited due to the small size of the sample, but there were similar levels of self-reported home practice between groups: In-person group: 6.5 times per participant/week (range = 1.4–13.4) and 28.8 min per participant/week (range = 4.3–154.7); and eHealth group: 6.0 times per participant/week (range = 2.9–9.7) and 30.6 min per participant/week (range = 6.6–107.8). Reported practices included all nine types of practices taught during MARS-A sessions (i.e., breathing meditation, body scan, mindful movement, eating meditation). These levels of individual practice, although much lower than those recommended (45 min per day) and observed (approximately 30 min per day) in adult MBIs [53], and lower than those reported in a recent in-person adolescent MBI study (median of 54 min per week) [11], provide some support that a number of different mindfulness practices were successfully integrated in participants' everyday life.

None of the participants recruited for this study (including potential participants that ultimately were not enrolled in the study) identified access to the technology required to participate in the eHealth group (computer/tablet, web camera, microphone, internet connection) as a barrier to participation. While there were some technical issues that impacted individuals and the entire group, such as mild delays (3–5 min) in establishing a stable internet connection for all members at the beginning of five of the eight eHealth sessions, loss of connection for a 30 s to 8 min on a total of 12 occasions for four of the eHealth participants, and a defective microphone requiring reliance on instant messaging functions for one of the participants during two of the sessions, along with some distractions from their own space (e.g., family talking loudly or a pet coming into the room), most online participants reported that the online platform was convenient and easy to use and shared that being at home, versus commuting, resulted in more ease for them before, during, and after the session. Although this was not reported by study participants, studies of MBIs provided remotely suggest that learning mindfulness skills in one's usual environment facilitates implementation of mindfulness skills and generalization to everyday life [54], with the added benefit of not having to plan additional time for transportation.

Study limitations: Due to a slower recruitment than anticipated, the sample size was small, and it is unclear if data saturation was reached. In addition, semi-structured interviews were short (less than thirty minutes), which could have limited the depth of participant reflections, and interviews took place immediately after the end of the MBI, which did not allow the capturing of any long-term effects of the intervention. In addition, interviews were conducted remotely through the same audio-video platform that was used for the delivery of the MBI in the eHealth group and was being trialed for feasibility. Finally, our study population was highly heterogeneous, limiting the possibility of applying findings to specific medical conditions.

5. Conclusions

Qualitative results from this study suggest that eHealth may be an acceptable and feasible mode of delivery for MBIs for adolescents with chronic illnesses. Given the small size and preliminary nature of our study, more research is needed to confirm these findings. Nonetheless, eHealth should be considered as an alternative option in future studies of MBIs for adolescents, and as a promising avenue to increase access to MBIs for youth who might not be able to access in-person programs.

Author Contributions: Conceptualization, N.C., M.K. and D.X.V.; Data curation, C.V.; Formal analysis, N.C., E.W., C.M.-H.and C.V.; Funding acquisition, N.C. and M.K.; Investigation, N.C. and C.V.; Methodology, N.C. and E.W.; Project administration, N.C. and C.V.; Supervision, S.A.K., M.K. and D.X.V.; Validation, C.M.-H. and C.V.; Visualization, N.C. and E.W.; Writing-original draft, N.C. and E.W.; Writing-review & editing, N.C., E.W., C.M.-H., S.A.K., C.V., M.K., J.L. and D.X.V.

Funding: This research was funded by the Mind and Life Institute (grant number 2016-1440-Chadi) and by a postgraduate medical research award from the University of Toronto (grant number 2016-Chadi).

Acknowledgments: The authors of this paper wish to acknowledge the contributions of Blathnaid McCoy, Abhaya Kulkarni, Nades Palaniyar, Danielle Ruskin, and Claire De Souza in drafting and submitting the initial study proposal.

Conflicts of Interest: The authors declare no conflict of interest. The funders had no role in the design of the study; in the collection, analyses, or interpretation of data; in the writing of the manuscript, and in the decision to publish the results.

Appendix A

Post-Intervention Semi-Structured Interview Guide

Participant ID: _____

Interviewer: _____

Date: _____

Start Time: _____ AM/PM   End Time: _____ AM/PM

Hello, my name is (insert research assistant's name). I am one of the research assistants for the Mindfulness research project you are participating in at SickKids Hospital. First, I would like to thank you for participating in the research project. Now that you have completed the eight-week mindfulness program, I would like to ask you a few questions about the program. Our research team is interested in hearing your opinion about things that went well or were helpful for you and things that could be changed to improve the program in the future. This conversation should not take more than 15 to 20 min of your time. Is this still a good time for you to conduct this interview? [If no: Can I call you back at another time? What is the best time to reach you?]

1. **What did you like the most about the program?** *Probe: What were some of the good things that came out of the mindfulness sessions?*
2. **What did you like the least about the program?** *Probes: Were there some parts of the program that you didn't like? Why? What ways could we improve on those parts?*
3. **What was the most useful part of the program for you?** *Probes: Are there some things that you learned the program that you think you will use in the future?*
4. **What did you think of the teens in your group?** *Probes: Did you enjoy being part of a group? If so, how or in what way? Was the size of the group too large/small? Did you find that you had enough/too much time to share your experience?*
5. (For participants in the eHealth arm) **What did you think of the iMeet platform?** *Probes: What issues, if any, did you have with the iMeet platform? What did you like/dislike about doing the program at home? Online/remotely?*
6. **How did you find your instructors?** *Probes: Is there something that your instructors could have done differently? What did you like/dislike about your instructors?*
7. **Did you practice mindfulness between the sessions? If yes, approximately how many times a week did you practice and for how long? If no, why not?** *Probe: What made it easy/difficult to practice at home? What were the barriers to home practice?*
8. (If yes at the previous question) **Which mindfulness practices did you do at home? Why did you choose this/these practice(s)?**
9. **What changes, if any, did you see in yourself after finishing the mindfulness program?** *Probes: Better sleep, feeling happier, more energy, less anxious/stressed, less pain, increased school/social event attendance*
10. **Would you recommend the mindfulness program to a friend or to another young person with a health condition?** *Probes: If no, why not? If yes, why would you recommend it?*
11. **Do you think that you will continue to practice mindfulness? Why or Why not?**
12. **Do you have any other comments that you would like to share with us about the program?** *Probes: positive/negative experiences? General thoughts and feelings about program?*

Thanks again for your time and your participation in the program.

References

1. Pinquart, M.; Teubert, D. Academic, physical, and social functioning of children and adolescents with chronic physical illness: A meta-analysis. *J. Pediatr. Psychol.* **2012**, *37*, 376–389. [CrossRef] [PubMed]
2. Christie, D.; Viner, R. Adolescent development. *BMJ* **2005**, *330*, 301–304. [CrossRef] [PubMed]
3. Chadi, N.; Amaria, K.; Kaufman, M. Expand your HEADS, follow the THRxEADS! *Paediatr. Child Health* **2017**, *22*, 23–25. [CrossRef] [PubMed]
4. Warschburger, P.; Hanig, J.; Friedt, M.; Posovszky, C.; Schier, M.; Calvano, C. Health-related quality of life in children with abdominal pain due to functional or organic gastrointestinal disorders. *J. Pediatr. Psychol.* **2014**, *39*, 45–54. [CrossRef] [PubMed]
5. Kabat-Zinn, J. *Wherever You Go, There You Are: Mindfulness Meditation in Everyday Life*, 10th ed.; Hachette Books: New York, NY, USA, 2005; ISBN 978-1401307783.
6. Zenner, C.; Herrnleben-Kurz, S.; Walach, H. Mindfulness-based interventions in schools-A systematic review and meta-analysis. *Front. Psychol.* **2014**, *5*, 603. [CrossRef] [PubMed]
7. Vo, D.X.; Doyle, J.; Christie, D. Mindfulness and Adolescence: A Clinical Review of Recent Mindfulness-Based Studies in Clinical and Nonclinical Adolescent Populations. *Adolesc. Med. State Art Rev.* **2014**, *25*, 455–472. [PubMed]
8. Zoogman, S.; Goldberg, S.B.; Hoyt, W.T.; Miller, L. Mindfulness Interventions with Youth: A Meta-Analysis. *Mindfulness* **2015**, *6*, 290–302. [CrossRef]
9. Ahola Kohut, S.; Stinson, J.; Davies-Chalmers, C.; Ruskin, D.; van Wyk, M. Mindfulness-Based Interventions in Clinical Samples of Adolescents with Chronic Illness: A Systematic Review. *J. Altern. Complement. Med.* **2017**. [CrossRef] [PubMed]
10. Webb, L.; Perry-Parrish, C.; Ellen, J.; Sibinga, E. Mindfulness instruction for HIV-infected youth: A randomized controlled trial. *AIDS Care* **2018**, *30*, 688–695. [CrossRef] [PubMed]
11. Ali, A.; Weiss, T.R.; Dutton, A.; McKee, D.; Jones, K.D.; Kashikar-Zuck, S.; Silverman, W.K.; Shapiro, E.D. Mindfulness-Based Stress Reduction for Adolescents with Functional Somatic Syndromes: A Pilot Cohort Study. *J. Pediatr.* **2017**, *183*, 184–190. [CrossRef] [PubMed]
12. Chadi, N.; McMahon, A.; Vadnais, M.; Malboeuf-Hurtubise, C.; Djemli, A.; Dobkin, P.L.; Lacroix, J.; Luu, T.M.; Haley, N. Mindfulness-based intervention for female adolescents with chronic pain: A pilot randomized trial. *J. Can. Acad. Child Adolesc. Psychiatry* **2016**, *25*, 159–168. [PubMed]
13. Malboeuf-Hurtubise, C.; Achille, M.; Hardouin, M.; Vadnais, M. Impact of a mindfulness-based randomized, wait-list controlled clinical trial intervention on mood, sleep and quality of life in teenagers with cancer. *Psychosom. Med.* **2014**, *76*, A30.
14. Ruskin, D.A.; Gagnon, M.M.; Kohut, S.A.; Stinson, J.N.; Walker, K.S. A Mindfulness Program Adapted for Adolescents With Chronic Pain: Feasibility, Acceptability, and Initial Outcomes. *Clin. J. Pain.* **2017**. [CrossRef] [PubMed]
15. Ruskin, D.; Harris, L.; Stinson, J.; Kohut, S.A.; Walker, K.; McCarthy, E. "I Learned to Let Go of My Pain". The Effects of Mindfulness Meditation on Adolescents with Chronic Pain: An Analysis of Participants' Treatment Experience. *Children* **2017**, *4*, 110. [CrossRef] [PubMed]
16. Waelde, L.; Feinstein, A.; Bhandari, R.; Griffin, A.; Yoon, I.; Golianu, B. A Pilot Study of Mindfulness Meditation for Pediatric Chronic Pain. *Children* **2017**, *4*, 32. [CrossRef] [PubMed]
17. Murray, G.; Leitan, N.D.; Berk, M.; Thomas, N.; Michalak, E.; Berk, L.; Johnson, S.L.; Jones, S.; Perich, T.; Allen, N.B.; et al. Online mindfulness-based intervention for late-stage bipolar disorder: Pilot evidence for feasibility and effectiveness. *J. Affect. Disord.* **2015**, *178*, 46–51. [CrossRef] [PubMed]
18. Boggs, J.M.; Beck, A.; Felder, J.N.; Dimidjian, S.; Metcalf, C.A.; Segal, Z.V. Web-based intervention in mindfulness meditation for reducing residual depressive symptoms and relapse prophylaxis: A qualitative study. *J. Med. Internet Res.* **2014**, *16*, e87. [CrossRef] [PubMed]
19. Cavalera, C.; Pagnini, F.; Rovaris, M.; Mendozzi, L.; Pugnetti, L.; Garegnani, M.; Molinari, E. A telemedicine meditation intervention for people with multiple sclerosis and their caregivers: Study protocol for a randomized controlled trial. *Trials* **2016**, *17*, 4. [CrossRef] [PubMed]
20. Mikolasek, M.; Berg, J.; Witt, C.M.; Barth, J. Effectiveness of Mindfulness- and Relaxation-Based eHealth Interventions for Patients with Medical Conditions: A Systematic Review and Synthesis. *Int. J. Behav. Med.* **2018**, *25*, 1–16. [CrossRef] [PubMed]

21. Sibinga, E.M.S.; Perry-Parrish, C.; Thorpe, K.; Mika, M.; Ellen, J.M. A Small Mixed-Method RCT of Mindfulness Instruction for Urban Youth. *Explore J. Sci. Heal.* **2014**, *10*, 180–186. [CrossRef] [PubMed]
22. Monshat, K.; Khong, B.; Hassed, C.; Vella-Brodrick, D.; Norrish, J.; Burns, J.; Herrman, H. A conscious control over life and my emotions: Mindfulness practice and healthy young people. A qualitative study. *J. Adolesc. Health* **2013**, *52*, 572–577. [CrossRef] [PubMed]
23. Kerrigan, D.; Johnson, K.; Stewart, M.; Magyari, T.; Hutton, N.; Ellen, J.M.; Sibinga, E.M.S. Perceptions, experiences, and shifts in perspective occurring among urban youth participating in a mindfulness-based stress reduction program. *Complement. Ther. Clin. Pract.* **2011**, *17*, 96–101. [CrossRef] [PubMed]
24. Caldwell, C. Mindfulness & Bodyfulness: A New Paradigm. *J. Contempl. Inq.* **2014**, *1*, 77–96.
25. Chadi, N.; Kaufman, M.; Weisbaum, E.; Malboeuf-Hurtubise, C.; Kohut, S.A.; Viner, C.; Locke, J.; Vo, D.X. In-Person Versus eHealth Mindfulness-Based Intervention for Adolescents With Chronic Illness: Protocol for a Randomized Controlled Trial. *JMIR Res. Protoc.* **2017**, *6*, e241. [CrossRef] [PubMed]
26. Sandelowski, M. Whatever happened to qualitative description? *Res. Nurs. Health* **2000**, *23*, 334–340. [CrossRef]
27. Thorne, S.; Kirkham, S.R.; MacDonald-Emes, J. Interpretive description: A noncategorical qualitative alternative for developing nursing knowledge. *Res. Nurs. Health* **1997**, *20*, 169–177. [CrossRef]
28. Caelli, K.; Ray, L.; Mill, J. 'Clear as Mud': Toward Greater Clarity in Generic Qualitative Research. *Int. J. Qual. Methods* **2003**, *2*, 1–13. [CrossRef]
29. Kahlke, R.M. Generic Qualitative Approaches: Pitfalls and Benefits of Methodological Mixology. *Int. J. Qual. Methods* **2014**, *13*, 37–52. [CrossRef]
30. Schwartz-Shea, P.; Yanow, D. *Interpretive Research Design: Concepts and Processes*; Routhledge: New York, NY, USA, 2012.
31. Vo, D.X.; Locke, J.J.; Johnson, A.; Marshall, S.K. The Effectiveness of the Mindful Awareness and Resilience Skills for Adolescents (MARS-A) Intervention on Adolescent Mental Health: A Pilot Clinical Trial. *J. Adolesc. Health* **2015**, *56*, S27. [CrossRef]
32. Biegel, G.M.; Brown, K.W.; Shapiro, S.L.; Schubert, C.M. Mindfulness-based stress reduction for the treatment of adolescent psychiatric outpatients: A randomized clinical trial. *J. Consult. Clin. Psychol.* **2009**, *77*, 855–866. [CrossRef] [PubMed]
33. Kabat-Zinn, J. *Full Catastrophe Living: Using the Wisdom of Your Body and Mind to Face Stress, Pain, and Illness*; Delta Trade Paperbacks: New York, NY, USA, 1991.
34. Teasdale, J.D.; Segal, Z.V.; Williams, J.M.; Ridgeway, V.A.; Soulsby, J.M.; Lau, M.A. Prevention of relapse/recurrence in major depression by mindfulness-based cognitive therapy. *J. Consult. Clin. Psychol.* **2000**, *68*, 615–623. [CrossRef] [PubMed]
35. Segal Williams, J.M.G.; Teasdale, J.D.; Segal, Z. *Mindfulness-Based Cognitive Therapy for Depression*; Guilford Press: New York, NY, USA, 2013.
36. Vo, D. *The Mindful Teen. Powerful Skill to Help You Handle Stress One Moment At a Time*; New Harbinger Publications: Vancouver, BC, Canada, 2015.
37. Ahola Kohut, S.; Stinson, J.; Forgeron, P.; van Wyk, M.; Harris, L.; Luca, S. A qualitative content analysis of peer mentoring video calls in adolescents with chronic illness. *J. Health Psychol.* **2016**, *23*, 788–799. [CrossRef] [PubMed]
38. Dierckx de Casterlé, B.; Gastmans, C.; Bryon, E.; Denier, Y. QUAGOL: A guide for qualitative data analysis. *Int. J. Nurs. Stud.* **2012**, *49*, 360–371. [CrossRef] [PubMed]
39. De Zoysa, N.; Ruths, F.A.; Walsh, J.; Hutton, J. Mindfulness Based Cognitive Therapy for Mental Health Professionals: A Long-Term Qualitative Follow-up Study. *Mindfulness* **2014**, *5*, 10–17. [CrossRef]
40. Bluth, K.; Campo, R.A.; Pruteanu-Malinici, S.; Reams, A.; Mullarkey, M.; Broderick, P.C. A School-Based Mindfulness Pilot Study for Ethnically Diverse At-Risk Adolescents. *Mindfulness* **2016**, *7*, 90–104. [CrossRef] [PubMed]
41. Dariotis, J.K.; Mirabal-Beltran, R.; Cluxton-Keller, F.; Gould, L.F.; Greenberg, M.T.; Mendelson, T. A Qualitative Evaluation of Student Learning and Skills Use in a School-Based Mindfulness and Yoga Program. *Mindfulness* **2016**, *7*, 76–89. [CrossRef] [PubMed]
42. McCown, D.; Reibel, D.; Micozzi, M.S. *Teaching Mindfulness: A Practical Guide for Clinicians and Educators*; Springer: Berlin, Germany, 2010; ISBN 9780387094830.

43. Crane, R.S.; Kuyken, W.; Hastings, R.P.; Rothwell, N.; Williams, J.M.G. Training Teachers to Deliver Mindfulness-Based Interventions: Learning from the UK Experience. *Mindfulness* **2010**, *1*, 74–86. [CrossRef] [PubMed]
44. Sansom-Daly, U.M.; Wakefield, C.E.; McGill, B.C.; Patterson, P. Ethical and Clinical Challenges Delivering Group-based Cognitive-Behavioural Therapy to Adolescents and Young Adults with Cancer Using Videoconferencing Technology. *Aust. Psychol.* **2015**, *50*, 271–278. [CrossRef]
45. Colgan, D.D.; Wahbeh, H.; Pleet, M.; Besler, K.; Christopher, M. A Qualitative Study of Mindfulness Among Veterans With Posttraumatic Stress Disorder: Practices Differentially Affect Symptoms, Aspects of Well-Being, and Potential Mechanisms of Action. *J. Evid.-Based Complement. Altern. Med.* **2017**, *22*, 482–493. [CrossRef]
46. Hyland, T. The Limits of Mindfulness: Emerging Issues for Education. *Br. J. Educ. Stud.* **2016**, *64*, 97–117. [CrossRef]
47. Van Dam, N.T.; van Vugt, M.K.; Vago, D.R.; Schmalzl, L.; Saron, C.D.; Olendzki, A.; Meissner, T.; Lazar, S.W.; Kerr, C.E.; Gorchov, J.; et al. Mind the Hype: A Critical Evaluation and Prescriptive Agenda for Research on Mindfulness and Meditation. *Perspect. Psychol. Sci.* **2018**, *13*, 36–61. [CrossRef] [PubMed]
48. Bluth, K.; Gaylord, S.A.; Campo, R.A.; Mullarkey, M.C.; Hobbs, L. Making Friends with Yourself: A Mixed Methods Pilot Study of a Mindful Self-Compassion Program for Adolescents. *Mindfulness* **2016**, *7*, 479–492. [CrossRef] [PubMed]
49. Lenhart, A. *Teens, Social Media and Technology Overview*; Pew Research Center: Washington, DC, USA, 2015.
50. Brown, K.W.; West, A.M.; Loverich, T.M.; Biegel, G.M. Assessing adolescent mindfulness: Validation of an adapted Mindful Attention Awareness Scale in adolescent normative and psychiatric populations. *Psychol. Assess.* **2011**, *23*, 1023–1033. [CrossRef] [PubMed]
51. Ramasubramanian, S. Mindfulness, stress coping and everyday resilience among emerging youth in a university setting: A mixed methods approach. *Int. J. Adolesc. Youth* **2017**, *22*, 308–321. [CrossRef]
52. Chadi, N.; Kaufman, M.; Weisbaum, E.; Malboeuf-Hurtubise, C.; Kohut, S.A.; Locke, J.; Vo, D.X. Comparison of an in-Person vs. Ehealth Mindfulness Meditation-Based Intervention for Adolescents with Chronic Medical Conditions: A Mixed Methods Study. *J. Adolesc. Health* **2018**, *62*, S12. [CrossRef]
53. Parsons, C.E.; Crane, C.; Parsons, L.J.; Fjorback, L.O.; Kuyken, W. Home practice in Mindfulness-Based Cognitive Therapy and Mindfulness-Based Stress Reduction: A systematic review and meta-analysis of participants' mindfulness practice and its association with outcomes. *Behav. Res. Ther.* **2017**, *95*, 29–41. [CrossRef] [PubMed]
54. Bazarko, D.; Cate, R.A.; Azocar, F.; Kreitzer, M.J. The Impact of an Innovative Mindfulness-Based Stress Reduction Program on the Health and Well-Being of Nurses Employed in a Corporate Setting. *J. Workplace Behav. Health* **2013**, *28*, 107–133. [CrossRef] [PubMed]

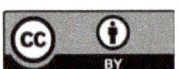 © 2018 by the authors. Licensee MDPI, Basel, Switzerland. This article is an open access article distributed under the terms and conditions of the Creative Commons Attribution (CC BY) license (http://creativecommons.org/licenses/by/4.0/).

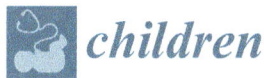

Review

A Review of Non-Pharmacological Treatments for Pain Management in Newborn Infants

Avneet K. Mangat [1,2], Ju-Lee Oei [3], Kerry Chen [4], Im Quah-Smith [5] and Georg M. Schmölzer [2,6,*]

1. Faculty of Science, University of Alberta, Edmonton, AB T6G 2R3, Canada; amangat@ualberta.ca
2. Centre for the Studies of Asphyxia and Resuscitation, Neonatal Research Unit, Royal Alexandra Hospital, Edmonton, AB T6G 2R3, Canada
3. School of Women's and Children's Health, University of New South Wales, Kensington, NSW 2031, Australia; j.oei@unsw.edu.au
4. Faculty of Medicine, University of New South Wales, Kensington, NSW 2033, Australia; kerry.chen@unsw.edu.au
5. School of Women's and Children's Health University of New South Wales, Kensington, NSW 2033, Australia; quahsmith@gmail.com
6. Department of Pediatrics, University of Alberta, Edmonton, AB T6G 2R3, Canada
* Correspondence: georg.schmoelzer@me.com; Tel.: +1-780-735-4660; Fax: +1-780-735-4072

Received: 2 August 2018; Accepted: 17 September 2018; Published: 20 September 2018

Abstract: Pain is a major problem in sick newborn infants, especially for those needing intensive care. Pharmacological pain relief is the most commonly used, but might be ineffective and has side effects, including long-term neurodevelopmental sequelae. The effectiveness and safety of alternative analgesic methods are ambiguous. The objective was to review the effectiveness and safety of non-pharmacological methods of pain relief in newborn infants and to identify those that are the most effective. PubMed and Google Scholar were searched using the terms: "infant", "premature", "pain", "acupuncture", "skin-to-skin contact", "sucrose", "massage", "musical therapy" and 'breastfeeding'. We included 24 studies assessing different methods of non-pharmacological analgesic techniques. Most resulted in some degree of analgesia but many were ineffective and some were even detrimental. Sucrose, for example, was often ineffective but was more effective than music therapy, massage, breast milk (for extremely premature infants) or non-invasive electrical stimulation acupuncture. There were also conflicting results for acupuncture, skin-to-skin care and musical therapy. Most non-pharmacological methods of analgesia provide a modicum of relief for preterm infants, but none are completely effective and there is no clearly superior method. Study is also required to assess potential long-term consequences of any of these methods.

Keywords: infant; premature; pain; acupuncture; skin-to-skin contact; sucrose; massage; musical therapy; breastfeeding

1. Introduction

Newborn infants admitted to an Neonatal Intensive Care Unit (NICU) undergo an average of 134 painful procedures within the first two weeks [1,2]. Even more concerning, some infants might experience more than 3000 painful procedures during the entire course of their NICU stay [3]. These procedures are often necessary to ensure best care, such as heel pricks for blood sampling or endotracheal suctioning. Some of these procedures are also performed repeatedly on the same infant and have been shown to cause adverse physiological consequences, such as hypoxemia, bradycardia and hypertension [1].

Apart from acute discomfort, there is now growing evidence, that painful (and particularly, repetitive) procedures may have adverse consequences on long-term neurological development. Animal models demonstrate that painful events in early life can increase the number of glucocorticoid receptors in the hippocampus, which may affect future stress response [4]. Pain may not even need to be chronic or repetitive to elicit adverse future outcomes. For example, infants have increased stress behavior during routine immunizations at 4–6 months if circumcision was conducted at birth without analgesia [5]. This highlights the lifelong implications of pain management during this critical period in life [1,6].

Pharmacological methods are the most frequently used means to ameliorate or prevent pain in infants. However, many analgesics have adverse effects. For example, opioids can have troublesome adverse effects including somnolence, and respiratory depression making it unsuitable for use in spontaneously breathing, opioid-naïve patients [7].

Adjuvants to pharmacological analgesia are therefore needed. Non-pharmacological analgesic methods include acupuncture, non-nutritive sucking (NNS), breastfeeding (BF), sucrose/glucose solution, skin-to-skin care (SSC), swaddling, therapeutic massage, musical therapy (MT) and facilitated tucking (Table 1). These methods utilize environmental, behavioral, and pharmacological approaches by activating a "gate control mechanism" that prevents the pain sensation from traveling to the central nervous system [8]. While evidence exists for non-pharmacological analgesic methods, the strategies are not used universally. We therefore aimed to summarize the current evidence about the efficacy, safety, and feasibility of non-pharmacological interventions for pain management in newborn infants to determine if they could be considered an alternative to other methods of analgesia, including medications.

Table 1. Non-pharmacological treatments for pain relief.

Environmental Control
Skin-to-skin care
Swaddling
Facilitated tucking
Therapeutic touch/massage
Musical therapy
Feeding Methods
Non-nutritive sucking
Breastfeeding
Other Interventions
Acupuncture
Sucrose/glucose solutions

2. Methods

PubMed and Google Scholar were systematically searched include the following search-terms "infants", "pain", "acupuncture", "skin-to-skin contact", "sucrose", "massage", "musical therapy" and "breastfeeding" between 1965 and 2018 (Appendix A). List of references of identified articles were manually searched. Articles were included if they described non-pharmacological techniques in preterm or term infants and excluded if they compared pharmacological and non-pharmacological intervention or there was no behavioral measurement of pain (e.g., PIPP (Premature Infant Pain Profile), or NIPS (Neonatal Infant Pain Scale)). Only human studies were included and no language restrictions were applied.

3. Results

A total of 26 studies describing acupuncture (n = 3), skin to skin care (n = 3), non-nutritive sucking (n = 1), swaddling (n = 3), sucrose/glucose solution (n = 3), massage (n = 4), musical therapy (n = 5), breastfeeding (n = 3) and facilitated tucking (n = 1) were identified (Table 2). A total of 10 studies were done in preterm infants, 12 studies were in term infants and four studies were done in preterm and term infants. It was not possible to make a distinction between preterm and term infants since many studies did not separate their samples by gestation.

Table 2. Randomized controlled trials for non-pharmacological methods of pain relief in infants.

First Author, Year	Population	Intervention	Other Intervention	Primary Outcome Intervention	Primary Outcome Control	p-Value
Shabani, 2016 [9]	Preterm ($n = 20$)	MT	N/A	Facial pain expressions M (SD): MT: 0.4 (0.1)	Control: 2.1 (0.4)	0.001
Seo, 2016 [10]	Term ($n = 56$)	SSC	N/A	PIPP M ± SD: SSC: 4.1 ± 2.3	Control: 6.3 ± 3.5	0.01
Freire, 2008 [11]	Preterm ($n = 95$)	SSC	Glucose	HR M ± SD: SSC: 5.1 ± 3.9 bpm Glucose: 9.9 ± 6.1 bpm	Control: 10.8 ± 6.5 bpm	SSC vs. glucose: 0.0001 SSC vs. control: 0.0001
Olsson, 2016 [12]	Preterm ($n = 10$)	SSC	N/A	PIPP M: 5.7	Control: 5.0	>0.05 (NS)
Efendi, 2018 [13]	Preterm ($n = 30$)	Pacifier and swaddling	N/A	Increase in pain score: Swaddle: 5.9 ± 2.2 to 6.1 ± 2.0	Control: 5.4 ± 1.8 to 7.7 ± 2.7	Swaddling: NS Control: 0.003
Erkut, 2017 [14]	Term ($n = 74$)	Swaddle	N/A	NIPS M ± SD: Swaddle: 1.6 ± 0.8	Control: 3.3 ± 1.5	0.01
Ho, 2016 [15]	Preterm ($n = 54$)	Swaddle	N/A	PIPP M ± SD: Swaddle: 7.0 ± 2.7	Control: 14.7 ± 2.9	<0.001
Axelin, 2006 [16]	Preterm ($n = 20$)	FT	N/A	NIPS Median (IQR): FT: 3 (2–6)	Control: 5 (2–7)	<0.001
Arikan, 2008 [17]	Preterm/term ($n = 175$)	Massage	Sucrose herbal tea, hydrolyzed formula	Crying time after procedure M ± SD: Massage: 4.4 ± 1.8 s Sucrose: 3.9 ± 1.5 s Tea: 3.2 ± 1.2 s Formula: 2.7 ± 1.1 s	Control: 5.3 ± 1.76 s	Comparing before and after procedure: $p < 0.001$ for all but control ($p > 0.05$)
Chik, 2017 [18]	Preterm/term ($n = 80$)	Massage	N/A	PIPP M (SD): Massage: 6 (3.3)	Control: 12 (4.3)	<0.001
Jain, 2006 [19]	Preterm ($n = 23$)	Massage	N/A	NIPS M (SD): Massage: 1.5 (0.9)	Control: 3.5 (1.6)	<0.001
Zhu, 2015 [20]	Term ($n = 250$)	MT	BF	NIPS M (SD): MT: not significant MT + BF: not significant BF: 3.1 (1.9)	Control: 6.4 (0.2)	BF vs. control: <0.001
Shah, 2017 [21]	Preterm/term ($n = 35$)	MT	Sucrose	PIPP median (IQR): MT: 6 (3–11) MT + sucrose: 3 (0–4)	Sucrose: 5 (3–10)	MT vs. sucrose: >0.05 MT + sucrose vs. sucrose: <0.001 MT + sucrose vs. MT: <0.001

Table 2. Cont.

First Author, Year	Population	Intervention	Other Intervention	Primary Outcome Intervention	Primary Outcome Control	p-Value
Zurita-Cruz, 2017 [22]	Term ($n = 144$)	BF	MS	Crying time Median (IQR): BF: 19 (0–136) MS: 41.5 (0–184)	Control: 41 (0–161)	BF vs. control: 0.007 Control vs. MS: >0.05
Erkul, 2017 [23]	Term ($n = 100$)	BF	N/A	NIPS M ± SD: BF: 1.9 ± 2.2	Control: 6.8 ± 0.7	<0.05
Simonse, 2012 [24]		BF	Bottle fed, sucrose	PIPP M (95%CI): BF: 7.0 (5.3–8.7) Bottle fed: 5.4 (3.7–7.1)	Sucrose: 5.3 (3.6–6.9)	BF vs. bottle fed: >0.05 BF vs. sucrose: >0.05
Baudesson, 2017 [25]	Preterm ($n = 33$)	MO	N/A	PIPP M (SD): MO: 7.3 (3.0)	Control: 10 (3.5)	0.03
Mitchell, 2016 [26]	Term ($n = 162$)	NESAP	Sucrose	PIPP M ± SD: NESAP: 5.0 ± 4.0 Sucrose: 4.0 ± 1.8 NESAP + sucrose: 3.6 ± 1.2	Control: 4.9 ± 4.0	<0.01
Chen, 2017 [27]	Preterm/term ($n = 30$)	MA	N/A	PIPP M ± SD: MA: 5.9 ± 3.7	Control: 8.3 ± 4.7	0.04
Abbasoglu, 2015 [28]	Preterm ($n = 32$)	Acupressure	N/A	PIPP M ± SD: Acupressure: 9.1 ± 2.0	Control: 9.6 ± 1.7	0.5
Lima, 2017 [29]	Term ($n = 78$)	NNS	Glucose	NIPS M ± SD: NNS: 33.9 ± 17.6	Glucose: 10.9 ± 11.3	<0.001
Gouin, 2018 [30]	Term ($n = 245$)	Sucrose	N/A	NIPS M ± SD: Sucrose: 2.3 ± 0.5	Control: 1.6 ± 0.5	0.6
Collados-Gómez, 2018 [31]	Preterm ($n = 66$)	Sucrose	EBM	PIPP Median (IQR): Sucrose: 6 (4–8)	EBM: 7 (4–9)	0.28

M: mean, SD: standard deviation, IQR: interquartile range, NS: not significant, HR: heart rate, SSC: skin-to-skin care, FT: facilitated tuck, MT: musical therapy, BF: breast feeding, MO: milk odor, NS: non-significant, NNS: non-nutritive sucking, NESAP: non-invasive electrical stimulation at acupuncture points, N/A: not/applicable, MS: milk substitute, EBM: expressed breastmilk, PIPP: Premature Infant Pain Profile, NIPS: Neonatal Infant Pain Scale, bpm: beats per minute.

3.1. Environmental Control

Creating a more comforting environment with SSC, swaddling, therapeutic touch/massage, music therapy and comfort positioning for the infant can produce analgesic effects. Cholecystokinin, a neuropeptide associated with analgesia, is released when the infant is exposed to familiar smell of the mother [32]. Therefore, providing an infant with SSC with the mother can have an analgesic effect [32]. Swaddling, the practice of wrapping infants in blankets and can help simulate the environment of the womb which may translate to analgesia [33,34]. Massage can potentially saturate the senses and decrease the pain signals that are sent to the central nervous system [35]. Music uses distraction to activate the infant's attention and thus distracts them from the pain and decreases their sensation of pain [9]. Holding the infant in a flexed position, which is known as facilitated tucking, can also have analgesic effects due to saturation of senses similar to massage therapy [35].

3.1.1. Skin-to-Skin Care

Overall, most studies reported decreased pain responses during SSC compared to placebo methods. Seo et al. reported 35% less pain and an 88% decrease in crying duration with SSC compared to controls during heel pricks [10]. Similarly, Freire et al. compared SSC with oral glucose solution or placebo for pain relief of 95 preterm infants during heel prick. The infants randomized to SSC had significantly lower heart rates (mean ± standard deviation (SD), 5 ± 4 vs. control 11 ± 7 vs. oral glucose 10 ± 6 beats per minute (bpm); $p = 0.0001$) and oxygen saturation variation (1.5 ± 1.7 vs. control 2.6 ± 1.5 vs. oral glucose 1.9 ± 1.5%; $p = 0.0012$) than those given glucose or to controls [11]. Olsson et al. reported similar pain scores between SSC and placebo during venepuncture of 10 preterm infants [12]. In summary, SSC might reduce pain in preterm and term infants.

3.1.2. Swaddling

Efendi et al. randomized 30 preterm infants to either swaddling and pacifier or control during painful procedures and demonstrated a significantly lower heart rate and pain scores in infants receiving swaddling and a pacifier [13]. As the study combined NNS and swaddling, it is therefore impossible to differentiate which of these methods might have provided pain relief. Other studies have reported that swaddling alone decreases pain during heel prick [14,15]. Erkut et al. reported a 50% pain reduction, a 30% decrease in duration of crying time, and a significantly increased oxygen saturation (mean ± SD, 97 ± 2 vs. control: 95 ± 2%, $p = 0.006$) in the swaddled group after a heel prick procedure in 74 term infants [14]. Ho et al. randomized 54 premature infants to swaddling or control and reported lower pain scores (7 ± 3 vs. control: 145 ± 3, $p < 0.001$), lower heart rate (162 ± 10 vs. control: 182 ± 17 bpm, $p < 0.001$), and higher oxygen saturation (96 ± 4 vs. control 87 ± 7%, $p < 0.001$) after heel prick [15]. These studies suggest that swaddling alone or combining with a pacifier has the potential to decrease pain in preterm and term infants.

3.1.3. Facilitated Tucking

Axelin et al. randomized 20 preterm infants to either control or facilitated tucking (flexed position by their parents) [16]. Overall, facilitated tucking reduced pain by 40% ($p < 0.001$) and crying time was significantly shorter 5 s vs. 17 s, $p = 0.024$ when compared to no tucking [16].

3.1.4. Therapeutic Touch/Massage

Two observational studies reported that massage therapy significantly reduced mean crying time (4.4 ± 1.8 vs. control: 5.3 ± 1.7 h/day, $p < 0.001$) in infants with infant colic [17] and decreased NIPS scores (3.9 vs. control: 4.8, $p = 0.002$) in term infants [34]. Two randomized trials reported that an upper limb massage significantly decreased pain responses during venipuncture in preterm and term infants [18,19]. Chik et al. randomized 80 infants and found significantly lower pain scores between the massage and control group (-6.0, $p < 0.001$) [18]. Similarly, Jain et al. found a 60% decrease in pain and a significant decrease in heart rate (mean ± SD: 149 ± 14 vs. control: 159 ± 13 bpm, p = 0.03) after venipuncture of 23 infants [19]. These studies suggest that a gentle massage prior a heel prick is safe and can decrease pain.

3.1.5. Musical Therapy

Using MT, a case study with five infants in a cardiac intensive care unit showed a decreased average heart rate in 4/5 infants in 66% of the sessions [36]. In addition, respiratory rate and blood pressure were also decreased, while oxygen saturation increased in some of the infants [36]. Furthermore, Olischar et al. reported more mature sleep-wake cycles in newborn infants > 32 weeks' gestation exposed to music when compared to controls suggesting a calming effect on quiet sleep [37]. These data suggest that MT has a stabilizing effect on physiological parameters and sleep, which could be translate to a decreased pain response. However, currently available evidence has conflicting results.

Shabani et al. randomized 20 preterm infants to MT or control during venous blood sampling and reported a significant decrease in heart rate (mean ± SD: 148 ± 4 vs. control 163 ± 4 bpm, p = 0.005) and an 80% decrease in the infants' mean facial pain expressions with MT [9]. Zhu et al. randomized 250 term infants to either MT, MT + BF, BF, or control and observed that the BF group had a 50% decrease in pain and a 70% decrease in duration of crying time [20]. In addition, no difference between BF or BF + MT was observed, suggesting that MT was ineffective for pain relief [20]. Shah et al. randomized 35 infants to MT, sucrose, or MT + sucrose using a cross-over design [21]. Overall, median interquartile range pain scores were significantly lower in the MT + sucrose group (3, 0–4) compared to MT (6, 3–11) or sucrose (5, 3–10) alone [21]. In addition, pain scores were similar between the MT and sucrose groups [21]. These data suggest that a combination of MT + sucrose provides improved pain relief compared to sucrose or music alone.

3.2. Feeding Methods

Breastfeeding and NNS are believed to support analgesia through the release of cholecystokinin (neuropeptide) [32,38]. With BF, cholecystokinin is believed to be released due to familiar odors of the mother [32]. Non-nutritive sucking has been associated with the activation of sensory nerves that can lead to the release of cholecystokinin which can then interact with opioids and produce analgesia [1].

3.2.1. Breastfeeding

Zurita-Cruz et al. randomized 144 infants to either BF, milk substitute, or no analgesia (control group) during vaccination and reported that infants who received BF had reduced pain and 50% reduction in median crying time compared with milk substitute or controls [22]. There were no significant differences in any of the parameters between the milk substitute and control groups suggesting that milk substitute was ineffective at decreasing pain [22]. Similarly, Erkul et al. randomized 100 infants to either BF or control prior vaccination and observed lower pain scores (mean ± SD: 1.9 ± 2.2 vs. 6.8 ± 0.7, p < 0.05), lower duration of crying (mean ± SD: 20.5 ± 16.2 vs. 45.1 ± 14.5 s, p = 0.005), lower heart rate (mean ± SD: 164 ± 17 vs. 172 ± 15 bpm, p < 0.05), and higher mean oxygen saturation (mean ± SD: 98 ± 3 vs. 94 ± 7%, p < 0.05) [23]. One may assume that there is a difference between the analgesic effects of BF compared to oral administering breast milk, due to BF having the additive analgesic effects from other factors such as parental presence and SSC. However, a randomized controlled trial of 71 preterm neonates reported a surprising distinction between BF and bottle feeding [24]. Bottle feeding significantly decreased the mean COMFORTneo pain score compared to breast feeding (BF: 19.0 vs. bottle-fed: 16.3, p = 0.03) [24]. The study also compared the analgesic effects of breast milk to sucrose and found no significant differences in PIPP scores eluding that both were just as effective [24]. It is also noteworthy that, in premature infants, even the smell of breast milk had a 50% reduction in pain scores during venipuncture and a decrease in percent of duration of crying (0.17 ± 0.6 vs. 9.7 ± 17.3 s, p = 0.04) after venipuncture [25]. These results are important in situations where breast feeding is not feasible in the NICU (e.g., mother not present) since the smell of breast milk has the potential to decrease pain.

3.2.2. Non-Nutritive Sucking

A case-control study compared infants who sucked on an adult's little finger ($n = 20$) with BF ($n = 20$) and without any analgesia ($n = 23$, control group) during venipuncture [39]. Overall outcomes with BF and NNS were similar (35 vs. 24%, $p > 0.05$) suggesting a similar efficacy in analgesia [39]. While NNS has some effect on pain relief further studies are needed to examine different approaches of NNS (e.g., use of finger or pacifier) or combination with glucose.

3.3. Other Interventions

3.3.1. Acupuncture

Body acupuncture and pain management is well known with the spinal pain pathways being recruited for attenuation of pain signaling in needle acupuncture. Manual acupuncture activates different afferent fibers (Aβ, Aδ, and C) and these signals ascend mainly through the spinal ventrolateral funiculus to the brain [26]. Many brain nuclei compose the network involved in processing acupuncture analgesia such as locus coeruleus and arcuate nucleus [26]. However, more recent research reveals the bigger impact of acupuncture on the individual. Now considered a complex sensory stimulation, acupuncture effects also include autonomic re-regulation and regulatory changes in functional connectivity centrally—mitigating the effects of physical and emotional trauma in the individual [40,41]. The non-invasive approach (no needling modalities of acupuncture such as low-level laser and magnet application), is more autonomically driven to gain direct access to central pain control centers [40]. Neuroimaging studies have confirmed the re-regulatory capacity of acupuncture centrally [42].

Several studies examined the effects of non-invasive acupuncture on neonatal pain [27,28,43]. Chen et al. randomized 30 term infants to either auricular non-invasive magnetic acupuncture or placebo to decrease infant pain during heel pricks [27]. The study reported a 30% reduction in pain in infants receiving magnetic acupuncture [27]. Abbasoglu et al. reported a 45% reduction in mean duration of crying with acupressure compared to control infants during heel pricks in 32 preterm infants, but no significant differences in pain score between groups [28]. Differences in these studies could have been due to the use of varying techniques (e.g., acupuncture or acupressure) or different acupuncture points. Future studies should distinguish between the optimal points and duration of treatment (e.g., duration of placement of acupuncture) and to elucidate the long-term implications of different methods of acupuncture.

3.3.2. Sucrose/Glucose Solutions

Oral sucrose solution is most commonly used as non-pharmacological interventions for pain management in newborn infants. Sucrose may exert its analgesic effects through endogenous opioid pathways or via an increase in dopamine and acetylcholine [1,44]. However, the evidence for pain relief is conflicting. Lima et al. reported a 40% reduction in pain scores and a 70% reduction in crying time with oral glucose compared to NNS in 78 healthy newborns during immunization [29]. Gouin et al. randomized 1–3 months old children undergoing a venipuncture to either sucrose or placebo and found similar pain scores (mean ± SD: sucrose 2.3 ± 0.5 vs. placebo 1.6 ± 0.5, $p = 0.6$), heart rate variability (mean ± SD: sucrose 33 ± 6 vs. placebo 24 ± 5 bpm, $p = 0.44$), and crying time (mean ± SD: sucrose 63 ± 3 vs. placebo 49 ± 5 sec, $p = 0.17$) for both groups [30]. Similarly, a randomized trial with 66 preterm infants > 28 weeks gestation administered expressed breast milk or oral sucrose for pain management during venipuncture [31]. Overall, similar pain scores with 7 (range 4–9) with expressed breast milk and 6 (range 4–8) with sucrose were observed [31]. These studies suggest that oral sucrose might not be effective in all infants and that expressed breast milk has similar analgesic effects. Furthermore, the analgesia effect of sucrose might be ineffective in infants' experience opioid withdrawal [45]. However, a recent study reported similar pain scores for opioid exposed and non-exposed infants suggesting that oral sucrose might be effective in both exposed and non-exposed infants [46].

There may, however, be negative effects of oral sucrose. Asmerom et al. randomized 131 premature infants undergoing a heel lance procedure to either control, placebo with NNS, or sucrose [47]. Although, a 22% decrease in median pain scores was observed with sucrose compared to control, increased markers of oxidative stress and increased use of adenosine triphosphate could indicate cellular injury in infants receiving sucrose. Furthermore, infants receiving sucrose had a significant increase in the heart rate from (mean ± SD): 155 ± 14 to 171 ± 155 bpm compared to infants the control (154 ± 13 to 155 ± 14 bpm) and placebo groups (156 ± 14 to 165 ± 15 bpm, $p < 0.001$) [47].

However, there might be also some positive long-term effects of sucrose on spatial learning and memory [48]. Rat models showed that chronic pain impaired short-term memory, but sucrose prevented such impairment and increased endorphin levels [48]. Sucrose also prevented a decrease levels of brain derived neurotropic factor, which occurs during chronic pain [48]. This conflicting evidence suggests that further studies are needed to examine long-term effects (e.g., long-term neurodevelopmental outcomes or obesity) of oral sucrose.

4. Discussion

Non-pharmacological techniques have the potential to provide pain relief for preterm and term infants. Most studies included in this review demonstrated an improvement in behavioral pain responses including facial expressions, duration of crying or latency to first cry, and physiological parameters (e.g., heart rate, oxygen saturation). This indicates that non-pharmacological techniques are beneficial and were successful at reducing pain. However, this finding was not reproducible in sucrose vs. placebo, breastmilk vs. sucrose, and breast feeding vs. musical therapy studies [20,30,31]. These contradictory results raise questions about the potential mechanism of these interventions. Further research is needed to determine the best non-pharmacological intervention, duration of the intervention, and dose response for optimal pain relief in newborn infants.

While sucrose is now considered the gold standard in non-pharmacological pain relief, the current evidence remains contradictory. Although, several studies identified a clear benefit of sucrose compared to other techniques (e.g., music, massage or NNS) [16,20,26,29], other studies reported lower pain score with alternative techniques including magnetic acupuncture or SSC [11,27]. The mechanism of sucrose has also been controversial. Many believe that sucrose decreases pain through opioid mechanisms but methadone-exposed newborn infants do not appear to be susceptible to the effects of sucrose, probably because of opioid-receptor blockade by methadone [45]. However, Marceau et al. reported that opioid exposed neonates had decreased pain responses with the use of sucrose which suggests additional other mechanisms for sucrose's analgesic effects [46]. There is also conflicting evidence regarding any long-term effects of sucrose. Rat models reported that sucrose increased endorphins and brain-derived neurotrophic factor, which up-regulates neurogenesis and restores memory functions [48-50]. Interestingly, an increase in oxidative stress markers, which might lead to cellular damage was also reported after sucrose administration [47]. This raises questions as to whether sucrose can be should be the gold standard for non-pharmacological pain relief and studies examining long-term effects are needed.

The main limitation of the studies included in this review was the differences in the way pain was assessed. In preterm infants, heart rate or oxygen saturation variations may also have been due to physiological immaturity, entirely unrelated to the painful procedure or to the intervention. There is no standardized approach to the measurement of pain and each study used different scores e.g., Premature Infant Pain Profile score, Neonatal Infant Pain Scale score, Douleur Aiguë du Nouveau-né scale (a French scale of neonatal pain) [24], Face, Legs, Activity, Cry and Consolability Pain Scale [30], which makes it impossible to compare studies in a meta-analysis.

There are also limitations to the effectiveness of the non-pharmacological methods depending on many factors. Studies suggest that gestational age might influence the response to non-pharmacological treatments. Studies comparing sucrose with breast milk reported similar pain scores in infants >28 weeks' gestation [23], while infants <28 weeks' gestation had significantly lower pain scores after oral sucrose but not after breast milk [31]. Skin-to-skin care, swaddling and facilitated tucking is limited to times when the infant's position is not crucial and is not suitable for emergency procedures or for procedures dependent on position (e.g., lumbar puncture). Breastfeeding also may not always be available (e.g., in NICU or mother not present). If the infant is very ill, a lot of the interventions may not be possible.

One of the major advantages to using these non-pharmacological methods is their high safety profile. Most importantly, all these interventions have a very favorable benefit to risk ratio, even if the benefits are modest—the risk is extremely low. Supervision and support from staff helps with safety concerns for SSC, swaddling, massage therapy, facilitated tucking and BF such as improper technique, holding or positioning [51]. When using laser acupuncture, the infant and acupuncturists must wear protective ear-gear as well as cover any reflective surface to prevent the laser from hitting one's eye. Yates et al. assessed the safety of non-invasive electrical stimulation at acupuncture points (NESAP) by observing skin reactions, vital signs and PIPP scores [52]. There were no significant changes found in these measures and no adverse events occurred, which concludes that NESAP is safe [52]. Some of the main challenges in implementation is reluctance from staff or parents, due to disbelief or the invasiveness of the procedure (e.g., use of needle acupuncture in infants).

The major benefit of non-pharmacological treatments includes (i) ease of use, (ii) apparent safety, (iii) feasibility, and (iv) ease of learning, which would allow universal implementation of any of these interventions. However, acupuncture using needle or laser would require training and experience about the specific acupuncture points, and lasers might not be readily available. The long-term effects of any non-pharmacological intervention have not been studied and is a major knowledge gap, that needs to be addressed.

5. Conclusions

Newborn infants in an NICU undergo many painful but necessary procedures during hospitalizations. The implications of the pain associated with these procedures and the types of pain relief given to the infants have considerable implication for both short- and long-term outcomes. The evidence for non-pharmacological analgesia is sparse and needs further study. While most appear to be safe and relatively effective, their effects on the long-term outcomes of the infants is unknown, especially when coupled with pharmacological analgesia.

Author Contributions: Conception and design: G.M.S., J.-L.O., I.Q.-S., A.K.M.; Collection and assembly of data: G.M.S., J.-L.O., I.Q.-S., A.K.M.; Analysis and interpretation of the data: G.M.S., J.-L.O., I.Q.-S., A.K.M., K.C.; Drafting of the article: G.M.S., J.-L.O., I.Q.-S., A.K.M., K.C.; Critical revision of the article for important intellectual content: G.M.S., J.-L.O., I.Q.-S., A.K.M., K.C.; Final approval of the article: G.M.S., J.-L.O., I.Q.-S., A.K.M., K.C.

Funding: We would like to thank the public for donating money to our funding agencies: G.M.S. is a recipient of the Heart and Stroke Foundation/University of Alberta Professorship of Neonatal Resuscitation, a National New Investigator of the Heart and Stroke Foundation Canada and an Alberta New Investigator of the Heart and Stroke Foundation Alberta. This research has been facilitated by the Women and Children's Health Research Institute through the generous support of the Stollery Children's Hospital Foundation.

Conflicts of Interest: The authors declare no conflict of interest.

Appendix A

Search of PubMed—last performed 4 June 2018
#1 infant (n = 1,119,189)
#2 infants (n = 1,159,867)
#3 preterm (n = 62,246)

#4	premature (n = 170,785)
#5	pain (n = 733,273)
#6	relief (n = 84,761)
#6	acupuncture (n = 28,139)
#7	skin-to-skin care (n = 47,999)
#8	non-nutritive sucking (n = 367)
#9	sucrose (n = 74,579)
#10	massage (n = 13,982)
#11	music (n = 22,562)
#12	breastfeeding (n = 49,518)
#13	non-pharmacological (n = 6513)

Search of Google Scholar—last performed 4 June 2018

#1	infant (n = 3,220,000)
#2	infants (n = 2,080,000)
#3	preterm (n = 1,010,000)
#4	premature (n = 2,840,000)
#5	pain (n = 3,770,000)
#6	relief (n = 2,390,000)
#6	acupuncture (n = 592,000)
#7	skin-to-skin care (n = 3,820,000)
#8	non-nutritive sucking (n = 21,900)
#9	sucrose (n = 2,640,000)
#10	massage (n = 773,000)
#11	music (n = 3,770,000)
#12	breastfeeding (n = 649,000)
#13	non-pharmacological (n = 2,540,000)

References

1. Cignacco, E.; Hamers, J.P.; Stoffel, L.; Lingen, R.A.; Gessler, P.; McDougall, J.; Nelle, M. The efficacy of non-pharmacological interventions in the management of procedural pain in preterm and term neonates. *Eur. J. Pain* **2007**, *11*, 139–152. [CrossRef] [PubMed]
2. Saad, H.H.; Bours, G.J.J.W.; Stevens, B.; Hamers, J.P.H. Assessment of pain in the neonate. *Semin. Perinatol.* **1998**, *22*, 402–416. [CrossRef]
3. Barker, D.P.; Rutter, N. Exposure to invasive procedures in neonatal intensive care unit admissions. *Arch. Dis. Child.-Fetal Neonatal Ed.* **1995**, *72*, 47–48. [CrossRef]
4. Meaney, M.J.; Aitken, D.H. The effects of early postnatal handling on hippocampal glucocorticoid receptor concentrations: Temporal parameters. *Brain Res.* **1985**, *354*, 301–304. [CrossRef]
5. Taddio, A.; Katz, J.; Ilersich, A.L.; Koren, G. Effect of neonatal circumcision on pain response during subsequent routine vaccination. *Lancet* **1997**, *349*, 599–603. [CrossRef]
6. American and Canadian Academy of Pediatrics. Prevention and management of pain and stress in the neonate. *Pediatrics* **2000**, *15*, 454–461.
7. Taddio, A. Opioid analgesia for infants in the neonatal intensive care unit. *Clin. Perinatol.* **2002**, *29*, 493–509. [CrossRef]
8. Melzack, R.; Wall, P.D. Pain mechanism: A new theory. *Science* **1965**, *150*, 971–979. [CrossRef] [PubMed]
9. Shabani, F.; Nayeri, N.D.; Karimi, R.; Zarei, K.; Chehrazi, M. Effects of music therapy on pain responses induced by blood sampling in premature infants: A randomized cross-over trial. *Iran. J. Nurs. Midwifery Res.* **2016**, *21*, 391–396. [PubMed]
10. Seo, Y.S.; Lee, J.; Ahn, H.Y. Effects of Kangaroo Care on Neonatal Pain in South Korea. *J. Trop. Pediatr.* **2016**, *62*, 246–249. [CrossRef] [PubMed]
11. Freire, N.B.; Garcia, J.B.; Lamy, Z.C. Evaluation of analgesic effect of skin-to-skin contact compared to oral glucose in preterm neonates. *Pain* **2008**, *139*, 28–33. [CrossRef] [PubMed]
12. Olsson, E.; Ahlsén, G.; Eriksson, M. Skin-to-skin contact reduces near-infrared spectroscopy pain responses in premature infants during blood sampling. *Acta Paediatr.* **2016**, *105*, 376–380. [CrossRef] [PubMed]

13. Efendi, D.; Rustina, Y.; Gayatri, D. Pacifier and swaddling effective in impeding premature infant's pain score and heart rate. *Enferm. Clin.* **2018**, *1*, 46–50. [CrossRef]
14. Erkut, Z.; Yıldız, S. The Effect of Swaddling on Pain, Vital Signs, and Crying Duration during Heel Lance in Newborns. *Pain Manag. Nurs.* **2017**, *18*, 328–336. [CrossRef] [PubMed]
15. Ho, L.P.; Ho, S.S.; Leung, D.Y.; So, W.K.; Chan, C.W. A feasibility and efficacy randomized controlled trial of swaddling for controlling procedural pain in preterm infants. *J. Clin. Nurs.* **2016**, *25*, 472–482. [CrossRef] [PubMed]
16. Axelin, A.; Salanteräa, S.; Lehtonenb, L. Facilitated tucking by parents' in pain management of preterm infants—A randomized crossover trial. *Early Hum. Dev.* **2006**, *8*, 241–247. [CrossRef] [PubMed]
17. Arikan, D.; Alp, H.; Gözüm, S.; Orbak, Z.; Cifçi, E.K. Effectiveness of massage, sucrose solution, herbal tea or hydrolysed formula in the treatment of infantile colic. *J. Clin. Nurs.* **2008**, *17*, 1754–1761. [PubMed]
18. Chik, Y.M.; Ip, W.Y.; Choi, K.C. The Effect of Upper Limb Massage on Infants' Venipuncture Pain. *Pain Manag. Nurs.* **2017**, *18*, 50–57. [CrossRef] [PubMed]
19. Jain, S.; Kumar, P.; McMillan, D.D. Prior leg massage decreases pain responses to heel stick in preterm babies. *J. Paediatr. Child Health* **2006**, *42*, 505–508. [CrossRef] [PubMed]
20. Zhu, J.; Hong-Gu, H.; Zhou, X.; Wei, H.; Gao, Y.; Ye, B.; Liu, Z.; Chan, S.W. Pain relief effect of breast feeding and music therapy during heel lance for healthy-term neonates in China: A randomized controlled trial. *Midwifery* **2015**, *31*, 365–372. [CrossRef] [PubMed]
21. Shah, S.R.; Kadage, S.; Sinn, J. Trial of Music, Sucrose, and Combination Therapy for Pain Relief during Heel Prick Procedures in Neonates. *J. Pediatr.* **2017**, *190*, 153–158.e2. [CrossRef] [PubMed]
22. Zurita-Cruz, J.N.; Rivas-Ruiz, R.; Gordillo-Álvarez, V.; Villasis-Keever, M.Á. Breastfeeding for acute pain control on infants: A randomized controlled trial. *Nutr. Hosp.* **2017**, *34*, 301–307. [CrossRef] [PubMed]
23. Erkul, M.; Efe, E. Efficacy of Breastfeeding on Babies' Pain During Vaccinations. *Breastfeed. Med.* **2017**, *12*, 110–115. [CrossRef] [PubMed]
24. Simonse, E.; Mulder, P.G.; van Beek, R.H. Analgesic effect of breast milk versus sucrose for analgesia during heel lance in late preterm infants. *Pediatrics* **2012**, *129*, 657–663. [CrossRef] [PubMed]
25. Baudesson de Chanville, A.; Brevaut-Malaty, V.; Garbi, A.; Tosello, B.; Baumstarck, K.; Gire, C. Analgesic Effect of Maternal Human Milk Odor on Premature Neonates: A Randomized Controlled Trial. *J. Hum. Lact.* **2017**, *33*, 300–308. [CrossRef] [PubMed]
26. Zhao, Z. Neural mechanism underlying acupuncture analgesia. *Prog. Neurobiol.* **2008**, *85*, 355–375. [CrossRef] [PubMed]
27. Chen, K.L.; Lindrea, K.B.; Quah-Smith, I.; Schmölzer, G.M.; Daly, M.; Schindler, T.; Oei, J.L. Magnetic noninvasive acupuncture for infant comfort (MAGNIFIC)—A single-blinded randomised controlled pilot trial. *Acta Paediatr.* **2017**, *106*, 1780–1786. [CrossRef] [PubMed]
28. Abbasoğlu, A.; Cabıoğlu, M.T.; Tuğcu, A.U.; İnce, D.A.; Tekindal, M.A.; Ecevit, A.; Tarcan, A. Acupressure at BL60 and K3 Points Before Heel Lancing in Preterm Infants. *EXPLORE J. Sci. Heal.* **2015**, *11*, 363–366. [CrossRef] [PubMed]
29. Lima, A.; Santos, V.; Nunes, M.; Barreto, J.; Ribeiro, C.; Carvalho, J.; Ribeiro, M. Glucose solution is more effective in relieving pain in neonates than non-nutritive sucking: A randomized clinical trial. *Eur. J. Pain* **2017**, *21*, 159–165. [CrossRef] [PubMed]
30. Gouin, S.; Gaucher, N.; Lebel, D.; Desjardins, M.P. A Randomized Double-Blind Trial Comparing the Effect on Pain of an Oral Sucrose Solution vs. Placebo in Children 1 to 3 Months Old Undergoing Simple Venipuncture. *J. Emerg. Med.* **2018**, *54*, 33–39. [CrossRef] [PubMed]
31. Collados-Gómez, L.; Ferrera-Camacho, P.; Fernandez-Serran, E.; Camacho-Vicente, V.; Flores-Herrero, C.; García-Pozo, A.; Jiménez-García, R. Randomised crossover trial showed that using breast milk or sucrose provided the same analgesic effect in preterm infants of at least 28 weeks. *Acta Paediatr.* **2018**, *107*, 436–441. [CrossRef] [PubMed]
32. Hebb, A.L.; Poulin, J.F.; Roach, S.P.; Zacharko, R.M.; Drolet, G. Cholecystokinin and endogenous opioid peptides: Interactive influence on pain, cognition, and emotion. *Prog. Neuropsychopharmacol. Biol. Psychiatry* **2005**, *29*, 1225–1238. [CrossRef] [PubMed]
33. Huang, C.M.; Tung, W.S.; Kuo, L.L.; Chang, Y.J. Comparison of pain responses of premature infants to the heelstick between containment and swaddling. *J. Nurs. Res.* **2004**, *12*, 31–35. [CrossRef] [PubMed]

34. Esfahani, M.S.; Sheykhi, S.; Abdeyazdan, Z.; Jodakee, M.; Boroumandfar, K. A comparative study on vaccination pain in the methods of massage therapy and mothers' breastfeeding during injection of infants referring to Navabsafavi Health Care Center in Isfahan. *Iran. J. Nurs. Midwifery Res.* **2013**, *18*, 494–498. [PubMed]
35. Bellieni, C.V.; Buonocore, G.; Nenci, A.; Franci, N.; Cordelli, D.M.; Bagnoli, F. Sensorial saturation: An effective analgesic tool for heel-prick in preterm infants. *Neonatology* **2001**, *80*, 15–18. [CrossRef] [PubMed]
36. Yurkovich, J.; Burns, D.S.; Harrison, T. The Effect of Music Therapy Entrainment on Physiologic Measures of Infants in the Cardiac Intensive Care Unit: Single Case Withdrawal Pilot Study. *J. Music Ther.* **2018**, *55*, 62–82. [CrossRef] [PubMed]
37. Olischar, M.; Shoemark, H.; Holton, T.; Weninger, M.; Hunt, R.W. The influence of music on aEEG activity in neurologically healthy newborns ≥32 weeks' gestational age. *Acta Paediatr.* **2011**, *100*, 670–675. [CrossRef] [PubMed]
38. Porter, R.H.; Winberg, J. Unique salience of maternal breast odors for newborn infants. *Neurosci. Biobehav. Rev.* **1999**, *23*, 439–449. [CrossRef]
39. Lima, A.H.; Hermont, A.P.; Friche, A.A.L. Analgesia in newborns: A case-control study of the efficacy of nutritive and non-nutritive sucking stimuli. *CoDAS* **2013**, *25*, 365–368. [CrossRef] [PubMed]
40. Napadow, V.; Ahn, A.; Longhurst, J.; Lao, L.; Stener-Victorin, E.; Harris, R.; Langevin, H.M. The status and future of acupuncture mechanism research. *J. Altern. Complement. Med.* **2008**, *14*, 861–869. [CrossRef] [PubMed]
41. Quah-Smith, I.; Sachdev, P.S.; Wen, W.; Chen, X.; Williams, M.A. The Brain Effects of Laser Acupuncture in Healthy Individuals: An fMRI Investigation. *PLoS ONE* **2010**, *5*, e12619. [CrossRef] [PubMed]
42. Cho, Z.H.; Oleson, T.D.; Alimi, D.; Niemtzow, R.C. Acupuncture: The search for biologic evidence with functional magnetic resonance imaging and positron emission tomography techniques. *J. Altern. Complement. Med.* **2002**, *8*, 399–401. [CrossRef] [PubMed]
43. Mitchell, A.J.; Hall, R.W.; Golianu, B.; Yates, C.; Williams, D.K.; Chang, J.; Anand, K.J. Does noninvasive electrical stimulation of acupuncture points reduce heelstick pain in neonates? *Acta Paediatr.* **2016**, *105*, 1434–1439. [CrossRef] [PubMed]
44. Holsti, L.; Grunau, R.E. Considerations for using sucrose to reduce procedural pain in preterm infants. *Pediatrics* **2010**, *125*, 1042–1047. [CrossRef] [PubMed]
45. Blass, E.M.; Ciaramitaro, V. A new look at some old mechanisms in newborns: Taste and tactile determinants of state, affect and action. *Monogr. Soc. Child Dev.* **1994**, *59*, 1–81. [CrossRef]
46. Marceau, J.R.; Murray, H.; Nanan, R.K. Efficacy of oral sucrose in infants of methadone-maintained mothers. *Neonatology* **2010**, *97*, 67–70. [CrossRef] [PubMed]
47. Asmerom, Y.; Slater, L.; Boskovic, D.S.; Bahjri, K.; Holden, M.S.; Phillips, R.; Deming, D.; Ashwal, S.; Fayard, E.; Angeles, D.M. Oral sucrose for heel lance increases adenosine triphosphate use and oxidative stress in preterm neonates. *J. Pediatr.* **2013**, *163*, 29–35. [CrossRef] [PubMed]
48. Nuseir, K.Q.; Alzoubi, K.H.; Alabwaini, J.; Khabour, O.F.; Kassab, M.I. Sucrose-induced analgesia during early life modulates adulthood learning and memory formation. *Physiol. Behav.* **2015**, *145*, 84–90. [CrossRef] [PubMed]
49. Siuciak, J.A.; Wong, V.; Perasall, D.; Weigand, S.J.; Lindsay, R.M. BDNF produces analgesia in the formalin test and modifies neuropeptide levels in rat brain and spinal cord areas associated with nociception. *Eur. J. Neurosci.* **1995**, *7*, 663–670. [CrossRef] [PubMed]
50. Zhang, H.; Torregrossa, M.M.; Jutkiewica, E.M. Endogenous opioids upregulate brain-derived neurotrophic factor mRNA through delta- and micro-opioid receptors independent of antidepressant-like effects. *Eur. J. Neurosci.* **2006**, *23*, 984–994. [CrossRef] [PubMed]
51. Feldman-Winter, L.; Goldsmith, J.P. Safe Sleep and Skin-to-Skin Care in the Neonatal Period for Healthy Term Newborns. *Pediatrics* **2016**, *138*, e20161889. [CrossRef] [PubMed]
52. Yates, C.C.; Mitchell, A.J.; Lowe, L.M.; Lee, A.; Hall, R.W. Safety of Noninvasive Electrical Stimulation of Acupuncture Points During a Routine Neonatal Heel Stick. *Med. Acupunct.* **2013**, *25*, 285–290. [CrossRef] [PubMed]

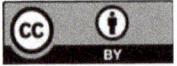

© 2018 by the authors. Licensee MDPI, Basel, Switzerland. This article is an open access article distributed under the terms and conditions of the Creative Commons Attribution (CC BY) license (http://creativecommons.org/licenses/by/4.0/).

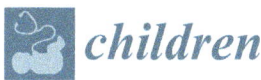

Review

Multidisciplinary Pain Management for Pediatric Patients with Acute and Chronic Pain: A Foundational Treatment Approach When Prescribing Opioids

Anava A. Wren [1], Alexandra C. Ross [2], Genevieve D'Souza [3], Christina Almgren [3], Amanda Feinstein [3], Amanda Marshall [4] and Brenda Golianu [3,*]

1. Department of Pediatrics, Division of Pediatric Gastroenterology, Hepatology and Nutrition, Stanford University, Palo Alto, CA 94305, USA; awren2@stanford.edu
2. Department of Pediatrics, Child and Adolescent Headache Program, University of California San Francisco, San Francisco, CA 94158, USA; alexandra.ross2@ucsf.edu
3. Department of Anesthesiology Perioperative and Pain Medicine, Stanford University, Palo Alto, CA 94305, USA; gdsouza@stanford.edu (G.D); calmgren@stanfordchildrens.org (C.A.); abfein@stanford.edu (A.F.)
4. Centre for Clinical Brain Sciences, University of Edinburgh, Edinburgh EH16 4SB, UK; a.marshall-15@sms.ed.ac.uk
* Correspondence: bgolianu@stanford.edu; Tel.: +1-650-723-5728

Received: 11 December 2018; Accepted: 13 February 2019; Published: 21 February 2019

Abstract: Opioid therapy is the cornerstone of treatment for acute procedural and postoperative pain and is regularly prescribed for severe and debilitating chronic pain conditions. Although beneficial for many patients, opioid therapy may have side effects, limited efficacy, and potential negative outcomes. Multidisciplinary pain management treatments incorporating pharmacological and integrative non-pharmacological therapies have been shown to be effective in acute and chronic pain management for pediatric populations. A multidisciplinary approach can also benefit psychological functioning and quality of life, and may have the potential to reduce reliance on opioids. The aims of this paper are to: (1) provide a brief overview of a multidisciplinary pain management approach for pediatric patients with acute and chronic pain, (2) highlight the mechanisms of action and evidence base of commonly utilized integrative non-pharmacological therapies in pediatric multidisciplinary pain management, and (3) explore the opioid sparing effects of multidisciplinary treatment for pediatric pain.

Keywords: multidisciplinary pain management strategies; opioid reduction therapy; non-pharmacological therapy; cognitive behavioral therapy; hypnosis; mindfulness-based stress reduction; acupuncture; pain rehabilitation

1. Introduction

Acute and chronic pain are common and often debilitating problems among both pediatric and adult populations according to the Institute of Medicine statement on Relieving Pain in America. The International Association of the Study of Pain (IASP) defines pain as an unpleasant sensory and emotional experience associated with actual or potential tissue damage or described in terms of such damage [1]. Acute pain is the expected physiological response to a noxious chemical, thermal, or mechanical stimulus, and usually accompanies surgery, traumatic injury, tissue damage, or inflammatory processes. It is self-limiting and typically resolves over days to weeks, but it can persist longer as healing occurs [2]. Chronic pain is defined as intractable pain that exists for three or more months despite adequate treatment [1,3].

Opioid therapy is the cornerstone of treatment for acute procedural and postoperative pain in pediatric populations, and is also regularly prescribed for severe and debilitating chronic pain conditions [4]. Despite the benefits of opioids for pain management, opioids have been associated with a range of side effects including respiratory depression, constipation, cognitive dysfunction, and psychiatric comorbidities [5–8]. Persistent opioid use is also associated with physical tolerance, dependence, and addiction [9], as well as heightened pain sensitization [10].

Given the potential for negative outcomes related to opioid use, there have been increased efforts to use multidisciplinary analgesia treatments (i.e., the concurrent use of treatment provided by practitioners from different disciplines) [11]. Combining pharmacological and integrative non-pharmacological therapies, which operate via different modes of action, has been shown to decrease opioid use and related adverse side effects in the perioperative period, as well as improve acute pain symptoms and emotional wellbeing [12]. When acute pain transforms to chronic pain, the consideration of multidisciplinary care may become even more central in facilitating patient comfort, decreasing reliance on opioid therapy, and improving functionality. Of note, in 2016, the CDC published recommended guidelines for prescribing opioids for adults with non-malignant chronic pain in the US stating [13]:

"Nonpharmacologic therapy and nonopioid pharmacologic therapy are preferred for chronic pain. Clinicians should consider opioid therapy only if expected benefits for both pain and function are anticipated to outweigh risks to the patient. If opioids are used, they should be combined with nonpharmacologic therapy and nonopioid pharmacologic therapy, as appropriate."

For patients 18 years and younger, there do not yet exist specific consensus guidelines on prescribing opioids for chronic pain [4,14,15]. Pediatric practitioners are advised to use their best judgment when using opioids after appropriate use of nonopioid alternatives. Opioids are not usually indicated as a first line therapy for primary pain disorders [16]. However, current evidence suggests that opioid prescriptions should not be curtailed for moderately to severely painful conditions [17,18].

Aims

Overall, multidisciplinary treatment is important to consider in the treatment of both acute and chronic pain. The aims of this paper are to: (1) provide a brief overview of a multidisciplinary pain management approach for pediatric patients with acute and chronic pain, (2) highlight the mechanisms of action and evidence base of commonly utilized integrative non-pharmacological therapies in pediatric multidisciplinary pain management, and (3) explore the opioid sparing effects of multidisciplinary treatments for pediatric pain.

This article will discuss the evidence base of several integrative non-pharmacological treatments (cognitive behavioral therapy, mindfulness, medical hypnosis, acupuncture) for the general pediatric practitioner to consider as part of a multidisciplinary treatment plan in the management of complex pain conditions. The therapies discussed were chosen as they are among the most frequently utilized integrative non-pharmacological therapies in pediatric pain clinics [19]. The aim of this review is not to be exhaustive of each integrative non-pharmacological therapy, but rather to provide an overview of the specific therapy, briefly review mechanisms of action as currently understood, and provide relevant research on the topic. While a systematic review of the aforementioned integrative non-pharmacological therapies is outside the scope of this current paper (for several excellent and relevant systematic reviews, please see Fisher et al., 2018 [20] and Kamper et al., 2015 [21]), the overarching goal of this paper is to educate the general pediatric practitioner in evidence-based integrative non-pharmacological therapies included in multidisciplinary pain management to optimize care for youth with acute and chronic pain conditions.

Throughout this paper, we review both pediatric and adult literature. A search was performed using Pubmed, Ovid, Embase, Prospero, Medline, and Cochrane Database on the following topics in both pediatric and adult literature from 2000 to 2018 (see Table 1). Inclusion criteria were: pediatric chronic pain and each of the following: multidisciplinary treatment, cognitive behavioral therapy, mindfulness, hypnosis, acupuncture, and pain rehabilitation. Opioids and opioid reduction therapy were also used as inclusion criteria with each modality. Exclusion criteria were: pediatric procedural pain, acute pediatric pain, pharmacological management of pediatric pain, and regional management of pediatric pain.

Table 1. Search data for pediatric pain articles and selected integrative non-pharmacological therapies (2000–2018).

Modalities	Ovid	Embase	Prospero	Cochrane	Pubmed	Number of Articles Screened	Number of Articles Reviewed
CBT	42	537	2	2	274	48	12
Mindfulness	37	53	2	17	26	45	25
Hypnosis	164	272	1	1	152	28	14
Acupuncture	149	357	2	24	132	32	14
Intensive Rehab	189	164	2	51	87	15	6
Multidisciplinary	324	1232	1	19	546	52	13

CBT = Cognitive Behavioral Therapy.

Regarding article selection criteria, studies were screened and identified by two authors (AW and AR for Cognitive Behavioral Therapy (CBT), mindfulness and hypnosis; CA and GD for multidisciplinary pain management, acupuncture and rehabilitation), and when a consensus could not be reached regarding the inclusion/exclusion of an article in this review BG mediated and made a final decision. The research team prioritized systematic reviews, non-systematic reviews, and randomized controlled studies of these therapies in pediatric pain. Where these were not available, we identified pilot studies in pediatric pain populations to provide the reader with the current state of science and preliminary evidence for a given integrative non-pharmacological therapy. Pediatric pain articles were supplemented with adult articles where systematic reviews were not available, and where studies investigating mechanisms of action were well elucidated in the adult literature and not studied in pediatrics. Of note, adult studies exploring potential mechanisms of action for integrative non-pharmacological therapies are not meant to imply that adult mechanisms are the same as pediatric mechanisms of action, but rather to inform the reader of the current evidence base of this emerging field of research. Due to limitations of space, the use of these interventions to address specific procedural and/or acute pain is not discussed.

2. Multidisciplinary Pain Management Overview

Evidence suggests that multidisciplinary analgesia treatments incorporating nonopioid pharmacological and integrative non-pharmacological therapies can be effective for both acute and chronic pain management, and can improve patients' quality of life and general wellbeing [13,21–24]. Integrative non-pharmacological therapies include modalities such as cognitive behavioral therapy (CBT), mindfulness, medical hypnosis, acupuncture, massage, and music therapy [25]. See Figure 1 for an overview of some elements of multidisciplinary pain management treatment.

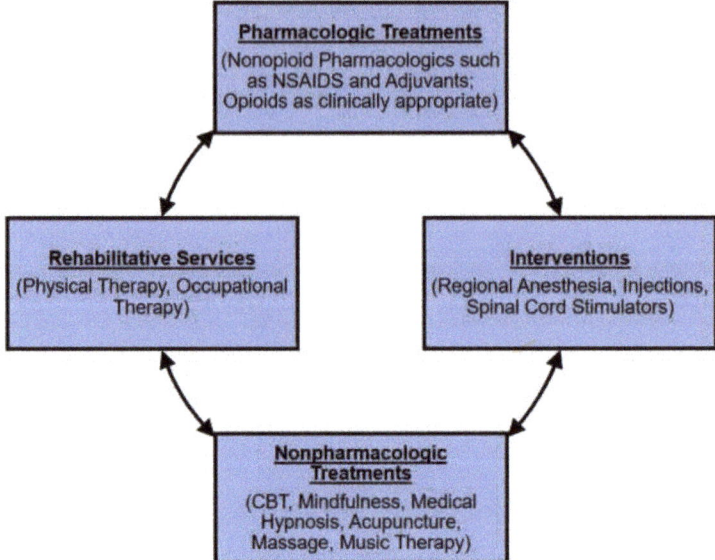

Figure 1. Multidisciplinary pain management treatment: key components in acute and chronic pain management. This figure displays the key treatment components in multidisciplinary treatment for both acute and chronic pain. In the acute setting, in addition to reduction of pain, the efficacy of multidisciplinary treatments is often measured by reduction in needed opioid doses to achieve comfort, while in the setting of chronic pain, the improvements obtained through a multidisciplinary approach are often measured by improvements in function. As is clinically appropriate, in both settings, pharmacologic treatments are combined with regional interventions [26], integrative non-pharmacological techniques, and rehabilitative services as is clinically appropriate to support pain management and improve patients' pain symptoms, functioning and quality of life. Multidisciplinary analgesia treatment aims to ensure patient comfort and wellbeing, while at the same time potentially decreasing the need for opioid use in pediatric populations [25].

2.1. Acute Multidisciplinary Pain Management

Multimodal treatment is defined as "the concurrent use of separate therapeutic interventions with different mechanisms of action within one discipline aimed at different pain mechanisms" [11]. This treatment approach involving multiple medications for pain management is considered optimal in the setting of acute pain (see Figure 2), where the primary goal is immediate analgesia sufficient to allow for the recovery from medical treatments/procedures with minimal side effects.

While acute pain management has historically emphasized the use of opioids, multimodal analgesia treatment incorporates opioid-sparing adjuvants targeting specific aspects of the nociceptive and neuropathic pain physiology. Nociceptive analgesics include acetaminophen, NSAIDS, and glucocorticoids. Neuropathic analgesics commonly include gabapentinoids, lidocaine, ketamine, and alpha 2 agonists. Regional anesthesia and injection of local anesthetics are also regularly utilized to allow targeted analgesia to a specific surgical area. These agents provide safe and effective analgesia and sedation and may help reduce the need for opioid therapies [27–29].

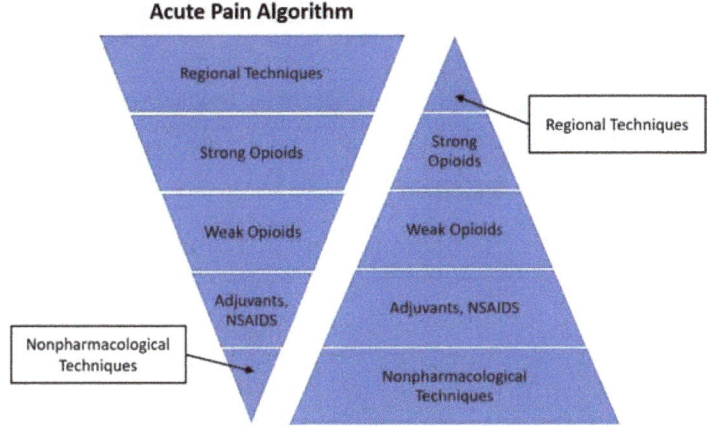

Figure 2. Multidisciplinary pain management: acute and chronic pain algorithms. In acute pain algorithms, the initial treatment begins with regional techniques or intravenous analgesia as a mainstay of therapy. As acute pain improves, therapies are then transitioned as appropriate to varying strengths of PO opioid medications, to adjuvants/NSAIDS, and ultimately integrative non-pharmacological strategies. For situations where severe pain is anticipated, adjuvants and integrative non-pharmacological strategies may be added on at the beginning of treatment, as an opioid sparing strategy, and to increase patient comfort. In chronic pain algorithms, treatment is delivered in the reverse order, beginning with integrative non-pharmacological techniques, then moving to adjuvants, and ultimately progressing to various strengths of opioids and regional techniques and stimulators as clinically appropriate.

Acute pharmacological interventions can be enhanced by the assistance of integrative non-pharmacological interventions (i.e., multidisciplinary treatment). In treatment of pediatric acute pain, the integration of a psychologist or child life specialist into the treatment team can support pain management efforts in the perioperative period by educating the patient in an age appropriate manner about medical procedures, a pain management plan, and implementing behavioral pain management interventions (e.g., distraction, play, active relaxation training) to reduce post-operative pain and anxiety [30]. An acupuncturist or massage therapist can also support acute pediatric pain management following medical procedures and surgeries [31,32]. Incorporating integrative non-pharmacological therapies into multidisciplinary analgesia treatments for acute pediatric pain has been shown to reduce perioperative anxiety and procedural pain [33,34], and thus has the potential to reduce pediatric patients' reliance on pharmacological interventions such as opioids and benzodiazepines. Preliminary evidence supports this notion, demonstrating that even in an acute medical setting such as the management of perioperative pain following a minimally invasive surgery for Pectus Excavatum repair (Nuss procedure) in adolescents, the addition of an integrative non-pharmacological therapy (in this example, self-hypnosis instruction preoperatively) can reduce pain, postoperative opioid use, and even length of hospital stay [35].

2.2. Chronic Multidisciplinary Pain Management

In the management of chronic pain, the emphasis shifts from immediate analgesia to extended pain management services and facilitation of function across domains (e.g., performance of activities of daily living). A multidisciplinary approach to chronic pain management (see Figure 2) has therefore increasingly become the standard of care in pediatric pain management settings. Chronic pain treatment places a central emphasis on integrative non-pharmacological techniques, minimizing side effects, and ideally providing the child skills they can use to more independently manage their symptoms.

Oftentimes, in pain management of complex patients, the utility of integrative non-pharmacological therapies is discussed only when all pharmaceutical therapy options have been exhausted. By then, the patient may begin to feel that medical care is somehow being limited or withdrawn, or that using integrative non-pharmacological therapies indicates that the "pain is in their head". This can lead to patients and families feeling resistant to learning and incorporating these essential integrative non-pharmacological pain management tools. In multidisciplinary chronic pain management, integrative non-pharmacological therapies are incorporated in early phases of treatment, along with appropriate pharmacological interventions to provide optimal care for complex pediatric patients.

Pharmacological interventions in this setting often include analgesics such as acetaminophen and nonsteroidal agents, gabapentinoids, clonidine, tricyclic antidepressants, and where appropriate serotonin-norepinephrine reuptake inhibitors. Another novel adjuvant therapy that deserves mention as a possible opioid sparing agent, cannabidiol (CBD), is gaining popularity in multimodal pain management. CBD is the nonpsychoactive cannabinoid identified in cannabis, while tetrahydrocannabinol or THC is responsible for the hallucinogenic side effects of cannabis [36]. Further research is needed to examine the efficacy and side effect profile of CBD in chronic pain management, and to elucidate side effects and risks.

Opioids are typically minimized in chronic pain management, as the analgesic benefits of opioids are often offset by their long-term negative side effects such as constipation, nausea, vomiting, and sedation, as well as the risk of tolerance, dependence, opioid-induced hyperalgesia, and addiction [5,6]. If opioids are deemed clinically necessary, weak opioids like Tramadol or Hydrocodone can be used in the initial treatment phase but stronger opioids may be needed with recalcitrant pain. Regional anesthesia also may play less of a role, as the duration of the local anesthetic and length of time a catheter can be safely inserted may not provide longer-term analgesic benefit.

3. Integrative Non-Pharmacological Therapies in Pediatric Multidisciplinary Pain Management

Incorporating integrative non-pharmacological interventions into pediatric multidisciplinary chronic pain management has been demonstrated to be feasible and effective and has become the gold standard of care [27,37–39]. These techniques aim to modulate psychological factors, improve coping abilities, and enhance emotional well-being. Specifically, these therapies are thought to target: cognitions (e.g., modifying the child's anxious thoughts related to distressing physical sensations), emotions (e.g., teaching the child emotion regulation strategies and distress tolerance skills to support reductions in negative emotional/somatic symptoms), behaviors (e.g., decreasing pain avoidance behaviors and increasing the use of coping skills), and sensory experiences (e.g., directly targeting pain perceptions through enhanced nervous system inhibitory processes) [37,40]. In contrast to short-term pharmacological management, which provide patients transitory benefit, integrative non-pharmacological techniques can lead to long-term results via changes in neural circuits that regulate habits, affect, and cognitive pain responses [41]. Directly addressing cognitive-affective processes may increase youths' coping repertoire of strategies to manage pain (short-term and long-term), regulate mood, improve psychological well-being and resiliency, and potentially buffer against opioid misuse.

For the purpose of this review, we focus on four frequently utilized interventions in U.S. pain clinics, which include three psychologically based interventions: cognitive behavioral therapy, mindfulness, and medical hypnosis. Acupuncture, an integrative medicine approach widely used in pain management clinics, is additionally reviewed [39,42–45]. Rehabilitative therapies, including physical and occupational therapy (PT, OT), are also an important part of the treatment of chronic pain and are regularly integrated into care to support pain management and increase function [39,46–49]. Of note, rehabilitative therapies are uniquely dependent on the condition being treated (e.g., back pain, ankle sprain, complex regional pain syndrome), and as such, a comprehensive review of PT and OT in pediatric pain was deemed outside the scope of this paper. Overall, there is growing evidence that integrative non-pharmacological techniques can provide lasting pain management benefits, [37] have the potential to decrease reliance on opioids [41], and may minimize side effects [50]. Recent evidence also suggests that interdisciplinary pain management programs can even support effective opioid weaning among youth with chronic pain [14,51]. The importance of integrating non-pharmacologic strategies into the care of youth with acute and chronic pain will be explored below. See Appendix A for a summary of select studies reviewed.

Lastly, it is important to highlight that the integrative non-pharmacological treatments reviewed below often require significant commitment and effort from both children and families, and while frequently effective, improvements typically occur over time. Some barriers to implementation include: patient and family "buy-in" to the proposed treatment; work, family, and scheduling demands; financial challenges; accessibility of local resources (e.g., no accessible providers trained in a particular treatment modality); and the general burden of care. Awareness, sensitivity, and attention to such issues are required on the part of providers to best support patients and families in structuring their multidisciplinary treatment plan.

3.1. Cognitive Behavioral Therapy

Cognitive behavioral therapy (CBT) is a form of psychotherapy that has empirical support across a wide range of child, adolescent, and adult populations and is considered an evidence-based intervention in multidisciplinary chronic pain management [52,53]. CBT is based on the premise that thoughts, emotions, and behaviors are closely connected, and how one perceives a situation can significantly influence emotional, behavioral, and physiological responses [54]. When considering CBT for the treatment of chronic pain, protocols often consist of behavioral strategies that encourage engagement in normal daily activities (e.g., activity pacing to increase functioning across domains), cognitive techniques that support challenging and reframing negative "self-talk" statements (e.g., acknowledging catastrophic pain-related thoughts—"This pain is ruining my life"—and using evidence to determine more helpful responses—"This pain is bothersome, but I can handle it and go forward"), and self-regulation skills that help decrease physiological arousal and increase relaxation and wellbeing (e.g., diaphragmatic breathing, progressive muscle relaxation). Acceptance and Commitment Therapy (ACT), an extension of CBT, aims to improve functioning by increasing the ability to act effectively in the presence of pain and distress (i.e., psychological flexibility) [55]. CBT strategies are effective with a wide age range when adapted to the specific developmental level of the child or adolescent [56].

Of note, in the adult literature, neuroimaging data suggest that cognitive reappraisal of pain, a central CBT strategy for patients with chronic pain, may impact pain experiences through top-down processes resulting in increased prefrontal cortex gray matter [57]. CBT has also been linked to increased activation in the ventrolateral prefrontal and lateral orbitofrontal cortices, providing additional support for the role of a cortical control mechanism in CBT [58]. Additionally, CBT for chronic pain has led to changes in somatosensory cortices, potentially reflecting alterations in the perception of noxious signals (i.e., adaptive responses to pain signals) [57].

3.1.1. Evidence for CBT and Pain Management

There is a strong evidence base for the effectiveness of CBT among adults with chronic pain. A meta-analysis of 25 randomized controlled trials of CBT for adults with chronic pain noted significant changes in patients' reported pain experiences, cognitive coping, and behavioral expressions of pain as compared to wait list controls [59].

CBT is also the most well-established psychological intervention among youth with chronic pain [20,60]. A growing evidence base of systematic reviews and meta-analyses have documented that behavioral and cognitive behavioral interventions can produce a medium to large effect on pain outcomes and small effect on disability in chronic pain populations (e.g., headache, abdominal pain). [37,61,62]. In one strong meta-analytic review of randomized controlled trials of psychological therapies for the management of chronic pain in children and adolescents, Palermo and colleagues noted positive effects of CBT on clinically significant pain reduction, with an odds ratio of 4.13 across 9 studies with 406 participants [61]. Recent research is also beginning to explore various models of treatment delivery for CBT for chronic pain including online modules [63] and group-based formats [64,65]. As compared to other evidence-based psychological therapies, CBT is currently the dominant therapeutic model implemented in both medical and non-medical settings and is viewed as well accepted by patients and providers alike [60].

3.1.2. CBT Summary

In sum, while additional research is needed (e.g., larger RCTs with varying treatment delivery modes and monitoring of longer-term follow-up), a growing body of literature demonstrates the efficacy of CBT protocols for children, teenagers, and adults with chronic pain. This evidence-based treatment is well accepted by patients and providers and is increasingly available to pediatric patients. Although youth in more remote areas may have limited access to cognitive behavioral interventions for chronic pain, the advent of web-based treatments holds promise for reaching a wider pediatric audience [63].

3.2. Mindfulness

Mindfulness has been described as the ability to be aware of the present moment and one's experiences (e.g., thoughts, emotions, body sensations) in a purposeful, non-judgmental manner [66]. Research demonstrates associations between mindfulness, psychological and physical well-being, and improved health outcomes [67–69]. Interventions and training programs targeting the cultivation of mindfulness (i.e., mindfulness-based interventions; MBIs) have received increasing attention in pain management in recent years. The primary goal of MBIs is to teach individuals mindfulness via a series of breathing, meditation, and movement exercises, all of which cultivate present-moment, compassionate awareness [66,70]. Bringing attention to the present in this manner aims to serve as a buffer from ruminating on bothersome physical symptoms such as pain, negative cognitions, and perceived stress that can contribute to the experience of pain [71–73].

Neuroimaging studies in adults have provided further support for the mechanisms by which mindfulness meditation practice can lead to change. Specifically, regions of the brain associated with sensory processing and the cognitive modulation of pain (e.g., thalamus, insula, anterior cingulate cortex, orbitofrontal cortex) [74,75] have high concentrations of opioid receptors, [75,76] prompting hypotheses that mindfulness practice may modulate the endogenous opioid system [77]. Other neuroimaging research proposes that mindfulness-induced analgesia is due to a more complex process engaging multiple brain networks and neurochemical mechanisms [78].

3.2.1. Evidence for MBIs and Pain Management

An increasing body of literature has demonstrated that mindfulness interventions are feasible and efficacious in adult pain populations. Systematic reviews and meta-analyses have documented that mindfulness-based protocols can significantly improve pain outcomes (e.g., pain severity, interference, and sensitivity), psychological distress (e.g., depression), and quality of life among adults [79–81].

In pediatric populations, pilot studies have demonstrated initial feasibility and acceptability of mindfulness-based interventions for children and adolescents experiencing a range of chronic pain conditions (e.g., musculoskeletal, neuropathic, headache, abdominal pain) [82–84]. These mindfulness protocols have also garnered preliminary empirical support for their efficacy in improving pain-related outcomes such as fibromyalgia symptoms, functional disability, cortisol levels, pain acceptance, and emotional distress among youth with pain symptoms [82–86]. The existing research is promising. For example, in one pilot randomized trial of a mindfulness-based intervention for female adolescents with chronic pain, patients reported improvements in coping with pain, and reductions in pre- and post-mindfulness session salivary cortisol levels ($p < 0.001$) [83]. The quality of this research; however, has varied from randomized controlled trials to pilot studies and is limited in generalizability by small sample sizes, lack of a control groups, and lack of random assignment [83,86–88].

Given the more robust body of literature supporting the use of mindfulness interventions with youth to address symptoms of anxiety and depression [89], MBIs have become increasingly popular and available in recent years. Many schools are beginning to implement skills-based learning for stress management, including mindfulness, bringing developmentally appropriate adaptations (e.g., teaching is varied and interactive) of the intervention directly to groups of children with little cost [90]. A recent well controlled sizable RCT compared the application of mindfulness-based stress reduction (MBSR) to a health education control group in 300 5th- to 8th-grade students in an urban public school setting and found significantly lower levels of somatization, depression, negative affect, negative coping, rumination, self-hostility, and post-traumatic symptom severity (all $p < 0.05$) as compared to control [91]. Attention to cultural and developmental aspects of the child and family are important in the successful implementation of these therapies as well. There is also increasing availability of mindfulness-based self-administered electronic resources that may help bring this intervention to the most underserved areas. While free or low cost and easily accessible, there is unfortunately little evidence yet available on the efficacy of these electronic resources [92].

3.2.2. Mindfulness Summary

Substantive findings support the use of mindfulness interventions among adults with chronic pain. While preliminary research among pediatric pain populations demonstrates feasibility and acceptability of MBI's among youth, further research to investigate adaptations of mindfulness protocols for children and adolescents with chronic pain is needed. Clinical judgment is recommended until published research can better guide the use of MBIs among youth with pain. That being said, mindfulness interventions may be low cost or free adjunctive treatments that have fewer side effects as compared to pharmacologic interventions.

3.3. Hypnosis

Hypnosis is another integrative non-pharmacological treatment increasingly used in multidisciplinary pain management. Hypnosis has been defined as a state of attentive and receptive concentration generating changes in individuals' experiences of themselves and their environment [93,94]. While hypnosis usually (but not always) involves relaxation, [95] this treatment modality differs from mindfulness meditation in the thoughtful and deliberate use of therapeutic suggestions to facilitate change in a targeted domain (in the case of hypnotic analgesia, the patient's sensory experience) [40].

Similar to the impact of opioids on the brain, hypnotic analgesia is hypothesized to enhance nervous system inhibitory processes that attenuate pain experiences [96] through a variety of brain areas involved in pain processing (for a detailed review, see Jensen and Patterson, 2015) [97]. Neuroimaging studies in adults conducted during hypnotic experiences have noted significant signal changes associated with sensation and perception (e.g., primary somatosensory cortex, thalamus, insula), as well as in sensorimotor integration pain systems (e.g., supplementary motor cortex) [97–99].

3.3.1. Evidence for Hypnosis and Pain Management

There is a growing evidence base supporting the efficacy of hypnotically induced analgesia, identifying medical hypnosis as a "well established treatment" for pain in adult populations [100,101]. A meta-analysis investigating hypnosis for acute and chronic pain management found that for 75% of patients across studies (18 studies; $n = 933$) hypnosis provided substantial pain relief and was shown to be superior to non-hypnotic psychological interventions [52].

While there is a significantly smaller pediatric research base, extant controlled studies indicate positive results for pain reduction using this treatment modality among pediatric populations.

Supportive findings for pain reduction have been noted in youth undergoing surgery, cancer patients, and young people diagnosed with irritable bowel syndrome (IBS) [102–105]. In one noteworthy randomized controlled trial of hypnosis for children with functional abdominal pain or IBS, hypnosis was demonstrated as highly superior to standard medical therapy in reducing both pain frequency and pain intensity ($p < 0.001$) [104]. Additionally, one recent randomized controlled trial examined self-hypnosis training for 22 self-selected adolescents hospitalized for the Nuss procedure [35]. The results of this study indicated that in addition to better pain control, self-hypnosis training was associated with use of fewer milligrams per hour of morphine equivalents throughout a patient's five-day hospitalization ($p = 0.005$). A smaller and earlier study exploring this same procedure (five treatment patients and five control patients) noted no significant difference between opioid use in these two groups, but did document a shorter hospital stay for adolescents in the self-hypnosis group [95]. Numerous uncontrolled trials report results that trend in a positive direction including additional trials of hypnosis for abdominal pain, cancer, headaches, and juvenile classic migraine [106–109].

National training for pediatric hypnosis exists to teach providers across disciplines (e.g., physicians, psychologists, nurses, child life specialists) to use hypnosis tools and integrate them into clinical practice. In-person provider training with a child and adolescent focus is recommended before implementing this modality. Notably, in many geographic locations, patients may not have access to a provider trained in pediatric hypnosis.

3.3.2. Hypnosis Summary

Like mindfulness-based interventions, hypnosis is a well-established integrative non-pharmacological intervention for chronic pain management among adults [100], and there is a smaller but growing research base for pediatric pain management and hypnosis [103,104]. While preliminary evidence is promising, more research will be necessary before providers can confidently assert that hypnosis aides in pain management in pediatric populations.

3.4. Acupuncture

Acupuncture is an ancient medical procedure that has been practiced in China and other East Asian countries for over 2000 years. The technique involves the placement of small needles at various locations in the body. Traditional explanations suggest that acupuncture works by activating and engaging movement in the body's own energy resources, termed "Qi" [110]. Traditionally, acupuncture has been employed for the prevention of disease, as well as an early intervention in emerging illness. As an adjunct to current medical practice, acupuncture is often employed late in the course of illness (e.g., to assist with pain, loss of function), as well as to support withdrawal from opioid therapy. Related therapies include electroacupuncture, acupressure, moxibustion (i.e., burning of an herb near an acupoint to create local warming), laser stimulation of acupoints, and non-invasive stimulation of acupoints utilizing a transcutaneous electrical nerve stimulator (TENS, referred to as TEAS).

Studies exploring the mechanisms of action involved in acupuncture to better understand how acupuncture can lead to improvements in symptoms such as pain and withdrawal have focused on several areas. First, fMRI studies have demonstrated that acupuncture can lead to changes in brain blood flow, including the activity of the default mode network (DMN), and normalization of activity in areas of the limbic system often referred to as the "pain matrix" (e.g., insula, anterior cingulate gyrus, prefrontal cortex) [47,111,112]. Other work has shown that acupuncture can stimulate endorphin release in the central nervous system [113]. Research has not elucidated exactly how the needling procedures lead to these changes in brain activity; however, one possible explanation suggests activation of the cholinergic anti-inflammatory pathway—a neural pathway that modulates the body's immune response to injury [114,115].

3.4.1. Evidence for Acupuncture and Pain Management

In 1997, the NIH conducted a Consensus Meeting, where studies of acupuncture were reviewed by an expert panel. It was determined that sufficient evidence was present to recommend acupuncture for the treatment of adult postoperative pain, postoperative dental pain, and nausea and vomiting [116]. Other promising indications included the treatment of addiction. Since that time, multiple clinical studies have demonstrated that acupuncture was efficacious in the treatment of chronic back pain, headaches, and osteoarthritis among adults [117–119].

Pediatric applications have centered on the use of acupuncture for both acute and chronic pain [120]. Of particular relevance, research has demonstrated that acupuncture can decrease acute postoperative pain among pediatric populations. In a prospective randomized controlled study, Lin and colleagues found that acupuncture led to a statistically significant reduction in pain and agitation ($p < 0.001$) among 60 children undergoing bilateral myringotomy and tympanostomy compared to a control condition [121]. Additionally, fewer youth required additional analgesia in the acupuncture versus control condition. In another randomized controlled trial, acupuncture led to significantly less pain ($p < 0.001$) following tonsillectomy compared to a sham acupuncture condition [122].

Acupuncture treatment may also be useful in reducing opioid-related withdrawal symptoms among pediatric populations. In a randomized controlled trial to treat Neonatal Abstinence Syndrome, acupuncture led to a shorter duration of morphine treatment (28 days vs. 39 days in the control group; $p = 0.019$) and hospital stay (35 vs. 50 days in the control group; $p = 0.048$) [123]. Another study demonstrated that a course of acupuncture was helpful in supporting infants wean off a high dose opioid infusion in the intensive care unit [43].

Several randomized studies have explored in more detail the effect of acupuncture on pediatric chronic pain. Gottschling and colleagues performed a randomized trial using laser acupuncture, a non-invasive type of acupuncture, with 43 children who suffered from either migraine or tension type headache. The mean number of headaches per month decreased by 6.4 days in the group which received acupuncture treatment, and by 1 day in the placebo group ($p < 0.001$). Secondary outcomes of headache severity likewise decreased and were statistically significant at all time points [124].

In a small randomized controlled trial comparing acupuncture with sham acupuncture, 14 adolescents with pelvic pain due to endometriosis experienced a 4.8 (SD 2.4) point reduction in pain (on an 11-point numeric rating scale) after 4 weeks, which differed significantly from the control group who experienced an average reduction of 1.4 (SD 2.1) ($p = 0.004$). Reduction in pain was found to persist six months post-intervention; however, after four weeks the differences were not clinically significant, suggesting continued acupuncture may be necessary for a more prolonged therapeutic effect [125].

3.4.2. Acupuncture Summary

Acupuncture appears to be an effective integrative non-pharmacological therapy in the management of acute postoperative pain and neonatal abstinence syndrome, and there is some preliminary evidence for chronic pediatric pain. Additional basic and clinical research is needed to adequately characterize the mechanisms of acupuncture and clinical effects on pain and withdrawal symptoms in pediatric populations. Given that acupuncture has been shown to be a well-tolerated and acceptable intervention among youth, feasible to implement in clinics, and has a low side effect profile, it should be considered for incorporation into multidisciplinary analgesia for youth with acute and chronic pain.

4. Intensive Interdisciplinary Pediatric Pain Rehabilitative Programs

As described above, the primary goal of pediatric pain management is functional restoration in concert with the management of discomfort. When multimodal analgesia and multidisciplinary outpatient care have not successfully met these goals, some youth are referred to comprehensive interdisciplinary pain programs. Interdisciplinary care involves "multimodal treatment provided by a multidisciplinary team collaborating in assessment and treatment using a shared biopsychosocial model and goals" [11]. This interdisciplinary approach involves escalation of intensity and quantity of standard therapies to better meet the need for this vulnerable population.

Intensive interdisciplinary pain treatment (IIPT) programs are becoming a popular treatment choice for children with chronic pain who exhibit significant functional disability and are unable to progress in an outpatient setting or for those who lack the proper resources in their local environment. IIPT involves patient and family participation in either an inpatient or outpatient day hospital setting with coordinated interventions among at least three disciplines including pain or rehabilitation physicians, psychologists, and physical and occupational therapists [38]. Logan et al. performed a longitudinal case series of 56 patients ages 8 to 18 suffering from Complex Regional Pain Syndrome (CRPS) and showed that an IIPT program led to improvements in functional disability, pain symptoms, medication use, and emotional functioning (all $p < 0.01$) [126]. Simons et al. showed that IIPT was superior to outpatient treatment with significantly larger improvements in functional disability, pain-related fear, and readiness to change among children with chronic pain [127]. Of note, Bruce et al. demonstrated that patients in a three-week IIPT program who were receiving opioids were able to be weaned off these medications and remained opioid-free at the 3-month follow-up [51]. While these results are promising, these studies require further investigation and corroboration. In the United States, 11 pediatric pain centers exist that offer this high level of coordinated treatment, varying in treatment duration (2–12 weeks) and daily treatment components [128].

5. Discussion

This article provides an overview of a multidisciplinary pain management approach for pediatric patients with acute and chronic pain, and highlights the evidence base of commonly utilized integrative non-pharmacological therapies for the treating pediatrician, primary health care pediatric provider, or non-pain pediatric specialist. The review explores a topic that is often overlooked in the medical literature, resulting in a noteworthy gap of knowledge among many providers caring for pediatric patients with complex medical and pain conditions. As such, this review aims to further inform providers about multidisciplinary pain management and highlight the role of integrative non-pharmacological therapies in medically complex situations by summarizing and synthesizing relevant literature. Currently, many patients often receive a medical cocktail including opioids, benzodiazepines, gabapentinoids, and other medications for pain management. The early incorporation of the integrative non-pharmacological therapies reviewed in this paper may help in lowering the doses of medications needed to attain comfort for this young and vulnerable population. Of note, there is preliminary evidence that some of the integrative non-pharmacological therapies reviewed, specifically hypnosis and acupuncture, may decrease the need for opioid therapy in inpatient populations (e.g., Nuss procedure, neonatal abstinence syndrome). While additional research is needed to explore the efficacy and generalizability of these results, these studies are encouraging and suggest that practitioners should specifically consider incorporating multidisciplinary pain management strategies where possible and feasible for patients for whom prolonged opioid therapy is being considered or prescribed for acute or chronic pain.

Additionally, many of the integrative non-pharmacological therapies reviewed consist of teaching skills that are applicable beyond an individual pain episode. The patient is taught to implement pain management skills themselves, which may increase the patient's personal efficacy, coping resources, and overall resilience. These integrative non-pharmacological therapies can provide effective pain relief and give patients the feeling that they are able to have some "control" over a difficult pain management problem. Through increased knowledge and familiarity with these therapies and multidisciplinary pain management, the general pediatric practitioner is better equipped to help pediatric patients feel empowered to explore evidence-based integrative non-pharmacological options, creating an integrative process of care that is holistic, safe, and effective.

Limitations

Although this paper is not a formal systematic review, it provides a thorough review of the literature that may be most pertinent to our intended audience—the general pediatric practitioner. The data base for the therapies described above in pediatric pain is still in its infancy, and therefore, few RCT's exist within several the integrative non-pharmacological topic areas described (see Table A1). In addition, the heterogeneity of study population and design precludes a systematic comparison that would be of value to the general reader. In some instances, there was no pediatric data available on a particular topic. While mechanisms of action may differ between adult and pediatric populations due to developmental effects, adult data was reviewed where it was available and felt to contribute to an understanding of a mechanism of action of the therapy.

6. Conclusions

Multidisciplinary pain management, including pharmacological and integrative non-pharmacological therapies, has been demonstrated to be efficacious in the treatment of both acute and chronic pain. Pharmacological interventions include opioids and opioid-sparing agents that target specific aspects of the nociceptive and neuropathic pain physiology. Simultaneously, integrative non-pharmacological interventions such as CBT, MBIs, hypnosis, and acupuncture target the cognitive-affective and physiologic components of the pain experience, and support the cultivation of coping tools that can lead to long-term improvements in pain, psychological functioning, and quality of life. Given extant research, the incorporation of multidisciplinary pain management treatment including both multimodal pharmacological and integrative non-pharmacological therapies is recommended early in the process of caring for youth experiencing acute and chronic pain.

Suggested future directions include performance of larger pediatric trials across integrative non-pharmacological pain interventions, assessing the potential synergistic nature of combined integrative non-pharmacological therapies, and conducting further research on the transition from acute to chronic pain management. It is also recommended that studies more directly explore the associations and effects of multidisciplinary treatment on the necessity for and use of opioid therapies in pediatric pain, especially in chronic pain management, and on the possible utility of these therapies in weaning from opioids and other therapies. Overall, additional societal resources are urgently needed to increase availability of multidisciplinary pain management services to all youth impacted by acute and chronic pain.

Author Contributions: Conceptualization, A.W., A.R. and B.G.; Methodology, A.W., A.R., B.G., G.D.; Diagrams, G.D.; Writing—Original Draft Preparation, all; Writing—Review & Editing, all.; Visualization, B.G.; Supervision, B.G.

Funding: This research received no external funding.

Conflicts of Interest: The authors declare no conflict of interest.

Appendix A

Table A1. Selection of important studies in pediatric integrative non-pharmacological therapies reviewed for this paper. From all the articles screened, the articles with the highest level of evidence are summarized below.

Therapy Type	Authors (Reference Number)	Study Type (Grade of Evidence)	Study Population	Outcome	Key Results
CBT	Eccleston et al. [37]	Cochrane systematic review (1)	Cochrane systematic review of psychological therapies (37 RCTs; 2111 participants, mean age 12.45, SD 2.2)	Pain intensity; Disability	Reduced headache pain (RR 2.47, CI 1.97–3.09, $p < 0.01$; Reduced disability in headache pain (SMD −0.49, CI −0.74 to −0.24, $p < 0.01$); Reduced nonheadache pain (SMD −0.57, CI −0.86 to −0.27, $p < 0.01$); Reduced disability in nonheadache pain (SMD −0.45, CI −0.71 to −0.19, $p < 0.01$
	Palermo et al. [61]	Meta-analysis (1)	Meta-analysis (25 RCTs; 1247 participants, 9–17 yo)	Pain intensity	Decreased headache (OR 6.1, CI 4.06 to 9.15, $p < 0.0001$); Decreased abdominal pain (OR 7.5, CI 3.29 to 17.16, $p < 0.001$)
	Fisher et al. [62]	Systematic review and meta-analysis (1)	Meta-analysis (37 RCTs; 1005 participants, mean age 9.4, SD 1.14)	Pain intensity; Disability	Decreased non-headache pain (SMD −0.60, CI −0.91 to −0.29, $p < 0.001$); Decreased nonheadache pain disability (SMD −0.27, CI −0.46 to −0.08, $p < 0.01$); Decreased headache (RR 2.9, CI 2.25 to 3.73, $p < 0.001$); Decreased headache at follow-up (RR 3.34, CI 2.02 to 5.53, $p < 0.001$
	Ruskin et al. [82]	Prospective pre-post interventional study (2)	21 adolescents, 12–18 yo with chronic pain	Feasibility; Acceptability	90.5% treatment completion rate; No dropouts; Compliance with home practice ($M = 60$ min/week); Would recommend group to a friend
Mindfulness	Chadi et al. [83]	RCT (2)	19 adolescents, 13.9–17.8 yo with chronic pain	Quality of life; Depression; Anxiety; Pain perception; Psychological distress; Salivary cortisol	No significant changes in quality of life, depression, anxiety, pain perception, or psychological distress; Cortisol levels decreased from an average of 3.37 (±1.72) pre-intervention nmol/L to 1.95 (±1.13) nmol/L post-intervention; Cohen's d = 0.77, $p < 0.001$).
	Ali et al. [84]	Pilot (3)	15 adolescents, 10–18 yo with fibromyalgia, chronic fatigue, musculoskeletal pain, headache, or abdominal pain	Functional disability; Fibromyalgia symptoms; Quality of life; Mindfulness	Decreased functional disability (33% improvement, $p = 0.026$); improved fibromyalgia symptoms (26% improvement, $p = 0.03$), and improved mindfulness (child: 12% improvement, $p = 0.02$; parent: 17% improvement, $p = 0.03$).
	Waelde et al. [85]	Pilot (3)	20 adolescents, 13–17 yo with chronic pain	Feasibility and Acceptability Parental assessment	Feasible and acceptable; Decreased parental worry about child ($p < 0.01$)
Hypnosis	Hesse et al. [86]	Pilot (3)	20 adolescent females, 11–16 yo, with recurrent headaches	Quality of Life; Pain acceptance; Depression	Improved quality of life, Parent assess PedsQL, $p = 0.049$; Improved child acceptance of pain, CPAQ-A $p = −0.005$; Improved child depression, CES-DC $p = 0.009$
	Manworren et al. [35]	RCT (2)	24 adolescents, 10–18 yo undergoing Nuss procedure	Pain intensity; Morphine equivalent/hour; Length of stay (LOS)	Lower mean pain intensity (−1.72, 95% CI 2.89–0.55, $p = 0.0047$); Lower maximum pain intensity (−2.27, 95% CI 3.73–0.82, $p = 0.0028$); Less morphine equivalents/hour (−0.13, 95% CI −0.25–0.00, $p = 0.046$); Shorter LOS ($p = 0.0013$)
Acupuncture	Tsao et al. [22]	RCT (2)	59 children, 3–12 yo undergoing tonsillectomy	Pain, Oral food intake	Improvement in pain control and oral intake ($p = 0.0065$ and 0.001, respectively)
	Raith et al. [123]	RCT (2)	28 newborns with neonatal abstinence syndrome	Duration of morphine treatment; Length of stay	Shorter duration of morphine treatment (28 days vs. 39 days; $p = 0.019$) and hospital stay (35 vs. 50 days, $p = 0.048$)

Table A1. *Cont.*

Therapy Type	Authors (Reference Number)	Study Type (Grade of Evidence)	Study Population	Outcome	Key Results
Rehabilitation	Hechler, et al. [38]	Systematic review (1)	10 studies (1020 adolescents, mean age 13.9, SD 1.5)	Pain intensity; Pain-related disability	Decreased pain intensity (d = −1.33, CI −2.28 to −0.38, p = 0.01); Decreased pain related disability (d = −1.09, CI −1.71 to −0.48, p < 0.001)
	Logan et al. [126]	Longitudinal case series (3)	56 children and adolescents, 8–18 yo with CRPS	Pain intensity; Functional disability; Subjective report of limb function, timed running, occupational performance, medication use, use of assistive devices, emotional functioning, anxiety and depression	Statistically significant improvements from admission to discharge in pain intensity, functional disability, subjective report of limb function, timed running, occupational performance, medication use, use of assistive devices, emotional functioning, anxiety, and depression. (all p < 0.01). (multiple outcomes)
	Simons et al. [127]	Comparative study (case-controlled) (3)	100 children and adolescents, mean age 13.9 (SD 2.17)	Functional disability; Fear of pain; Readiness to change	Improved functional disability (p = 0.00); Improved fear of pain (p = 0.00); Increased readiness to change (precontemplation p = 0.01, action/maintenance p = 0.00) (multiple outcomes)
	Bruce et al. [51]	Prospective longitudinal case series (3)	171 adolescents 12–18, mean age 15.3 (SD 1.73)	Functional disability; depressive symptoms; catastrophizing; Changes in opioid medication	Improved functional disability (p < 0.001) Improved depressive symptoms (p < 0.0001) Improved catastrophizing (p < 0.0001) Reduced pain severity (p = 0.0001) Decreased opioid medication (Out of 30 patients on opioids, 21 were weaned off medication, 1 did not finish program)

Notes: RCT, randomized controlled trials; SD, standard deviation; RR, risk ratio; CI, confidence interval; SMD, standardized mean difference; yo, years old; OR, odds ratios; M, mean; PedsQL, Pediatric Quality of Life Inventory; CPAQ-A, Chronic Pain Acceptance Questionnaire–Activity Engagement; CES-DC, Center for Epidemiological Studies of Depression Scale for Children; LOS, length of stay; d, effect sizes; CRPS, complex regional pain syndrome.

References

1. Pain terms: A list with definitions and notes on usage. Recommended by the IASP Subcommittee on Taxonomy. *Pain* **1979**, *6*, 249.
2. Anwar, K. Pathophysiology of pain. *Dis. Mon.* **2016**, *62*, 324–329. [CrossRef] [PubMed]
3. IASP Pain Terminology. International Association for the Study of Pain Committee on Taxonomy. Available online: http://www.iasp-pain.org/Taxonomy#Pain (accessed on 1 December 2018).
4. Slater, M.E.; De Lima, J.; Campbell, K.; Lane, L.; Collins, J. Opioids for the management of severe chronic nonmalignant pain in children: A retrospective 1-year practice survey in a children's hospital. *Pain Med.* **2010**, *11*, 207–214. [CrossRef] [PubMed]
5. Berde, C.; Nurko, S. Opioid side effects—Mechanism-based therapy. *N. Engl. J. Med.* **2008**, *358*, 2400–2402. [CrossRef] [PubMed]
6. Moore, R.A.; McQuay, H.J. Prevalence of opioid adverse events in chronic non-malignant pain: Systematic review of randomised trials of oral opioids. *Arthritis Res. Ther.* **2005**, *7*, R1046–R1051. [CrossRef] [PubMed]
7. Gomes, T.; Mamdani, M.M.; Dhalla, I.A.; Paterson, J.M.; Juurlink, D.N. Opioid dose and drug-related mortality in patients with nonmalignant pain. *Arch. Intern. Med.* **2011**, *171*, 686–691. [CrossRef] [PubMed]
8. Grunkemeier, D.M.; Cassara, J.E.; Dalton, C.B.; Drossman, D.A. The narcotic bowel syndrome: Clinical features, pathophysiology, and management. *Clin. Gastroenterol. Hepatol.* **2007**, *5*, 1126–1139. [CrossRef]
9. Fudin, J.; Raouf, M.; Wegrzyn, E.L. *Opioid Dosing Policy: Pharmacological Considerations Regarding Equianalgesic Dosing*; American Academy of Integrative Pain Management: Lenexa, KS, USA, 2017.
10. Lee, M.; Silverman, S.M.; Hansen, H.; Patel, V.B.; Manchikanti, L. A comprehensive review of opioid-induced hyperalgesia. *Pain Physician* **2011**, *14*, 145–161.
11. Task Force on Multimodal Pain Treatment Defines Terms for Chronic Pain Care. Available online: http://www.iasp-pain.org/PublicationsNews/NewsDetail.aspx?ItemNumber=6981 (accessed on 1 December 2018).
12. Friedrichsdorf, S.J. Contemporary pediatric palliative care: Myths and barriers to integration into clinical care. *Curr. Pediatr. Rev.* **2016**, *13*, 8–12. [CrossRef]
13. Dowell, D.; Haegerich, T.M.; Chou, R. CDC guideline for prescribing opioids for chronic pain—United States, 2016. *MMWR Recomm. Rep.* **2016**, *65*, 1–49. [CrossRef]
14. Dash, G.F.; Wilson, A.C.; Morasco, B.J.; Feldstein Ewing, S.W. A Model of the Intersection of Pain and Opioid Misuse in Children and Adolescents. *Clin. Psychol. Sci.* **2018**, *6*, 629–646. [CrossRef] [PubMed]
15. Schechter, N.L.; Walco, G.A. The Potential Impact on Children of the CDC Guideline for Prescribing Opioids for Chronic Pain: Above All, Do No Harm. *JAMA Pediatr.* **2016**, *170*, 425–426. [CrossRef] [PubMed]
16. Friedrichsdorf, S.J.; Giordano, J.; Desai Dakoji, K.; Warmuth, A.; Daughtry, C.; Schulz, C.A. Chronic Pain in Children and Adolescents: Diagnosis and Treatment of Primary Pain Disorders in Head, Abdomen, Muscles and Joints. *Children (Basel)* **2016**, *3*, 42. [CrossRef] [PubMed]
17. Chung, C.P.; Callahan, S.T.; Cooper, W.O.; Dupont, W.D.; Murray, K.T.; Franklin, A.D.; Hall, K.; Dudley, J.A.; Stein, C.M.; Ray, W.A. Outpatient Opioid Prescriptions for Children and Opioid-Related Adverse Events. *Pediatrics* **2018**, *142*. [CrossRef] [PubMed]
18. Krane, E.J.; Weisman, S.J.; Walco, G.A. The National Opioid Epidemic and the Risk of Outpatient Opioids in Children. *Pediatrics* **2018**, *142*. [CrossRef] [PubMed]
19. Lin, Y.C.; Lee, A.C.; Kemper, K.J.; Berde, C.B. Use of complementary and alternative medicine in pediatric pain management service: A survey. *Pain Med.* **2005**, *6*, 452–458. [CrossRef] [PubMed]
20. Fisher, E.; Law, E.; Dudeney, J.; Palermo, T.M.; Stewart, G.; Eccleston, C. Psychological therapies for the management of chronic and recurrent pain in children and adolescents. *Cochrane Database Syst. Rev.* **2018**, *9*. [CrossRef]
21. Kamper, S.J.; Apeldoorn, A.T.; Chiarotto, A.; Smeets, R.J.; Ostelo, R.W.; Guzman, J.; van Tulder, M.W. Multidisciplinary biopsychosocial rehabilitation for chronic low back pain: Cochrane systematic review and meta-analysis. *BMJ* **2015**, *350*, h444. [CrossRef]
22. Lee, C.; Crawford, C.; Swann, S. Active Self-Care Therapies for Pain (PACT) Working Group. Multimodal, integrative therapies for the self-management of chronic pain symptoms. *Pain Med.* **2014**, *15* Suppl. 1, S76–S85. [CrossRef]

23. Nicol, A.L.; Hurley, R.W.; Benzon, H.T. Alternatives to opioids in the pharmacologic management of chronic pain syndromes: A narrative review of randomized, controlled, and blinded clinical trials. *Anesth. Analg.* **2017**, *125*, 1682–1703. [CrossRef]
24. Gardiner, P.; Lestoquoy, A.S.; Gergen-Barnett, K.; Penti, B.; White, L.F.; Saper, R.; Fredman, L.; Stillman, S.; Lily Negash, N.; Adelstein, P.; et al. Design of the integrative medical group visits randomized control trial for underserved patients with chronic pain and depression. *Contemp. Clin. Trials* **2017**, *54*, 25–35. [CrossRef] [PubMed]
25. Tick, H.; Nielsen, A.; Pelletier, K.R.; Bonakdar, R.; Simmons, S.; Glick, R.; Ratner, E.; Lemmon, R.L.; Wayne, P.; Zador, V.; et al. Evidence-Based Nonpharmacologic Strategies for Comprehensive Pain Care: The Consortium Pain Task Force White Paper. *Explore (NY)* **2018**, *14*, 177–211. [CrossRef] [PubMed]
26. Waldman, S. *Pain Management*, 2nd ed.; Elsevier: Philadelphia, PA, USA, 2011; ISBN 9781437736038.
27. Odell, S.; Logan, D.E. Pediatric pain management: The multidisciplinary approach. *J. Pain Res.* **2013**, *6*, 785–790. [CrossRef] [PubMed]
28. Gritsenko, K.; Khelemsky, Y.; Kaye, A.D.; Vadivelu, N.; Urman, R.D. Multimodal therapy in perioperative analgesia. *Best Pract. Res. Clin. Anaesthesiol.* **2014**, *28*, 59–79. [CrossRef] [PubMed]
29. Brooks, M.R.; Golianu, B. Perioperative management in children with chronic pain. *Paediatr. Anaesth.* **2016**, *26*, 794–806. [CrossRef] [PubMed]
30. Panella, J.J. Preoperative care of children: Strategies from a child life perspective. *AORN J.* **2016**, *104*, 11–22. [CrossRef] [PubMed]
31. Suresh, S.; Wang, S.; Porfyris, S.; Kamasinski-Sol, R.; Steinhorn, D.M. Massage therapy in outpatient pediatric chronic pain patients: Do they facilitate significant reductions in levels of distress, pain, tension, discomfort, and mood alterations? *Paediatr. Anaesth.* **2008**, *18*, 884–887. [CrossRef]
32. Wang, S.M.; Escalera, S.; Lin, E.C.; Maranets, I.; Kain, Z.N. Extra-1 acupressure for children undergoing anesthesia. *Anesth. Analg.* **2008**, *107*, 811–816. [CrossRef]
33. Brewer, S.; Gleditsch, S.L.; Syblik, D.; Tietjens, M.E.; Vacik, H.W. Pediatric anxiety: Child life intervention in day surgery. *J. Pediatr. Nurs.* **2006**, *21*, 13–22. [CrossRef]
34. Yip, P.; Middleton, P.; Cyna, A.M.; Carlyle, A.V. Non-pharmacological interventions for assisting the induction of anaesthesia in children. *Cochrane Database Syst. Rev.* **2009**, CD006447. [CrossRef]
35. Manworren, R.C.B.; Girard, E.; Verissimo, A.M.; Ruscher, K.A.; Santanelli, J.P.; Weiss, R.; Hight, D. Hypnosis for postoperative pain management of thoracoscopic approach to repair pectus excavatum: Retrospective analysis. *J. Pediatr. Surg. Nurs.* **2015**, *4*, 60–69. [CrossRef]
36. Jensen, B.; Chen, J.; Furnish, T.; Wallace, M. Medical marijuana and chronic pain: A review of basic science and clinical evidence. *Curr. Pain Headache Rep.* **2015**, *19*, 50. [CrossRef] [PubMed]
37. Eccleston, C.; Palermo, T.M.; Williams, A.C.; Lewandowski, H.A.; Morley, S.; Fisher, E.; Law, E. Psychological therapies for the management of chronic and recurrent pain in children and adolescents. *Cochrane Database Syst. Rev.* **2014**, CD003968. [CrossRef] [PubMed]
38. Hechler, T.; Kanstrup, M.; Holley, A.L.; Simons, L.E.; Wicksell, R.; Hirschfeld, G.; Zernikow, B. Systematic review on intensive interdisciplinary pain treatment of children with chronic pain. *Pediatrics* **2015**, *136*, 115–127. [CrossRef] [PubMed]
39. Lee, B.H.; Scharff, L.; Sethna, N.F.; McCarthy, C.F.; Scott-Sutherland, J.; Shea, A.M.; Sullivan, P.; Meier, P.; Zurakowski, D.; Masek, B.J.; et al. Physical therapy and cognitive-behavioral treatment for complex regional pain syndromes. *J. Pediatr.* **2002**, *141*, 135–140. [CrossRef] [PubMed]
40. Kuttner, L. Pediatric hypnosis: Pre-, peri-, and post-anesthesia. *Paediatr. Anaesth.* **2012**, *22*, 573–577. [CrossRef] [PubMed]
41. Garland, E.L. Disrupting the downward spiral of chronic pain and opioid addiction with mindfulness-oriented recovery enhancement: A review of clinical outcomes and neurocognitive targets. *J. Pain Palliat. Care Pharmacother.* **2014**, *28*, 122–129. [CrossRef]
42. Agoston, A.M.; Sieberg, C.B. Nonpharmacologic treatment of pain. *Semin. Pediatr. Neurol.* **2016**, *23*, 220–223. [CrossRef]
43. Golianu, B.; Seybold, J.; Almgren, C. Acupuncture helps reduce need for sedative medications in neonates and infants undergoing treatment in the intensive care unit. *Med. Acupunct.* **2014**, *26*, 279–285. [CrossRef]

44. Schmitt, Y.S.; Hoffman, H.G.; Blough, D.K.; Patterson, D.R.; Jensen, M.P.; Soltani, M.; Carrougher, G.J.; Nakamura, D.; Sharar, S.R. A randomized, controlled trial of immersive virtual reality analgesia, during physical therapy for pediatric burns. *Burns* **2011**, *37*, 61–68. [CrossRef]
45. Brown, M.L.; Rojas, E.; Gouda, S. A Mind-body approach to pediatric pain management. *Children (Basel)* **2017**, *4*, 50. [CrossRef] [PubMed]
46. Rabin, J.; Brown, M.; Alexander, S. Update in the treatment of chronic pain within pediatric patients. *Curr. Probl. Pediatr. Adolesc. Health Care* **2017**, *47*, 167–172. [CrossRef] [PubMed]
47. Dhond, R.P.; Yeh, C.; Park, K.; Kettner, N.; Napadow, V. Acupuncture modulates resting state connectivity in default and sensorimotor brain networks. *Pain* **2008**, *136*, 407–418. [CrossRef] [PubMed]
48. Jiang, H.; White, M.P.; Greicius, M.D.; Waelde, L.C.; Spiegel, D. Brain activity and functional connectivity associated with hypnosis. *Cereb. Cortex* **2017**, *27*, 4083–4093. [CrossRef] [PubMed]
49. Kucyi, A.; Salomons, T.V.; Davis, K.D. Cognitive behavioral training reverses the effect of pain exposure on brain network activity. *Pain* **2016**, *157*, 1895–1904. [CrossRef] [PubMed]
50. Becker, W.C.; Dorflinger, L.; Edmond, S.N.; Islam, L.; Heapy, A.A.; Fraenkel, L. Barriers and facilitators to use of non-pharmacological treatments in chronic pain. *BMC Fam. Pract.* **2017**, *18*, 41. [CrossRef] [PubMed]
51. Bruce, B.K.; Ale, C.M.; Harrison, T.E.; Bee, S.; Luedtke, C.; Geske, J.; Weiss, K.E. Getting back to living: Further evidence for the efficacy of an interdisciplinary pediatric pain treatment program. *Clin. J. Pain* **2017**, *33*, 535–542. [CrossRef]
52. Chambless, D.L.; Hollon, S.D. Defining empirically supported therapies. *J. Consult. Clin. Psychol.* **1998**, *66*, 7–18. [CrossRef]
53. Butler, A.C.; Chapman, J.E.; Forman, E.M.; Beck, A.T. The empirical status of cognitive-behavioral therapy: A review of meta-analyses. *Clin. Psychol. Rev.* **2006**, *26*, 17–31. [CrossRef]
54. Beck, J.S. *Cognitive Behavior Therapy: Basics and Beyond*; Guilford Press: New York, NY, USA, 2011.
55. Wicksell, R.K.; Greco, L.A. Acceptance and commitment therapy for pediatric chronic pain. In *Acceptance and Mindfulness Treatments for Children and Adolescents: A Practitioner's Guide*; New Harbinger Publications: Oakland, CA, USA, 2008; pp. 89–113. ISBN 978-1-57224-541-9.
56. Grave, J.; Blissett, J. Is cognitive behavior therapy developmentally appropriate for young children? A critical review of the evidence. *Clin. Psychol. Rev.* **2004**, *24*, 399–420. [CrossRef]
57. Seminowicz, D.A.; Shpaner, M.; Keaser, M.L.; Krauthamer, G.M.; Mantegna, J.; Dumas, J.A.; Newhouse, P.A.; Filippi, C.G.; Keefe, F.J.; Naylor, M.R. Cognitive-behavioral therapy increases prefrontal cortex gray matter in patients with chronic pain. *J. Pain* **2013**, *14*, 1573–1584. [CrossRef] [PubMed]
58. Jensen, K.B.; Kosek, E.; Wicksell, R.; Kemani, M.; Olsson, G.; Merle, J.V.; Kadetoff, D.; Ingvar, M. Cognitive Behavioral Therapy increases pain-evoked activation of the prefrontal cortex in patients with fibromyalgia. *Pain* **2012**, *153*, 1495–1503. [CrossRef] [PubMed]
59. Williams, A.C.; Eccleston, C.; Morley, S. Psychological therapies for the management of chronic pain (excluding headache) in adults. *Cochrane Database Syst. Rev.* **2012**, *11*, CD007407. [CrossRef] [PubMed]
60. Coakley, R.; Wihak, T. Evidence-based psychological interventions for the management of pediatric chronic pain: New directions in research and clinical practice. *Children (Basel)* **2017**, *4*, 9. [CrossRef] [PubMed]
61. Palermo, T.M.; Eccleston, C.; Lewandowski, A.S.; Williams, A.C.; Morley, S. Randomized controlled trials of psychological therapies for management of chronic pain in children and adolescents: An updated meta-analytic review. *Pain* **2010**, *148*, 387–397. [CrossRef] [PubMed]
62. Fisher, E.; Heathcote, L.; Palermo, T.M.; de C Williams, A.C.; Lau, J.; Eccleston, C. Systematic review and meta-analysis of psychological therapies for children with chronic pain. *J. Pediatr. Psychol.* **2014**, *39*, 763–782. [CrossRef] [PubMed]
63. Palermo, T.M.; Wilson, A.C.; Peters, M.; Lewandowski, A.; Somhegyi, H. Randomized controlled trial of an Internet-delivered family cognitive-behavioral therapy intervention for children and adolescents with chronic pain. *Pain* **2009**, *146*, 205–213. [CrossRef]
64. Huestis, S.E.; Kao, G.; Dunn, A.; Hilliard, A.T.; Yoon, I.A.; Golianu, B.; Bhandari, R.P. Multi-Family Pediatric Pain Group Therapy: Capturing Acceptance and Cultivating Change. *Children (Basel)* **2017**, *4*, 106. [CrossRef]
65. Coakley, R.; Wihak, T.; Kossowsky, J.; Iversen, C.; Donado, C. The Comfort Ability Pain Management Workshop: A Preliminary, Nonrandomized Investigation of a Brief, Cognitive, Biobehavioral, and Parent Training Intervention for Pediatric Chronic Pain. *J. Pediatr. Psychol.* **2018**, *43*, 252–265. [CrossRef]
66. Kabat-Zinn, J. *Wherever You Go, There You Are*; Hyperion: New York, NY, USA, 1994.

67. Black, D.S.; Slavich, G.M. Mindfulness meditation and the immune system: A systematic review of randomized controlled trials. *Ann. N. Y. Acad. Sci.* **2016**, *1373*, 13–24. [CrossRef]
68. Grossman, P.; Niemann, L.; Schmidt, S.; Walach, H. Mindfulness-based stress reduction and health benefits. A meta-analysis. *J. Psychosom. Res.* **2004**, *57*, 35–43. [CrossRef]
69. Ahola Kohut, S.; Stinson, J.; Davies-Chalmers, C.; Ruskin, D.; van Wyk, M. Mindfulness-based interventions in clinical samples of adolescents with chronic illness: A systematic review. *J. Altern. Complement. Med.* **2017**, *23*, 581–589. [CrossRef] [PubMed]
70. Baer, R.A. Mindfulness training as a clinical intervention: A conceptual and empirical review. *Clin. Psychol. Sci. Pract.* **2003**, *10*, 125–143. [CrossRef]
71. Garland, E.L.; Froeliger, B.; Zeidan, F.; Partin, K.; Howard, M.O. The downward spiral of chronic pain, prescription opioid misuse, and addiction: Cognitive, affective, and neuropsychopharmacologic pathways. *Neurosci. Biobehav. Rev.* **2013**, *37*, 2597–2607. [CrossRef] [PubMed]
72. Garland, E.L.; Gaylord, S.A.; Palsson, O.; Faurot, K.; Douglas Mann, J.; Whitehead, W.E. Therapeutic mechanisms of a mindfulness-based treatment for IBS: Effects on visceral sensitivity, catastrophizing, and affective processing of pain sensations. *J. Behav. Med.* **2012**, *35*, 591–602. [CrossRef] [PubMed]
73. Holzel, B.K.; Lazar, S.W.; Gard, T.; Schuman-Olivier, Z.; Vago, D.R.; Ott, U. How does mindfulness meditation work? Proposing mechanisms of action from a conceptual and neural perspective. *Perspect. Psychol. Sci.* **2011**, *6*, 537–559. [CrossRef] [PubMed]
74. Zeidan, F.; Martucci, K.T.; Kraft, R.A.; Gordon, N.S.; McHaffie, J.G.; Coghill, R.C. Brain mechanisms supporting the modulation of pain by mindfulness meditation. *J. Neurosci.* **2011**, *31*, 5540–5548. [CrossRef] [PubMed]
75. Zeidan, F.; Vago, D.R. Mindfulness meditation-based pain relief: A mechanistic account. *Ann. N. Y. Acad. Sci.* **2016**, *1373*, 114–127. [CrossRef]
76. Wager, T.D.; Scott, D.J.; Zubieta, J.K. Placebo effects on human mu-opioid activity during pain. *Proc. Natl. Acad. Sci. USA* **2007**, *104*, 11056–11061. [CrossRef]
77. Sharon, H.; Maron-Katz, A.; Ben Simon, E.; Flusser, Y.; Hendler, T.; Tarrasch, R.; Brill, S. Mindfulness meditation modulates pain through endogenous opioids. *Am. J. Med.* **2016**, *129*, 755–758. [CrossRef]
78. Zeidan, F.; Adler-Neal, A.L.; Wells, R.E.; Stagnaro, E.; May, L.M.; Eisenach, J.C.; McHaffie, J.G.; Coghill, R.C. Mindfulness-meditation-based pain relief is not mediated by endogenous opioids. *J. Neurosci.* **2016**, *36*, 3391–3397. [CrossRef] [PubMed]
79. Veehof, M.M.; Trompetter, H.R.; Bohlmeijer, E.T.; Schreurs, K.M. Acceptance- and mindfulness-based interventions for the treatment of chronic pain: A meta-analytic review. *Cogn. Behav. Ther.* **2016**, *45*, 5–31. [CrossRef] [PubMed]
80. Hilton, L.; Hempel, S.; Ewing, B.A.; Apaydin, E.; Xenakis, L.; Newberry, S.; Colaiaco, B.; Maher, A.R.; Shanman, R.M.; Sorbero, M.E.; et al. Mindfulness meditation for chronic pain: Systematic review and meta-analysis. *Ann. Behav. Med.* **2017**, *51*, 199–213. [CrossRef] [PubMed]
81. Anheyer, D.; Haller, H.; Barth, J.; Lauche, R.; Dobos, G.; Cramer, H. Mindfulness-based stress reduction for treating low back pain: A systematic review and meta-analysis. *Ann. Intern. Med.* **2017**, *166*, 799–807. [CrossRef] [PubMed]
82. Ruskin, D.A.; Gagnon, M.M.; Kohut, S.A.; Stinson, J.N.; Walker, K.S. A mindfulness program adapted for adolescents with chronic pain: Feasibility, acceptability, and initial outcomes. *Clin. J. Pain* **2017**. [CrossRef] [PubMed]
83. Chadi, N.; McMahon, A.; Vadnais, M.; Malboeuf-Hurtubise, C.; Djemli, A.; Dobkin, P.L.; Lacroix, J.; Luu, T.M.; Haley, N. Mindfulness-based intervention for female adolescents with chronic pain: A pilot randomized trial. *J. Can. Acad. Child Adolesc. Psychiatry* **2016**, *25*, 159–168. [PubMed]
84. Ali, A.; Weiss, T.R.; Dutton, A.; McKee, D.; Jones, K.D.; Kashikar-Zuck, S.; Silverman, W.K.; Shapiro, E.D. Mindfulness-based stress reduction for adolescents with functional somatic syndromes: A pilot cohort study. *J. Pediatr.* **2017**, *183*, 184–190. [CrossRef] [PubMed]
85. Waelde, L.C.; Feinstein, A.B.; Bhandari, R.; Griffin, A.; Yoon, I.A.; Golianu, B. A pilot study of mindfulness meditation for pediatric chronic pain. *Children (Basel)* **2017**, *4*, 32. [CrossRef]

86. Hesse, T.; Holmes, L.G.; Kennedy-Overfelt, V.; Kerr, L.M.; Giles, L.L. Mindfulness-based intervention for adolescents with recurrent headaches: A pilot feasibility study. *Evid. Based Complement. Alternat. Med.* **2015**, *2015*, 508958. [CrossRef]
87. Jastrowski Mano, K.E.; Salamon, K.S.; Hainsworth, K.R.; Anderson Khan, K.J.; Ladwig, R.J.; Davies, W.H.; Weisman, S.J. A randomized, controlled pilot study of mindfulness-based stress reduction for pediatric chronic pain. *Altern. Ther. Health Med.* **2013**, *19*, 8–14.
88. Ruskin, D.; Lalloo, C.; Amaria, K.; Stinson, J.N.; Kewley, E.; Campbell, F.; Brown, S.C.; Jeavons, M.; McGrath, P.A. Assessing pain intensity in children with chronic pain: Convergent and discriminant validity of the 0 to 10 numerical rating scale in clinical practice. *Pain Res. Manag.* **2014**, *19*, 141–148. [CrossRef] [PubMed]
89. Zoogman, S.; Goldberg, S.B.; Hoyt, W.T.; Miller, L. Mindfulness interventions with youth: A meta-analysis. *Mindfulness* **2015**, *6*, 290–302. [CrossRef]
90. Zenner, C.; Herrnleben-Kurz, S.; Walach, H. Mindfulness-based interventions in schools-a systematic review and meta-analysis. *Front. Psychol.* **2014**, *5*, 603. [CrossRef] [PubMed]
91. Sibinga, E.M.; Webb, L.; Ghazarian, S.R.; Ellen, J.M. School-Based Mindfulness Instruction: An RCT. *Pediatrics* **2016**, *137*. [CrossRef] [PubMed]
92. Mani, M.; Kavanagh, D.J.; Hides, L.; Stoyanov, S.R. Review and Evaluation of Mindfulness-Based iPhone Apps. *JMIR Mhealth Uhealth* **2015**, *3*, e82. [CrossRef] [PubMed]
93. Hilgard, E.R. *Hypnotic Susceptibility*; Harcourt, Brace & World Inc.: New York, NY, USA, 1965.
94. Spiegel, H.; Spiegel, D. *Trance and Treatment: Clinical Uses of Hypnosis*; American Psychistric Publishing: Washington, DC, USA, 1987; ISBN 978-1585621903.
95. Lobe, T.E. Perioperative hypnosis reduces hospitalization in patients undergoing the Nuss procedure for pectus excavatum. *J. Laparoendosc. Adv. Surg. Tech. A* **2006**, *16*, 639–642. [CrossRef] [PubMed]
96. Gruzelier, J.H. A working model of the neurophysiology of hypnosis: A review of the evidence. *Contemp. Hypn.* **1998**, *15*, 3–21. [CrossRef]
97. Jensen, M.P.; Patterson, D.R. Hypnotic approaches for chronic pain management: Clinical implications of recent research findings. *Am. Psychol.* **2014**, *69*, 167–177. [CrossRef]
98. Crawford, H.J.; Horton, J.E.; Harrington, G.C.; Vendemia, J.M.C.; Plantec, M.B.; Jung, S.; Shamro, C.; Downs, J.H., III. Hypnotic analgesia (Disattending pain) impacts neuronal network activation: An fMRI study of noxious somatosensory TENS stimuli. *Neuroimage* **1998**, *7*, S436. [CrossRef]
99. Rainville, P.; Duncan, G.H.; Price, D.D.; Carrier, B.; Bushnell, M.C. Pain affect encoded in human anterior cingulate but not somatosensory cortex. *Science* **1997**, *277*, 968–971. [CrossRef]
100. Montgomery, G.H.; DuHamel, K.N.; Redd, W.H. A meta-analysis of hypnotically induced analgesia: How effective is hypnosis? *Int. J. Clin. Exp. Hypn.* **2000**, *48*, 138–153. [CrossRef] [PubMed]
101. Adachi, T.; Fujino, H.; Nakae, A.; Mashimo, T.; Sasaki, J. A meta-analysis of hypnosis for chronic pain problems: A comparison between hypnosis, standard care, and other psychological interventions. *Int. J. Clin. Exp. Hypn.* **2014**, *62*, 1–28. [CrossRef] [PubMed]
102. Lambert, S.A. The effects of hypnosis/guided imagery on the postoperative course of children. *J. Dev. Behav. Pediatr.* **1996**, *17*, 307–310. [CrossRef] [PubMed]
103. Liossi, C.; Hatira, P. Clinical hypnosis versus cognitive behavioral training for pain management with pediatric cancer patients undergoing bone marrow aspirations. *Int. J. Clin. Exp. Hypn.* **1999**, *47*, 104–116. [CrossRef] [PubMed]
104. Vlieger, A.M.; Menko-Frankenhuis, C.; Wolfkamp, S.C.; Tromp, E.; Benninga, M.A. Hypnotherapy for children with functional abdominal pain or irritable bowel syndrome: A randomized controlled trial. *Gastroenterology* **2007**, *133*, 1430–1436. [CrossRef] [PubMed]
105. Vlieger, A.M.; Rutten, J.M.; Govers, A.M.; Frankenhuis, C.; Benninga, M.A. Long-term follow-up of gut-directed hypnotherapy vs. standard care in children with functional abdominal pain or irritable bowel syndrome. *Am. J. Gastroenterol.* **2012**, *107*, 627–631. [CrossRef]
106. Anbar, R.D. Self-hypnosis for the treatment of functional abdominal pain in childhood. *Clin. Pediatr. (Phila)* **2001**, *40*, 447–451. [CrossRef]
107. Olness, K. Imagery (self-hypnosis) as adjunct therapy in childhood cancer: Clinical experience with 25 patients. *Am. J. Pediatr. Hematol. Oncol.* **1981**, *3*, 313–321.

108. Kohen, D.P.; Zajac, R. Self-hypnosis training for headaches in children and adolescents. *J. Pediatr.* **2007**, *150*, 635–639. [CrossRef]
109. Olness, K.; MacDonald, J.T.; Uden, D.L. Comparison of self-hypnosis and propranolol in the treatment of juvenile classic migraine. *Pediatrics* **1987**, *79*, 593–597.
110. Lin, Y.C.; Wan, L.; Jamison, R.N. Using integrative medicine in pain management: An evaluation of current evidence. *Anesth. Analg.* **2017**, *125*, 2081–2093. [CrossRef]
111. Hui, K.K.; Liu, J.; Marina, O.; Napadow, V.; Haselgrove, C.; Kwong, K.K.; Kennedy, D.N.; Makris, N. The integrated response of the human cerebro-cerebellar and limbic systems to acupuncture stimulation at ST 36 as evidenced by fMRI. *Neuroimage* **2005**, *27*, 479–496. [CrossRef]
112. Napadow, V.; Kettner, N.; Liu, J.; Li, M.; Kwong, K.K.; Vangel, M.; Makris, N.; Audette, J.; Hui, K.K. Hypothalamus and amygdala response to acupuncture stimuli in Carpal Tunnel Syndrome. *Pain* **2007**, *130*, 254–266. [CrossRef] [PubMed]
113. Wang, S.M.; Kain, Z.N.; White, P. Acupuncture analgesia: I. The scientific basis. *Anesth. Analg.* **2008**, *106*, 602–610. [CrossRef] [PubMed]
114. Oke, S.L.; Tracey, K.J. The inflammatory reflex and the role of complementary and alternative medical therapies. *Ann. N. Y. Acad. Sci.* **2009**, *1172*, 172–180. [CrossRef] [PubMed]
115. Chavan, S.S.; Tracey, K.J. Regulating innate immunity with dopamine and electroacupuncture. *Nat. Med.* **2014**, *20*, 239–241. [CrossRef] [PubMed]
116. NIH consensus conference: Acupuncture. *JAMA* **1998**, *280*, 1518–1524. [CrossRef]
117. Haake, M.; Muller, H.H.; Schade-Brittinger, C.; Basler, H.D.; Schafer, H.; Maier, C.; Endres, H.G.; Trampisch, H.J.; Molsberger, A. German Acupuncture Trials (GERAC) for chronic low back pain: Randomized, multicenter, blinded, parallel-group trial with 3 groups. *Arch. Intern. Med.* **2007**, *167*, 1892–1898. [CrossRef]
118. Zhao, L.; Chen, J.; Li, Y.; Sun, X.; Chang, X.; Zheng, H.; Gong, B.; Huang, Y.; Yang, M.; Wu, X.; et al. The long-term effect of acupuncture for migraine prophylaxis: A randomized clinical trial. *JAMA Intern. Med.* **2017**, *177*, 508–515. [CrossRef]
119. Berman, B.M.; Lao, L.; Langenberg, P.; Lee, W.L.; Gilpin, A.M.; Hochberg, M.C. Effectiveness of acupuncture as adjunctive therapy in osteoarthritis of the knee: A randomized, controlled trial. *Ann. Intern. Med* **2004**, *141*, 901–910. [CrossRef]
120. Golianu, B.; Yeh, A.M.; Brooks, M. Acupuncture for pediatric pain. *Children (Basel)* **2014**, *1*, 134–148. [CrossRef] [PubMed]
121. Lin, Y.C.; Tassone, R.F.; Jahng, S.; Rahbar, R.; Holzman, R.S.; Zurakowski, D.; Sethna, N.F. Acupuncture management of pain and emergence agitation in children after bilateral myringotomy and tympanostomy tube insertion. *Paediatr. Anaesth.* **2009**, *19*, 1096–1101. [CrossRef] [PubMed]
122. Tsao, G.J.; Messner, A.H.; Seybold, J.; Sayyid, Z.N.; Cheng, A.G.; Golianu, B. Intraoperative acupuncture for posttonsillectomy pain: A randomized, double-blind, placebo-controlled trial. *Laryngoscope* **2015**, *125*, 1972–1978. [CrossRef] [PubMed]
123. Raith, W.; Schmolzer, G.M.; Resch, B.; Reiterer, F.; Avian, A.; Koestenberger, M.; Urlesberger, B. Laser acupuncture for neonatal abstinence syndrome: A randomized controlled trial. *Pediatrics* **2015**, *136*, 876–884. [CrossRef] [PubMed]
124. Gottschling, S.; Meyer, S.; Gribova, I.; Distler, L.; Berrang, J.; Gortner, L.; Graf, N.; Shamdeen, M.G. Laser acupuncture in children with headache: A double-blind, randomized, bicenter, placebo-controlled trial. *Pain* **2008**, *137*, 405–412. [CrossRef] [PubMed]
125. Wayne, P.M.; Kerr, C.E.; Schnyer, R.N.; Legedza, A.T.; Savetsky-German, J.; Shields, M.H.; Buring, J.E.; Davis, R.B.; Conboy, L.A.; Highfield, E.; et al. Japanese-style acupuncture for endometriosis-related pelvic pain in adolescents and young women: Results of a randomized sham-controlled trial. *J. Pediatr. Adolesc. Gynecol.* **2008**, *21*, 247–257. [CrossRef] [PubMed]
126. Logan, D.E.; Carpino, E.A.; Chiang, G.; Condon, M.; Firn, E.; Gaughan, V.J.; Hogan, M.; Leslie, D.S.; Olson, K.; Sager, S.; et al. A day-hospital approach to treatment of pediatric complex regional pain syndrome: Initial functional outcomes. *Clin. J. Pain* **2012**, *28*, 766–774. [CrossRef]

127. Simons, L.E.; Sieberg, C.B.; Pielech, M.; Conroy, C.; Logan, D.E. What does it take? Comparing intensive rehabilitation to outpatient treatment for children with significant pain-related disability. *J. Pediatr. Psychol.* **2013**, *38*, 213–223. [CrossRef]
128. American Pain Society. Pain in Infants, Children, and Adolescents SIG. Available online: http://americanpainsociety.org/get-involved/shared-interest-groups/pediatric-adolescent-pain (accessed on 1 December 2018).

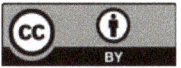

© 2019 by the authors. Licensee MDPI, Basel, Switzerland. This article is an open access article distributed under the terms and conditions of the Creative Commons Attribution (CC BY) license (http://creativecommons.org/licenses/by/4.0/).

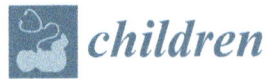

Review

Pharmacological Strategies for Decreasing Opioid Therapy and Management of Side Effects from Chronic Use

Genevieve D'Souza [1], Anava A. Wren [2], Christina Almgren [1], Alexandra C. Ross [1], Amanda Marshall [1] and Brenda Golianu [1,*]

[1] Department of Anesthesia, Perioperative and Pain Medicine, Stanford University, Palo Alto, CA 94304, USA; gdsouza@stanford.edu (G.D.); calmgren@stanfordchildrens.org (C.A.); alexandra.cram.ross@gmail.com (A.C.R.); 11am203@queensu.ca (A.M.)
[2] Department of Pediatrics, Division of Pediatric Gastroenterology, Hepatology and Nutrition, Stanford University, Palo Alto, CA 94304, USA; awren2@stanford.edu
* Correspondence: bgolianu@stanford.edu; Tel.: +1-650-723-5728

Received: 24 August 2018; Accepted: 3 December 2018; Published: 5 December 2018

Abstract: As awareness increases about the side effects of opioids and risks of misuse, opioid use and appropriate weaning of opioid therapies have become topics of significant clinical relevance among pediatric populations. Critically ill hospitalized neonates, children, and adolescents routinely receive opioids for analgesia and sedation as part of their hospitalization, for both acute and chronic illnesses. Opioids are frequently administered to manage pain symptoms, reduce anxiety and agitation, and diminish physiological stress responses. Opioids are also regularly prescribed to youth with chronic pain. These medications may be prescribed during the initial phase of a diagnostic workup, during an emergency room visit; as an inpatient, or on an outpatient basis. Following treatment for underlying pain conditions, it can be challenging to appropriately wean and discontinue opioid therapies. Weaning opioid therapy requires special expertise and care to avoid symptoms of increased pain, withdrawal, and agitation. To address this challenge, there have been enhanced efforts to implement opioid-reduction during pharmacological therapies for pediatric pain management. Effective pain management therapies and their outcomes in pediatrics are outside the scope of this paper. The aims of this paper were to: (1) Review the current practice of opioid-reduction during pharmacological therapies; and (2) highlight concrete opioid weaning strategies and management of opioid withdrawal.

Keywords: opioid therapy; weaning of opioids; withdrawal; assessment of withdrawal

1. Introduction

There is growing public concern regarding the use and risks related to prescription opioid therapy [1]. Historically, opioid therapy has been a central component to clinical pain management in most pediatric hospitals. Opioids are frequently prescribed for the management of pain related to acute conditions, as well as for sedation and management of agitation among patients receiving intensive care. Research in both adults and children has demonstrated that opioids are effective and potent in the acute management of pain [2,3]. Opioids increase descending modulation, and reduce descending facilitation in pain pathways of the central nervous system [4]. Opioids also target affective centers of the brain that impact emotional states, which can alter pain perception [5].

With long term use, however, physiological dependence and tolerance increase due to internalization of receptors and other adaptive processes [6]. Efficacy of clinical pain control decreases requiring increasing doses of analgesic agents, corresponding to increases in side effect profiles [6]. The range of side effects include respiratory depression, constipation, cognitive dysfunction, and psychiatric comorbidities such as anxiety and depression [7–10]. Additionally, chronic opioid use can lead to physical tolerance and dependence, and carries the risk of addiction [11]. Opioid use can also have the unexpected result of increased sensitization to pain (i.e., opioid induced hyperalgesia), though this is a rare phenomenon [12].

Understanding the appropriate use and side effect profiles of opioids, and effective tapering strategies, is vital to delivering safe pain management to pediatric patients. A search in Pubmed was performed on the following topics in both pediatric and adult literature: Opioid dependence, tolerance, withdrawal, and weaning from 2000 to 2018. Articles focused on pediatric data were chosen. Adult data was reviewed and utilized when pediatric data was lacking. Where data was pediatric-focused, specific references were made in the text. All other references refer to adult data.

The aims of this paper were to: (1) Review the current practice of opioid-reduction during pharmacological therapies; and (2) highlight concrete opioid weaning strategies, and management of opioid withdrawal. We reviewed and defined opioid dependence, withdrawal, tolerance and addiction, assessment of opioid withdrawal utilizing age appropriate withdrawal scales, and utilization of wean strategies and pharmacological aids to assist in safe reduction in therapy. This article did not address the use of opioids for pain management specifically or aim to assess pain management outcomes of opioid therapy.

2. Opioid-Reduction Weaning Protocols in Pediatric Patients

Effective medical management of patients receiving opioids can be addressed by appropriate assessment of pain, an accurate understanding of opioids and related side effects and withdrawal, and implementation of opioid reduction strategies including opioid weaning protocols and opioid-sparing adjuvants. Opioid withdrawal may occur in 0–100% of children who are exposed to opioids. Prevalence ranged from 45 to 86% in one recent review [13], while in another study 68% of patients experienced withdrawal [14].

Pediatric weaning protocols are highly variable. In a recent survey of pediatric healthcare providers, only 27% of respondents utilized a written protocol for opioid tapering, 22% consulted a pain management team regarding weaning of opioids, and the majority seldom or never consulted a pharmacist [15]. In another survey of pediatric congenital heart disease centers, only 25% of sites used a standardized clinical pathway when weaning opioid medications [16]. In the RESTORE study—a randomized controlled multicenter study of protocolized sedation of 1225 pediatric patients—Curley et al. demonstrated that the use of protocolized weaning of opioid medication was associated with shorter durations of opioid treatment (9 vs. 10 days, $p = 0.01$), and more study days spent in the calm and awake states (86% vs. 75%, $p = 0.004$) [14].

Common management strategies described in small pediatric studies include the use of methadone, addition of alpha 2 agonists, and protocolized reduction in dosing [17]. The most common weaning strategies involved decreases of 10–20% per day [13]. Identification of high-risk patients can help prevent iatrogenic withdrawal [18]. These include young age, pre-existing cognitive impairment, higher mean preweaning opioid dose, duration of opioid treatment, use of three or more sedative medications, and higher nurse to patient ratio.

The developmental aspects of opioid therapy deserve some consideration. The endogenous opioid system is highly expressed by developing neural cells, and can influence both neuronal as well as glial maturation [19]. While opioids do not directly trigger maturational events, they modulate ongoing cellular processes. These potentially detrimental effects must be balanced against the effects of untreated pain and physiologic stress, which have been associated with adverse outcomes and may also affect subsequent development [20], as well as ongoing clinical care of critically ill children [21]. Research on long-term neurocognitive effects of opioids on children is limited, and confounded by multiple co-existing morbidities [22].

The use of synthetic or short acting opioids may cause greater tolerance in preterm and term neonates. For example, patients receiving fentanyl while on extracorporeal membrane oxygenation (ECMO) require longer durations of opioid weaning compared to neonates who have received morphine during their treatment [23]. Additionally, neonates have immature kidney and liver functions leading to the accumulation of morphine metabolites, notably morphine-3-glucuronide, which can lead to antagonism of analgesia, as well as morphine-6-glucuronide, which is a more potent analgesic in comparison to morphine and may lead to excessive sedation [24].

Therefore, the treating physician must be aware of developmental concerns from pharmacokinetic to pharmacodynamic perspectives, as well as the developmental needs of the child from a neurological and psychological perspective at each phase of the treatment, and weaning processes. The use of appropriate and well timed adjuvant therapies, both pharmacological and nonpharmacological, may help minimize the need for sedatives and analgesics at various stages of the treatment process [25].

3. Opioids and Common Side Effects

The mechanisms of opioid analgesia include inhibiting the transmission of noxious input from the periphery to the central nervous system, and facilitating the descent of the inhibitory system that can decrease noxious input and affective modulation [26,27]. While opioids are very effective at the acute management of pain, some pediatric patients develop physiologic dependence or withdrawal following as little as seven days of opioid therapy [28]. Tolerance and addiction are other potential physiological effects of opioids. See Table 1 for a summary of potential physiological effects described below.

Table 1. Summary of physiological effects [29–31].

Term	Definition	Causative Mechanism
Dependence	A physiologic and biochemical adaptation of neurons such that removing a drug precipitates withdrawal or abstinence syndrome	Activation of second-messenger protein kinases; changes in neurotransmitter levels; changes in neuronal networks
Withdrawal	A clinical syndrome that manifests after stopping or reversing a drug after prolonged exposure to that drug	Superactivation of AC; opioid receptor coupling to G_s protein; activation of excitatory amino acid receptors
Tolerance	Decreasing clinical effects of a drug after prolonged exposure to it	Upregulation of the cAMP pathway; desensitization of opioid receptors
Addiction	A chronic, relapsing syndrome of psychological dependence and craving a drug for its psychedelic, sedative, or euphoric effects; characterized by compulsion, loss of control, and continued use of a substance despite harmful effects	Activation of dopaminergic reward systems in nucleus accumbens; mechanisms associated with tolerance and dependence

3.1. Dependence and Withdrawal

Dependence is an involuntary physiological response that occurs when there is an adaptation to the opioid, which is manifested by withdrawal symptoms when the opioid is abruptly discontinued [30,32]. Common neurologic signs of dependence in children include anxiety, agitation, grimacing, insomnia, increased muscle tone, abnormal tremors, and choreoathetoid movements. Gastrointestinal symptoms include vomiting, diarrhea, and poor appetite, while autonomic signs include tachypnea, tachycardia, fever, sweating, and hypertension [21].

In children, there are still many unanswered questions regarding the long term effects of opioid tolerance and withdrawal [33]. Sirnes et al., in a preliminary study, found that school-age children who had been exposed to prenatal opioids, showed Functional Magnetic Resonance Imaging (fMRI) changes and possible impaired executive function task performance [34]. Although some preliminary animal data suggests that there may be a faster onset of dependence in younger rats, it is unclear whether this applies to pediatric patients, and more studies are needed in this area [21].

The onset of withdrawal is dependent on the characteristics of the opioid the child was exposed to. For shorter acting opioids, such as oxycodone or hydrocodone, the symptoms may start as soon as 12 h after the last dose and peak over the next one or two days. In contrast, when stopping a longer acting opioid such as methadone, the signs of withdrawal may not be seen for more than 24 h and can last up to 10 days [35].

Studies have shown that children at increased risk of iatrogenic withdrawal syndrome include those who are less than six months old, have had a higher cumulative opioid dose or longer duration of exposure, have been exposed to three or more sedative classes (e.g., opioids, benzodiazepines, dexmedetomidine, and ketamine), or have a pre-existing cognitive impairment [18]. Of note, in neonatal abstinence syndrome, newborn infants may be dependent on opioids or benzodiazepines due to in-utero exposure. Following birth, they must be closely observed for signs of withdrawal, and treated as appropriate [18].

In older children, symptoms of delirium—a neurocognitive disorder due to a somatic illness or its treatment—can mimic those of withdrawal such as tachycardia, tachypnea, agitation, irritability, muscle tension, and sleep disturbances [36]. Children who are critically ill or in the Intensive Care Unit (ICU) are at risk of delirium secondary to the multiple sedative agents used, the severity of illness, changes in metabolic dysfunction or infection. Environmental factors such as changes in sleep can be additive [37,38]. One study found that children who received benzodiazepines were at a five-times greater risk of developing delirium than those that did not receive benzodiazepines [39]. Several delirium scoring tools have been developed, such as the Pediatric Confusion Assessment Method for ICU in children over five years of age (modified version of the adult assessment tool) [37]. Several symptoms of delirium such as tachycardia, tachypnea, and agitation are scored on both the withdrawal and delirium scales making definitive diagnostic determination difficult. Appropriate treatment of delirium may include, but is notlimited to, the treatment of any underlying withdrawal.

3.2. Tolerance

Tolerance is a state of physiological adaptation that occurs after prolonged exposure to an opioid. With tolerance, the patient requires progressively larger doses of the opioid to achieve the same effect. Complex intracellular neural mechanisms, including opioid receptor desensitization and down-regulation, are believed to be key mechanisms underlying opioid tolerance [40]. Tolerance can occur as soon as three days after opioid exposure [41]. In critically ill children, the effects can be profound. One multicenter study found that 16% of mechanically ventilated children required doubling of their opioid doses after seven days, and 20% doubled their requirement after 14 days [42]. In spite of potentially rapid development of tolerance in the pediatric population, especially in the case of life-limiting illnesses such as oncologic conditions or other severe illnesses, the rapid escalation and resultant tolerance to keep severely ill pediatric patients comfortable is often justified. [43,44].

3.3. Opioid Induced Hyperalgesia

Research has shown that the administration of higher doses of opioids over longer periods of time does not always lead to improved pain control, rather it can result in hyperalgesia. A recent study found that the regular use of opioids for more than 90 days led to increased pain sensitivity [45]. The exact mechanisms by which patients developcentral sensitization found in opioid induced hyperalgesia is still unknown, but possible contributing factors include characteristics of the opioids being used, changes in corticotrophin releasing factors, suppressed reuptake or increased release of excitatory neurotransmitters, changes in glial cells, and genetic variability [46,47]. Opioid induced hyperalgesia (OIH) is less commonly addressed in pediatric literature. One case report from 2012 noted the development of OIH in a nine year-old receiving opioids for flare of polyarticular juvenile idiopathic arthritis. The child was treated by stopping the opioid. Subsequently, pain and hyperalgesia decreased [48]. Treatment for OIH often involves the reduction or elimination of the opioid to monitor for resolution of symptoms. Ongoing adult research is evaluating ketamine and methadone, which have NMDA receptor antagonist activity, to determine if these medications decrease the likelihood of developing OIH or help resolve symptoms [12].

3.4. Addiction

Chronic opioid use also has the potential to lead to addiction. Addiction, as defined by the American Pain Society and the American Society of Addiction Medicine, is a chronic neurobiological disease with genetic, psychosocial, and environmental factors contributing to its development and presentation [31]. Addiction is characterized by the inability to consistently abstain from an addictive stimulus, impairment in behavioral control, craving, diminished recognition of significant problems with one's behaviors and interpersonal relationships, and a dysfunctional emotional response.

Research has demonstrated that approximately one in four adults receiving chronic opioid therapy in a primary care setting suffers from opioid addiction [49–51]. To our knowledge, there are no published data detailing rates of opioid addiction among youth. Interestingly, in a Canadian study examining methadone maintenance therapy, initial age of opioid use was associated with increased physical and psychological comorbidities. Individuals with an age-of-onset of opioid use younger than 18 years were found to be at higher odds of having a physical or psychiatric comorbid disorder, compared to individuals with an age-of-onset of 31 years or older [52]. Future research should explore rates and risk factors of opioid addiction among pediatric populations, as well as risk factors for addiction. Appropriate treatment of comorbid disorders in patients who are being considered for opioid therapy is recommended to minimize the risk of opioid addiction.

4. Assessment of Opioid Withdrawal

Assessment of opioid withdrawal is central to developing and applying effective opioid-reduction during pharmacological treatments. A number of scales have been developed to help providers distinguish between signs of neonatal withdrawal and iatrogenic withdrawal, and to help determine when treatment might be required. The Finnegan neonatal abstinence scale, and its recent modification, allows clinicians to accurately assess clinical symptoms of neonatal withdrawal [53]. Scores >8 indicate the necessity for further evaluation for treatment.

The Withdrawal Assessment Tool-1 (WAT-1) scores youth on symptoms of withdrawal including tremors, increased muscle tone, repetitive movements, loose stools, and vomiting. This tool was originally validated for children six months to eight years of age [32]; however, more recent studies have found WAT-1 to be reliable for youth up to 17 years of age [54].

The Sophia Observation withdrawal Symptoms scale scores infants and children three months or older on withdrawal symptoms within a four-hour period. Scores >4 should be evaluated further for withdrawal. This scale was found to have a sensitivity of 83%, and specificity of 95% in critically ill children in the Pediatric Intensive Care Unit (PICU) [55]. Only the Sophia Observation withdrawal scale and WAT-1 have been specifically developed to evaluate iatrogenic withdrawal in a range of ages and settings [54].

5. Opioid Weaning Treatments

Although there is no certainty about whether an individual patient will experience symptoms of withdrawal, some general guidelines are helpful for the clinician to consider in developing an individualized opioid-reduction program.

For opioid therapy lasting less than seven days, no gradual reduction in dose is necessary as patients are at a lower risk of withdrawal. The opioid infusion may be discontinued without a taper, and patients should be monitored for signs and symptoms of withdrawal. Additional factors placing a patient at increased risk for withdrawal following opioid therapy lasting less than seven days include higher cumulative dose of opioids and prior exposure to opioids.

When opioid therapy has been delivered for more than seven days, or symptoms of withdrawal are present, gradual opioid weaning is usually necessary. Opioid weaning protocols aim to gradually decrease plasma concentrations of the drug to prevent symptoms of opioid withdrawal syndrome. As no definite outcome-based evidence exists to support an ideal weaning protocol, therapy should be based on the individual treatment response, and should consider the length of opioid exposure and the total daily opioid dose (TDD) [56]. One suggested weaning schedule is to decrease the TDD by 10–20% everyday, while monitoring for signs and symptoms of withdrawal. Oral morphine, methadone, clonidine, and transdermal fentanyl have all been used in opioid weaning programs.

Methadone is often the most suitable medication for weaning due to the long half-life and convenience of oral dosing [57,58]. To account for cross tolerance, the converted methadone dosage may need to be reduced by 30–50%. The total daily dose of methadone is then divided into four equal doses to be given every 6 h (q6hr). Initial q6hr dosing is for 24 h only—this is functionally a "loading dose" to rapidly increase serum levels of methadone. Due to the long half-life of methadone, the dosing interval will change to every 12 h after the initial 24 h period, with close observation for possible sedation. Once a steady state is reached, methadone can then be tapered by 10–20% every other day, observing for symptoms of withdrawal. Of note, methadone is not suitable for children with prolonged QT corrected (QTc). A baseline EKG is recommended prior to initiating therapy with methadone. In these critically ill children, the TDD of their current opioid may be decreased by 10–20% daily until the wean is accomplished, or the patient may be transitioned to another oral or intravenous opioid (e.g., morphine, hydromorphone). See Table 2 for sample opioid weaning schedules.

Table 2. Sample Opioid Weaning Schedules.

Weaning schedules	
IV morphine dose	Methadone total daily dose
<0.05 mg/kg/h	0.3 mg/kg/day
0.05–0.1 mg/kg/h	0.4 mg/kg/day
0.11–0.2 mg/kg/h	0.6 mg/kg/day
0.21–0.4 mg/kg/h	0.8 mg/kg/day
>0.4 mg/kg/h	1 mg/kg/day
IV fentanyl dose	Methadone total daily dose
1 µg/kg/h	0.05 mg/kg/day
2 µg/kg/h	0.1 mg/kg/day
3 µg/kg/h	0.15 mg/kg/day
4 µg/kg/h	0.2 mg/kg/day

Transitioning to enteral methadone should be considered as early as clinically feasible. The bioavailability of enteral methadone is 75–80% that of intravenous methadone, thus it is not usually necessary to adjust dosing for this difference. If converting from high doses of opioid infusions, it is recommended that intravenous infusions be tapered to lower doses (e.g., ≤0.2 mg/kg/h morphine equivalent) before transitioning to methadone.

When weaning patients from opioids, withdrawal and related symptoms often occur and can be distressing for children. Clonidine can be useful in treating these symptoms of opioid withdrawal.

Duffet et al. performed a prospective randomized control trial (RCT) on 50 pediatric patients undergoing reduction of opioid therapy and studied the use of parenteral clonidine 5 µg/kg, administered every 6 h [59]. No significant effect on withdrawal symptoms was observed. Thirteen patients experienced hypotension or bradycardia requiring intervention; however, the relationship to the study group was unclear.

The use of clonidine as a prophylactic for withdrawal syndromes was studied in 10 consecutive patients undergoing single-state laryngotracheal reconstruction [60]. No significant side effects were noted. A study of plasma concentrations of whole vs. cut patches showed that the delivered dose from whole patches was found to be 7 ± 1.7 µg/kg/day (plasma concentration 0.55 ± 0.3 ng/mL), while cut patches delivered a lower dose but with increased variability, 6.4 ± 3 µg/kg/day (plasma concentration 1 ± 1.1 ng/mL) [61]. A recent review suggested that, while oral and transdermal clonidine have a potential role in the management of sedation and withdrawal in critically ill infants and children, and were relatively well tolerated, the use of cut transdermal patches should be avoided [62]. Further prospective studies were recommended. No data exists on the weaning of clonidine dose following its use as an adjuvant for opioid withdrawal [53]. The recommendations noted below are a result of developed clinical practice at our institution.

Sample Clonidine Dosing and Weaning Schedule

1. Start with clonidine 4–8 µg/kg/day oral (per os (PO)) divided every 4 h. If not taking oral intake (nil per os (NPO)), give clonidine 1 µg/kg IV q4h.
2. Concurrently initiate opioid weaning by reducing daily opioid dose by 5–10% of baseline dose.
3. After 48 h on oral or parenteral clonidine without adverse blood pressure effects, convert to clonidine patch 5–10 µg/kg/day, rounding up or down to nearest 50 µg increment.
4. The minimum patient weight for patch use is typically about 5 kg. Although doses as high as 2 µg/kg may be tolerated, the physical patch size makes it difficult to use in smaller children. Therefore, for children ≤5 kg, use oral or intravenous (i.v.) clonidine.
5. Once ready to wean, reduce the clonidine patch size by 50 µg/day two times a week until the dose is reduced to the 100 µg/day patch size for children >10 kg, or 50 µg/day patch size for children <10 kg. Then leave this last patch on for 14 days and discontinue afterwards.
6. Clonidine weaning may occur concomitantly with opioid weaning, provided the opioid parenteral morphine equivalent dose is less than 0.3 mg/kg/day.

For excessive withdrawal (WAT-1 > 3), the total as needed (pro re nata (PRN)) morphine requirement may be added to the daily methadone dose, and the taper resumed once symptoms are controlled consistently. For excessive sedation, a dose of methadone should be held, and the total daily methadone dose decreased by 10–20%. Ondansetron 0.1 mg/kg up to 4 mg every 6 h may be used to treat nausea related to withdrawal [63]. Patients should be assessed for QT prolongation, particularly if other QT-prolonging medications are being used [64]. Co-administration of benzodiazepines with opioids is frequently practiced in the context of intensive care sedation or in acute postoperative pain management settings. When discontinuation is planned, the benzodiazepines may need concurrent weaning, often alternating with the opioid wean, as described in a recent review by Fenn et al. [13]. Care should be taken due to the risk of over sedation when opioids and benzodiazepines are co-administered. Conversely, when benzodiazepines are reduced rapidly, withdrawal, agitation, and other potentially life-threatening side effects such as seizures may occur. The use of a flexible patient-centered approach is important where weaning of multiple medications is needed [65].

6. Adjuvant Therapies for Opioid Reduction Therapy

When implementing opioid-reduction pharmacological treatments, adjuvant therapies are regularly considered for possible integration into treatment regimens. Adjuvant analgesics target specific aspects of nociceptive and neuropathic pain physiology, reducing pain and opioid consumption [25]. Nociceptive analgesics include acetaminophen, non-steroidal anti-inflammatory drugs (NSAIDS), and glucocorticoids. Neuropathic analgesics commonly include gabapentinoids, lidocaine, ketamine, alpha-2-agonists, and rare use of tricyclic antidepressants and serotonin and norepinephrine reuptake inhibitors. Low dose ketamine may be helpful as an adjuvant to assist in weaning off opioid therapy [66].

Cannabidiol (CBD) is another adjuvant therapy that is increasingly considered for chronic pain management treatments. CBD is one of the active cannabinoids identified in cannabis. CBD does not appear to have the hallucinogenic/intoxication side effects of another major component of cannabis, tetrahydrocannabinol (THC) [67]. Randomized controlled studies are needed to further examine the efficacy of medical cannabis and its potential use in opioid weaning therapy.

Integrating adjuvant therapies with nonpharmacological therapies such as cognitive behavioral therapy, mindfulness, hypnosis, and acupuncture is commonly employed during opioid-reduction pharmacological treatments to optimize patient comfort, functional well-being, and quality of life. Consultation with a pain management specialists can facilitate this integrative opioid reduction approach.

7. Conclusions

Opioid use has risen significantly in the past two decades. Although opioids are an effective means of managing acute pain, risks associated with opioids are plentiful and may outweigh such benefits, especially when treating chronic pain. Having an accurate understanding of opioid-related side effects, age appropriate tools for assessment of withdrawal, and opioid reduction strategies, may help to minimize symptoms of withdrawal and safely reduce or discontinue opioid therapy.

As outlined above, opioids can be safely tapered in both acute and chronic settings by gradually reducing the total opioid dose or, if appropriate, transitioning to a long acting opioid such as methadone, followed by a gradual weaning protocol and close observation for symptoms of withdrawal. Opioid-sparing adjuvants, including acetaminophen, non-steroidal agents, gabapentinoids, benzodiazepines, ketamine and alpha-1-agonists, can also provide safe and effective analgesia and sedation, and may reduce the necessity and/or dose of opioid therapy. Alpha-1-agonists in particular may help in management of withdrawal symptoms. Opioid reduction utilizingpharmacological protocols provides a safe and efficacious way to decrease opioid therapy when this is appropriate, and minimizes related adverse side effects.

Author Contributions: Conceptualization, All; Methodology, All; Investigation, All; Tables, G.D.; Writing-Original Draft Preparation, All; Writing-Review & Editing, All; Supervision, B.G.

Funding: This research received no external funding.

Conflicts of Interest: The authors declare no conflict of interest.

References

1. Blendon, R.J.; Benson, J.M. The public and the opioid-abuse epidemic. *N. Engl. J. Med.* **2018**, *378*, 407–411. [CrossRef] [PubMed]
2. Fields, H.L. The doctor's dilemma: Opiate analgesics and chronic pain. *Neuron* **2011**, *69*, 591–594. [CrossRef] [PubMed]
3. Krane, E.J.; Weisman, S.J.; Walco, G.A. The national opioid epidemic and the risk of outpatient opioids in children. *Pediatrics* **2018**, *142*. [CrossRef] [PubMed]
4. Ossipov, M.H.; Morimura, K.; Porreca, F. Descending pain modulation and chronification of pain. *Curr. Opin. Support. Palliat. Care* **2014**, *8*, 143–151. [PubMed]
5. Nummenmaa, L.; Tuominen, L. Opioid system and human emotions. *Br. J. Pharmacol.* **2017**, *175*, 2737–2749. [CrossRef]
6. Koch, T.; Hollt, V. Role of receptor internalization in opioid tolerance and dependence. *Pharmacol. Ther.* **2008**, *117*, 199–206. [CrossRef]
7. Berde, C.; Nurko, S. Opioid side effects—Mechanism-based therapy. *N. Engl. J. Med.* **2008**, *358*, 2400–2402. [CrossRef]
8. Moore, R.A.; McQuay, H.J. Prevalence of opioid adverse events in chronic non-malignant pain: Systematic review of randomised trials of oral opioids. *Arthritis Res. Ther.* **2005**, *7*, R1046–R1051. [CrossRef]
9. Gomes, T.; Mamdani, M.M.; Dhalla, I.A.; Paterson, J.M.; Juurlink, D.N. Opioid dose and drug-related mortality in patients with nonmalignant pain. *Arch. Intern. Med.* **2011**, *171*, 686–691. [CrossRef] [PubMed]
10. Grunkemeier, D.M.; Cassara, J.E.; Dalton, C.B.; Drossman, D.A. The narcotic bowel syndrome: Clinical features, pathophysiology, and management. *Clin. Gastroenterol. Hepatol.* **2007**, *5*, 1126–1139. [CrossRef]

11. Fudin, J.; Raouf, M.; Wegrzyn, E.L. *Opioid Dosing Policy: Pharmacological Considerations Regarding Equianalgesic Dosing*; American Academy of Integrative Pain Management: Lenexa, KS, USA, 2017.
12. Lee, M.; Silverman, S.M.; Hansen, H.; Patel, V.B.; Manchikanti, L. A comprehensive review of opioid-induced hyperalgesia. *Pain Phys.* **2011**, *14*, 145–161.
13. Fenn, N.E., 3rd; Plake, K.S. Opioid and benzodiazepine weaning in pediatric patients: Review of current literature. *Pharmacotherapy* **2017**, *37*, 1458–1468. [CrossRef]
14. Curley, M.A.; Wypij, D.; Watson, R.S.; Grant, M.J.; Asaro, L.A.; Cheifetz, I.M.; Dodson, B.L.; Franck, L.S.; Gedeit, R.G.; Angus, D.C.; et al. Protocolized sedation vs. usual care in pediatric patients mechanically ventilated for acute respiratory failure: A randomized clinical trial. *JAMA* **2015**, *313*, 379–389. [CrossRef]
15. Deborah, F.; Ameringer, S.W. Survey of opioid tapering practices of pediatric healthcare providers: A national perspective. *J. Opioid Manag.* **2017**, *13*, 59–64.
16. O'Connell, C.; Ziniel, S.; Hartwell, L.; Connor, J. Management of Opioid and Sedative Weaning in Pediatric Congenital Heart Disease Patients: Assessing the State of Practice. *Dimens. Crit. Care Nurs.* **2017**, *36*, 116–124.
17. Chiu, A.W.; Contreras, S.; Mehta, S.; Korman, J.; Perreault, M.M.; Williamson, D.R.; Burry, L.D. Iatrogenic Opioid Withdrawal in Critically Ill Patients: A Review of Assessment Tools and Management. *Ann. Pharmacother.* **2017**, *51*, 1099–1111. [CrossRef]
18. Best, K.M.; Wypij, D.; Asaro, L.A.; Curley, M.A. Randomized evaluation of sedation titration for respiratory failure study investigators. Patient, process, and system predictors of iatrogenic withdrawal syndrome in critically ill children. *Crit. Care Med.* **2017**, *45*, e7–e15. [CrossRef]
19. Hauser, K.F.; Knapp, P.E. Opiate drugs with abuse liability hijack the endogenous opioid system to disrupt neuronal and glial maturation in the central nervous system. *Front. Pediatr.* **2017**, *5*, 294. [CrossRef]
20. Holsti, L.; Weinberg, J.; Whitfield, M.F.; Grunau, R.E. Relationships between adrenocorticotropic hormone and cortisol are altered during clustered nursing care in preterm infants born at extremely low gestational age. *Early Hum. Dev.* **2007**, *83*, 341–348. [CrossRef]
21. Anand, K.J.; Willson, D.F.; Berger, J.; Harrison, R.; Meert, K.L.; Zimmerman, J.; Carcillo, J.; Newth, C.J.; Prodhan, P.; Dean, J.M.; et al. Tolerance and withdrawal from prolonged opioid use in critically ill children. *Pediatrics* **2010**, *125*, e1208–e1225. [CrossRef]
22. Jain, G.; Mahendra, V.; Singhal, S.; Dzara, K.; Pilla, T.R.; Manworren, R.; Kaye, A.D. Long-term neuropsychological effects of opioid use in children: A descriptive literature review. *Pain Phys.* **2014**, *17*, 109–118. [CrossRef]
23. Franck, L.S.; Vilardi, J.; Durand, D.; Powers, R. Opioid withdrawal in neonates after continuous infusions of morphine or fentanyl during extracorporeal membrane oxygenation. *Am. J. Crit. Care* **1998**, *7*, 364–369.
24. Suresh, S.; Anand, K.J. Opioid tolerance in neonates: A state-of-the-art review. *Paediatr. Anaesth.* **2001**, *11*, 511–521. [CrossRef]
25. Brooks, M.R.; Golianu, B. Perioperative management in children with chronic pain. *Paediatr. Anaesth.* **2016**, *26*, 794–806. [CrossRef]
26. Bannister, K.; Kucharczyk, M.; Dickenson, A.H. Hopes for the future of pain control. *Pain Ther.* **2017**, *6*, 117–128. [CrossRef]
27. D'Mello, R.; Dickenson, A.H. Spinal cord mechanisms of pain. *Br. J. Anaesth.* **2008**, *101*, 8–16. [CrossRef]
28. Best, K.M.; Boullata, J.I.; Curley, M.A. Risk factors associated with iatrogenic opioid and benzodiazepine withdrawal in critically ill pediatric patients: A systematic review and conceptual model. *Pediatr. Crit. Care Med.* **2015**, *16*, 175–183. [CrossRef]
29. Heit, H.A. Addiction, physical dependence, and tolerance: Precise definitions to help clinicians evaluate and treat chronic pain patients. *J. Pain Palliat. Care Pharmacother.* **2003**, *17*, 15–29. [CrossRef]
30. Galinkin, J.; Koh, J.L.; Committee on Drugs; Section On Anesthesiology and Pain Medicine; American Academy of Pediatrics. Recognition and management of iatrogenically induced opioid dependence and withdrawal in children. *Pediatrics* **2014**, *133*, 152–155. [CrossRef]
31. American Society of Addiction Medicine. Public Policy Statement: Definition of Addiction. Available online: https://www.asam.org/advocacy/find-a-policy-statement/view-policy-statement/public-policy-statements/2011/12/15/the-definition-of-addiction (accessed on 14 June 2018).
32. Franck, L.S.; Scoppettuolo, L.A.; Wypij, D.; Curley, M.A. Validity and generalizability of the Withdrawal Assessment Tool-1 (WAT-1) for monitoring iatrogenic withdrawal syndrome in pediatric patients. *Pain* **2012**, *153*, 142–148. [CrossRef]

33. Maguire, D.J.; Taylor, S.; Armstrong, K.; Shaffer-Hudkins, E.; Germain, A.M.; Brooks, S.S.; Cline, G.J.; Clark, L. Long-term outcomes of infants with neonatal abstinence syndrome. *Neonatal Netw.* **2016**, *35*, 277–286. [CrossRef]
34. Sirnes, E.; Griffiths, S.T.; Aukland, S.M.; Eide, G.E.; Elgen, I.B.; Gundersen, H. Functional MRI in prenatally opioid-exposed children during a working memory-selective attention task. *Neurotoxicol. Teratol.* **2018**, *66*, 46–54. [CrossRef]
35. American Society of Addiction Medicine. National Practice Guideline for the Use of Medications in the Treatment of Addiction Involving Opioid Use. Available online: https://www.asam.org/docs/default-source/practice-support/guidelines-and-consensus-docs/asam-national-practice-guideline-supplement.pdf?sfvrsn=24 (accessed on 5 September 2018).
36. Harris, J.; Ramelet, A.S.; van Dijk, M.; Pokorna, P.; Wielenga, J.; Tume, L.; Tibboel, D.; Ista, E. Clinical recommendations for pain, sedation, withdrawal and delirium assessment in critically ill infants and children: An ESPNIC position statement for healthcare professionals. *Intensive Care Med.* **2016**, *42*, 972–986. [CrossRef]
37. Madden, K.; Burns, M.M.; Tasker, R.C. Differentiating delirium from sedative/hypnotic-related iatrogenic withdrawal syndrome: Lack of specificity in pediatric critical care assessment tools. *Pediatr. Crit. Care Med.* **2017**, *18*, 580–588. [CrossRef]
38. Thorn, R.P. Pediatric delirium. *Am. J. Psychiatry Resid. J.* **2017**, *12*, 6–8.
39. Traube, C.; Silver, G.; Gerber, L.M.; Kaur, S.; Mauer, E.A.; Kerson, A.; Joyce, C.; Greenwald, B.M. Delirium and mortality in critically ill children: Epidemiology and outcomes of pediatric delirium. *Crit. Care Med.* **2017**, *45*, 891–898. [CrossRef]
40. Williams, J.T.; Ingram, S.L.; Henderson, G.; Chavkin, C.; von Zastrow, M.; Schulz, S.; Koch, T.; Evans, C.J.; Christie, M.J. Regulation of mu-opioid receptors: Desensitization, phosphorylation, internalization, and tolerance. *Pharmacol. Rev.* **2013**, *65*, 223–254. [CrossRef]
41. Jenkins, I.A. Tolerance and addiction; the patient, the parent or the clinician? *Paediatr. Anaesth.* **2011**, *21*, 794–799. [CrossRef]
42. Anand, K.J.; Clark, A.E.; Willson, D.F.; Berger, J.; Meert, K.L.; Zimmerman, J.J.; Harrison, R.; Carcillo, J.A.; Newth, C.J.; Bisping, S.; et al. Opioid analgesia in mechanically ventilated children: Results from the multicenter Measuring Opioid Tolerance Induced by Fentanyl study. *Pediatr. Crit. Care Med.* **2013**, *14*, 27–36. [CrossRef]
43. Slater, M.E.; De Lima, J.; Campbell, K.; Lane, L.; Collins, J. Opioids for the management of severe chronic nonmalignant pain in children: A retrospective 1-year practice survey in a children's hospital. *Pain Med.* **2010**, *11*, 207–214. [CrossRef]
44. McCulloch, R.; Collins, J.J. Pain in children who have life-limiting conditions. *Child. Adolesc. Psychiatr. Clin. N. Am.* **2006**, *15*, 657–682. [CrossRef]
45. Samuelsen, P.J.; Nielsen, C.S.; Wilsgaard, T.; Stubhaug, A.; Svendsen, K.; Eggen, A.E. Pain sensitivity and analgesic use among 10,486 adults: The Tromso study. *BMC Pharmacol. Toxicol.* **2017**, *18*, 45. [CrossRef]
46. Weber, L.; Yeomans, D.C.; Tzabazis, A. Opioid-induced hyperalgesia in clinical anesthesia practice: What has remained from theoretical concepts and experimental studies? *Curr. Opin. Anaesthesiol.* **2017**, *30*, 458–465. [CrossRef]
47. Bannister, K.; Dickenson, A.H. Opioid hyperalgesia. *Curr. Opin. Support. Palliat. Care* **2010**, *4*, 1–5. [CrossRef]
48. Vijayan, V.; Moran, R.; Elder, M.E.; Sukumaran, S. Acute-onset opioid-induced hyperalgesia in a child with juvenile idiopathic arthritis. *J. Clin. Rheumatol.* **2012**, *18*, 349–351. [CrossRef]
49. Banta-Green, C.J.; Merrill, J.O.; Doyle, S.R.; Boudreau, D.M.; Calsyn, D.A. Opioid use behaviors, mental health and pain—Development of a typology of chronic pain patients. *Drug Alcohol. Depend.* **2009**, *104*, 34–42. [CrossRef]
50. Boscarino, J.A.; Rukstalis, M.; Hoffman, S.N.; Han, J.J.; Erlich, P.M.; Gerhard, G.S.; Stewart, W.F. Risk factors for drug dependence among out-patients on opioid therapy in a large US health-care system. *Addiction* **2010**, *105*, 1776–1782. [CrossRef]
51. Fleming, M.F.; Balousek, S.L.; Klessig, C.L.; Mundt, M.P.; Brown, D.D. Substance use disorders in a primary care sample receiving daily opioid therapy. *J. Pain* **2007**, *8*, 573–582. [CrossRef]

52. Naji, L.; Dennis, B.B.; Bawor, M.; Varenbut, M.; Daiter, J.; Plater, C.; Pare, G.; Marsh, D.C.; Worster, A.; Desai, D.; et al. The association between age of onset of opioid use and comorbidity among opioid dependent patients receiving methadone maintenance therapy. *Addict. Sci. Clin. Pract.* **2017**, *12*, 9. [CrossRef]
53. Zimmermann-Baer, U.; Notzli, U.; Rentsch, K.; Bucher, H.U. Finnegan neonatal abstinence scoring system: Normal values for first 3 days and weeks 5-6 in non-addicted infants. *Addiction* **2010**, *105*, 524–528. [CrossRef]
54. Hardesty, A.; Letzkus, L.; Miller, J.; Turner, L.; Conaway, M. Determining the reliability of the Withdrawal Assessment Tool-1 incomparison to the Neonatal Drug Withdrawal Scoring System. *Clin. Nurs. Stud.* **2015**, *3*, 66–71.
55. Ista, E.; de Hoog, M.; Tibboel, D.; Duivenvoorden, H.J.; van Dijk, M. Psychometric evaluation of the Sophia Observation withdrawal symptoms scale in critically ill children. *Pediatr. Crit. Care Med.* **2013**, *14*, 761–769. [CrossRef]
56. Dervan, L.A.; Yaghmai, B.; Watson, R.S.; Wolf, F.M. The use of methadone to facilitate opioid weaning in pediatric critical care patients: A systematic review of the literature and meta-analysis. *Paediatr. Anaesth.* **2017**, *27*, 228–239. [CrossRef]
57. Siddappa, R.; Fletcher, J.E.; Heard, A.M.; Kielma, D.; Cimino, M.; Heard, C.M. Methadone dosage for prevention of opioid withdrawal in children. *Paediatr. Anaesth.* **2003**, *13*, 805–810. [CrossRef]
58. Giby, K.; Vaillancourt, R.; Varughese, N.; Vadeboncoeur, C.; Pouliot, A. Use of methadone for opioid weaning in children: Prescribing practices and trends. *Can. J. Hosp. Pharm.* **2014**, *67*, 149–156. [CrossRef]
59. Duffett, M.; Choong, K.; Foster, J.; Cheng, J.; Meade, M.O.; Menon, K.; Cook, D.J. Clonidine in the sedation of mechanically ventilated children: A pilot randomized trial. *J. Crit. Care* **2014**, *29*, 758–763. [CrossRef]
60. Deutsch, E.S.; Nadkarni, V.M. Clonidine prophylaxis for narcotic and sedative withdrawal syndrome following laryngotracheal reconstruction. *Arch. Otolaryngol. Head Neck Surg.* **1996**, *122*, 1234–1238. [CrossRef]
61. Zuppa, A.F.; Tejani, S.M.; Cullen, E.J., Jr.; Nadkarni, V.M. Plasma Concentrations Following Application of Whole versus Cut Transdermal Clonidine Patches To Critically Ill Children. *J. Pediatr. Pharmacol. Ther.* **2004**, *9*, 43–48. [CrossRef]
62. Capino, A.C.; Miller, J.L.; Johnson, P.N. Clonidine for Sedation and Analgesia and Withdrawal in Critically Ill Infants and Children. *Pharmacotherapy* **2016**, *36*, 1290–1299. [CrossRef]
63. Gan, T.J.; Diemunsch, P.; Habib, A.S.; Kovac, A.; Kranke, P.; Meyer, T.A.; Watcha, M.; Chung, F.; Angus, S.; Apfel, C.C.; et al. Consensus guidelines for the management of postoperative nausea and vomiting. *Anesth. Analg.* **2014**, *118*, 85–113. [CrossRef]
64. Tobias, J.D. Tolerance, withdrawal, and physical dependency after long-term sedation and analgesia of children in the pediatric intensive care unit. *Crit. Care Med.* **2000**, *28*, 2122–2132. [CrossRef]
65. Siden, H.B.; Collin, K. Three patients and their drugs: A parallel case paper on paediatric opiate use and withdrawal. *Paediatr. Child. Health* **2005**, *10*, 163–168. [CrossRef]
66. Quinlan, J. The use of a subanesthetic infusion of intravenous ketamine to allow withdrawal of medically prescribed opioids in people with chronic pain, opioid tolerance and hyperalgesia: Outcome at 6 months. *Pain Med.* **2012**, *13*, 1524–1525. [CrossRef]
67. Jensen, B.; Chen, J.; Furnish, T.; Wallace, M. Medical marijuana and chronic pain: A review of basic science and clinical evidence. *Curr. Pain Headache Rep.* **2015**, *19*, 50. [CrossRef]

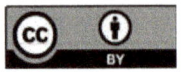

© 2018 by the authors. Licensee MDPI, Basel, Switzerland. This article is an open access article distributed under the terms and conditions of the Creative Commons Attribution (CC BY) license (http://creativecommons.org/licenses/by/4.0/).

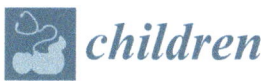

Opinion

The Elephant in the Room: The Need for Increased Integrative Therapies in Conventional Medical Settings

Missy Hall [1,*], Susanne M. Bifano [1], Leigh Leibel [2], Linda S. Golding [3] and Shiu-Lin Tsai [4]

1   Child Life Department, New York-Presbyterian Morgan Stanley Children's Hospital Columbia University Medical Center, 3959 Broadway, New York, NY 10032, USA; sub9053@nyp.org
2   Division of Hematology/Oncology, Columbia University Medical Center, 161 Ft. Washington Ave, Suite 922, New York, NY 10032-3789, USA; LL3125@cumc.columbia.edu
3   Pastoral Care, New York-Presbyterian Milstein Columbia University Medical Center, 622 W. 168th St., New York, NY 10032-3789, USA; lig9048@nyp.org
4   Division of Pediatric Emergency Medicine, Department of Emergency Medicine, Columbia University College of Physicians and Surgeons, 3959 Broadway, CHN-W116, New York, NY 10032; st166@cumc.columbia.edu
*   Correspondence: mmh9010@nyp.org; Tel.: +1-212-305-7952

Received: 15 October 2018; Accepted: 10 November 2018; Published: 16 November 2018

Abstract: Pediatric integrative therapy programs are essential to the treatment and well-being of patients. Identifying an effective integrative therapy model within conventional pediatric medical settings, however, often proves difficult. Our goal in this article is to explore varied solutions to increase access and inclusion of integrative therapies in an effort to promote best practice and holistic care. The main methods applied in this article are vignettes that illustrate how the integrative therapies in a metropolitan academic hospital successfully treat the patient by complementing conventional medicine. This leads to comprehensive care. The central finding of the article proposes viable solutions to increase interdisciplinary collaboration both internally within the institution and externally. Integrative therapists detail how they were able to increase visibility and yield best practice through increased educational initiatives and interdisciplinary collaboration.

Keywords: Integrative therapies; art therapy; music therapy; yoga therapy; acupuncture; pastoral care; creative arts therapy; pediatrics

---

1. Introduction

And so these men of Indostan, disputed loud and long,

each in his own opinion, exceeding stiff and strong,

Though each was partly in the right, and all were in the wrong!

So, oft in theologic wars, the disputants, I ween,

Rail on in utter ignorance, of what each other mean,

And prate about an Elephant

Not one of them has seen!

John Godfried Saxe [1]

The parable of the blind men and the elephant has long illustrated the importance of considering multiple viewpoints in order to see the full picture. The story tells of a group of blind men who are asked to characterize an elephant by touching a different part of its body, such as the tail, the ear, or the trunk. The result is that the elephant is universally mischaracterized because each man makes assumptions based on his partial interaction with the animal. The moral of the parable is that in order to attain a comprehensive version of the truth, we must first acknowledge our limitations and seek out other perspectives.

This parable mirrors conventional healthcare. Current medical practice routinely emphasizes treating the "diagnosis" at the expense of the patient. Doing so results in clinical "blindness" that inhibits best practice and limits comprehensive care.

For this reason, conventional medicine is increasingly trending toward interdisciplinary practice [2–4]. This practice acknowledges the patient and the person thereby targeting and treating the whole system.

One way to increase interdisciplinary practice is to promote integrative health care. This involves combining standard medical treatment with mind-body practices. This holistic approach to health care includes treating all parts of the patient, including the "mental, emotional, functional, spiritual, social and community aspects" [5].

Mind and body practices are centered around the patient-practitioner relationship and incorporate all available evidence-based therapies to treat the patient [6]. Acupuncturists, yoga therapists, and creative arts therapists engage in non-traditional mind-body practices that fall under this umbrella. Yoga therapists and creative arts therapists are mental health clinicians trained in psychotherapy and the psychology of their modality (yoga, art, music, dance, and poetry).

At NewYork-Presbyterian Morgan Stanley Children's Hospital, Columbia University Medical Center, mind-body therapies serve a variety of diverse populations. In an effort to advance integrative health care within this major metropolitan academic institution, these writers embarked upon several hospital-wide initiatives to educate the medical community on evidence-based mind-body interventions. To change culture, they organized a full day conference entitled Creative Arts Therapies Conversations in Healthcare and Therapeutic Transformations (CAT CHATTs): *"What Does Health Look Like in Healthcare Today? Sustaining Identity as an Integrative Therapist in Medicine"*. They invited art, music, dance-movement and yoga therapists, chaplains, physicians, social workers, nurses, psychiatrists, and acupuncturists from major academic institutions to present and discuss numerous ways integrative therapists yield best practice, mitigate effects of invasive procedures, treat physical and emotional pain, and increase communication among staff and with family members for responsible care. This event was supported by NewYork-Presbyterian Morgan Stanley Children's Hospital (NYP MSCH) and attended by approximately 100 professionals representing all levels of health care providers across New York State. Feedback from evaluations was overwhelmingly favorable and highlighted the need to make integrative healthcare a universal practice in conventional medical settings.

The following are vignettes from five different integrative clinicians at our urban teaching hospital. They serve to illustrate how integrative therapies are effective and evidence-based disciplines that when used in conjunction with standard medical treatment can promote best practice. All patients' names and identifiers have been changed or replaced with initials to maintain anonymity and privacy.

2. Acupuncture in the Pediatric Emergency Department

"Doc, need you in room 23 stat! We have an eight-year-old boy with paraphimosis since last night and clinic just sent him to us for reduction!" It's now 1:30 p.m. and the foreskin has been in the retracted position since CJ showered last night over 15 h ago. CJ appeared anxious and tearful due to pain from a swollen and red foreskin. After placing him in a Trendelenburg position, topical 2% Lidocaine and D50W plus ice were placed on the area to decrease pain and swelling. Next, intranasal Fentanyl was administered for pain and a child life specialist was at the bedside, providing breathing coaching and an iPad for distraction. The first attempt to release the foreskin was met with such pain and crying that the procedure was aborted. Urology was in the operating room, unavailable to assist. Should I give CJ another dose of opioids? Inject local anesthetics, but risk causing further swelling and emotional trauma? In this case, I offered the family auricular acupuncture to decrease CJ's pain and anxiety.

Oftentimes, children who are in pain or waiting to undergo a painful procedure are already afraid and anxious. In order to break this tension and dispel their trepidation of acupuncture, I would often jokingly say, "The acupuncture needle is the biggest one in our whole emergency room"! and then dramatically pull out a tiny needle as everyone laughs. To introduce acupuncture to CJ and his family, I first showed them how filamentous the acupuncture needle is by bending it along my finger. Next, I mimicked the pin prick needle sensation by gently pinching the dorsum of his hand while saying, "You might feel the acupuncture needle like a little pinch". This process helped to put CJ and his family more at ease and they agreed to give acupuncture a try. To further empower CJ at this time when he may feel especially vulnerable, I said, "Let me know if the needle bothers you. We can stop anytime you like". Using the Battlefield auricular acupuncture protocol [7], CJ calmly allowed me to place five needles in his right auricle. Within minutes we were able to perform a second attempt and successfully reduced the paraphimosis manually, thus avoiding surgery. CJ, his parents, and our emergency medical team were all very happy with the outcome.

This case demonstrates how a child benefited from a collaborative effort using standard pain medications and other non-pharmacologic therapies, including breathing techniques, distraction with iPad, and acupuncture. This multimodal, integrated approach resulted in a successful outcome-something no single therapy could have accomplished.

Acupuncture has been used in China for thousands of years to treat pain [8] and is recognized by the National Institutes of Health as a safe and effective therapy for pain [9]. The mechanisms for acupuncture analgesia have been extensively studied and include the involvement of the autonomic nervous system, endogenous endorphin release, brain region modulation, connective tissue and local needling effects [10–13]. While many caretakers have heard of acupuncture, most have never heard of its use in pediatrics and are pleasantly surprised when acupuncture is offered in the Pediatric Emergency Department (PED).

Acupuncture is often offered to pediatric patients undergoing radiation and chemotherapy on the Hematology-Oncology service at NYP MSCH because it mitigates symptoms, including nausea, vomiting, pain, and anxiety [14–16]. For children with sickle cell pain crisis who present to the MSCH PED, acupuncture is sometimes used in conjunction with standard pharmaceuticals to help decrease pain and anxiety [17], and the amount of opioids needed.

Nursing and physician colleagues in the PED have witnessed first-hand the positive result of acupuncture. For this reason they frequently refer patients for acupuncture when standard of care, including pharmaceuticals, fails to achieve sufficient pain relief. In a study conducted at NYP MSCH PED, patients were treated with acupuncture for diverse painful conditions, including headaches, otitis externa, torticollis, constipation, dysmenorrhea, and knee and ankle sprains. Acupuncture was well accepted, with 96% of patients and families reporting satisfaction with acupuncture and 52% achieving complete pain resolution. Unlike pharmaceuticals, acupuncture offers the additional advantage of low adverse side effects, and avoids medication interactions. Given our nation's opioid crisis, the integrative practices at NYP MSCH PED conform to the recommendations from the Centers for Disease Control and Prevention and the U.S Food and Drug Administration that nonpharmacologic therapies, including acupuncture, be offered to treat patients with pain [18,19].

It is gratifying to be able to relieve a patient's pain and suffering; to see a child's face change from a grimace to a smile. The practice of acupuncture has afforded me opportunities to show families and colleagues that medication alone is not always the solution, nor is it the only answer. With growing evidence on its efficacy and high safety profile, acupuncture may one day become an invaluable staple in our therapeutic armament to help treat pain in pediatrics.

3. Pastoral Care as an Integrating Practice

Ravi is a two-and-a-half-year-old boy with a hyphenated Jewish and Italian last name. He has been on the Neurology Unit for one month with seizures. Ravi's skin is very dark in contrast to everyone else in the room who has very white skin. Ravi is stiff, his limbs are at odd angles, his head is fixed, and he is silent except for occasional moans. Mom and Dad tell me they adopted Ravi after many in vitro attempts and know there is epilepsy in his African-American family of origin. They adore him and Mom talks about how articulate and talented he is. In terms of religious affiliation, Mom is of Jewish heritage and non-practicing. Dad was raised Catholic, but non-practicing, and has for some time sought spiritual expression in Buddhism.

As a chaplain, I am attuned to the different languages and styles people use to describe their values, the ways in which they cope, or do not. I am curious about how this couple navigates their different spiritual languages. These parents are at their wits' end and I feel like they are leaking out of the boundaries of their bodies. I am a witness to the leaks; and I am a bucket to catch and hold them. Perhaps the collection will be helpful for later reflection for Mom and Dad, but for now I am a bucket brigade with big ears. Over the course of an hour, Mom unfurls a rage aria; they hate the hospital and everyone in it and are furious at how long it is taking for a diagnosis. Next, she laments, revealing she is terrified that their boy will never be their boy again. She cannot bear considering this loss and she declares herself "desperate" for anything that will help, "even Jewish prayer". We both smile at "even Jewish prayer" as she tells me she never learned much about her Jewish heritage and is not sure what it might offer. I hear her curiosity expressed in the face of her desperation as a desire to connect to something, to claim something that is both a birth right and a tribal right, perhaps as intense as her desire to be a mother. I feel her words of anger and sorrow pierce my own body and consider the options. How to craft a communication from the depths of her soul to ... God? She wants to regain her equanimity, but feels she cannot if she is going to continue to advocate effectively for Ravi. A prayer for healing, but for whom? I center the prayer on text written by a 19th century Moroccan rabbi because his origins are as far-flung as the circumstances. Dad is restrained, but cries when we pray in Hebrew and English around Ravi.

Board certified hospital chaplains are responsible for assessing and supporting the emotional, religious, and/or spiritual needs of patients, families, and staff. In addition to supporting these needs, we are trained to listen and to help people access, re-access, or even develop new coping resources regardless of religious or spiritual affiliations. Chaplains help people remember who they are when they are not in the hospital. The conversations can be confessional, investigative, witnessing, and always confidential unless there is potential harm to self or others. Formal research in evidence-based chaplaincy is still in its infancy, however, existing research points to the power of narrative [20] and the value of pastoral care interventions focused on supporting the spiritual needs of primary caregivers of children with life-limiting illnesses [21].

Some weeks later, Ravi has suffered a brain hemorrhage and cardiac arrest, and is in the ICU. He is sedated on a ventilator, his cognitive condition unknown. Over the weeks, Mom and Dad's spiritual engagement has consisted of meditation with a Buddhist chaplain and a perfunctory wave to the ICU chaplain. When I see them, their eyes are blank and their vitality is sapped. While Ravi has been steadily losing his muscle tone, his parents have begun to lose their person tone. They have so profoundly passed beyond the boundaries of their bodies that they have quietly imploded, and the outlines of who they are in the world as employees, co-workers, friends, and parents are slowly being erased. They tell me they are using meditation to have a moment to "shut down" their thinking and seek a moment of refuge "to not feel". They are no longer seeking refuge in spiritual resources because they see no purpose. Ravi has become a stranger to them, and they to themselves. They appear as shadows.

Pastoral care in the hospital setting is about identity recalibration. The chaplain looks for the shards of a shattered identity and the ways in which to help reunite them. The intention is to pause the chaos and co-create with the patient, or family, or staff a pathway through the obstacles to find and reclaim a sense of self.

In Ravi's case, however, there is no clear pathway to reunion, nor definitive resolution. The tragedy of this story is multi-layered. I cannot fix the situation. Instead, I listen to the loss and reflect back the confusion. I hold the myriad of desperate emotions flying around the room and help them to integrate this part of their life story while rebuilding their person tone through reflection of the unwanted emotions they are fiercely trying to shed. I intervene in the moment as each conversation unfolds and I can only hope that my practice in some way helps them to begin to find meaning in the shadows.

4. Art Therapy and the Practice of Mirroring Medical Trauma

"Ewww, Alan's toilet has that thing hanging there with his urine in it, that's gross". Alan's older brother was referring to the urinal. Alan is a tiny 10-year-old boy who speaks in a small inaudible voice, occupying little space in his room, contrary to his older brother and sister. His mother, nervous in nature, and his father, calm yet distant, routinely accompany him to the clinic where he receives treatments for his astrocytoma.

I was consulted to assess for and provide art therapy services throughout Alan's long and arduous treatment course. Initially he presented with flat affect, withholding of feelings and what appeared to be an absorption of his mother's anxiety that was present during every medical encounter.

The creative process of art making mirrors life itself. Both process and product serve as a bridge from an individual's inner world to the outside. Art therapists actively look and listen for imagery, symbols and metaphors, and use them to help explore pre-conscious content with patients. The process of exploring art media, creating and talking about the art offers patients increased opportunities to find more compatible relationships to potentially overwhelming thoughts and feelings [22,23].

Hospitalized children may not have the words to express what they are thinking or feeling, or these words may not do their experience justice. Art, then, serves as a translator to communicate internalized emotions to the important people in the room. Images offer children opportunities to externalize their content safely while the art therapist helps them find personal meaning in their work [24]. Finding meaning, in turn helps to alleviate feelings of anxiety, depression and pain that often accompany children with chronic illnesses [25–27].

Alan reported that his G-tube feedings resulted in "excruciating" pain, the primary symptom which led to his current hospitalization. In our first art therapy session, Alan approached the art making inauspiciously, carefully and with unwavering focus. He chose art materials with intention, requesting to work with non-traditional media, and repurposing mundane objects that he altered into a three-dimensional environment.

Typically, children select paints, pastels or clay to form their visual expressions. Alan used a paint brush container as the central sculptural component in his artwork where he used string to attach plastic aquatic figurines from the top allowing them to dangle inside. In art therapy, these two attributes of using non-traditional materials and repurposing objects (e.g., the process of transforming ordinary objects to significantly alter their appearance or use) indicate flexibility, creative problem solving and adaptability.

"That's not an art material Alan, choose something that is in her [my] basket". His mother's reprimands appeared to imply that Alan's behavior was impolite or defying the rules- in contrast to what I assessed to be a series of creative and resilient solutions. I wondered if this was a mother's instinct to protect her child and find control in this desperate situation.

Adhering a plastic transparent circular container (paint brush cleaner) to the center of a green painted circular cardboard base, Alan began to redefine and transform the objects.

Midway through the session, the oncology attending physician humbly entered the room. Alan's mother stood up to meet him at the foot of the bed, his words stacking like bricks in her arms as he delivered the unresolved news about Alan's G-tube infection. Upon his exit, Alan's mother and father murmured their discouragement and concern for Alan's unexplainable pain.

Shortly after this, the surgical team arrived. "Looks like fun", a resident commented to Alan about his art. Alan gave no response. Surrounded by the team, his infected G-tube site was examined. I transitioned to the back of the room to be with his siblings who were observing from a distance. "Ewwwww", exclaimed his sister, "I just saw Alan's feeding tube site, gross".

Alan remained quiet, frozen and naked.

As the team discussed their impressions with the parents, Alan continued with his art, selecting a variety of jungle animal figurines and gluing more than twenty tigers, elephants, giraffes and hippos around the perimeter of the circular base, encircling the large ominous container in the center.

"That's too many animals, save some for the other children", prompted Alan's mother once again. Alan's expressive non-verbal voice is scolded, minimized and criticized as if to say, 'Don't take up that much space, stop taking from others and use unforbidden objects. Stay quiet and unseen.'

Unexpectedly, Alan's roar pierced the room bringing everyone to a halt. "STOP!" He yelled in response to his brother's persistent attempt to look at his feeding tube site. "Why can't I see it?" he whined. He silenced the pervasive buzz in the room, "Because I don't trust you!"

"Whom do you trust?" I asked.

His mother and father stood frozen, holding their son's eyes with their own. Tears poured down Alan's cheeks, "I'm scared". His parents, like bookends, stood on alternate sides of him. "There's a hole in my side". Alan's fear, resounding and exposed, was now unavoidable.

Alan's art- a depiction of animals surrounding the 'watering hole'- communicated 'observation', 'vigilance' and 'feeding', all of which were prominent themes from his medical experience. In this moment he was surrounded by teams peering at his feeding tube, his family verbally and visually poking at an area which was the very hole that fed and sustained him. Throughout his exam he exhibited a hypervigilance to incoming danger (i.e., the medical team and his feeds). The container that water is poured into is the focal point in his art piece and a reflection of his own body. Occupying all dimensions of space, the animals' small stillness reflects the vulnerable unknown. The myriad of feelings elicited from the imagery mirror different aspects of Alan and his experience during this pre-surgical exam and a visit from his physician. Alan's voicelessness in his treatment was finally unleashed in this compelling moment, providing him an uncensored expression of his fears. Had the surgical team been in the room when Alan was able to clearly verbalize his fears, it's possible that the team may have listened and responded differently throughout the exam. And alternatively, the response, "Looks like fun" to Alan's 'watering hole' sculpture would not minimize his expression but rather validate it with "Looks like you have a lot to say".

As an art psychotherapist, I enter into symbolic and metaphoric language to meet the child in his/her inner world. It is humbling to be invited into this space and experience his/her story through imagery and expressive language. The presence of disease in the body can be without symptoms. So too, meaningful messages can exist in a child, and like that of disease, the meaning can be unknown until it is ready to be revealed. In the case of Alan, the unknown became a shared space for Alan, his illness, his art, and me.

5. Music Therapy and Interdisciplinary Co-treatments to Creatively Address Complex Medical Needs

"We can beat the bad man, make him go away, if we sing loud enough...All the way up to GOD!" Josiah was a typically developing vivacious seven-year-old boy with a history of prolonged hospitalization and chronic illness awaiting heart transplant. During the first month of his admission, Josiah appeared to exhibit increased signs of anxiety and regression so the interdisciplinary team asked me to assess him for music therapy services. Music therapy as defined by the American Music Therapy Association is "the clinical and evidence-based use of music interventions to accomplish individualized goals within a therapeutic relationship" [28].

In our first session, I quickly established rapport with Josiah through active music making and musical improvisation (e.g., playing extemporized musical rhythms, tempos, dynamics, and melodies composed in the moment without previous preparation on varied rhythmic and harmonic instruments, including drums, guitar, xylophones, and shakers). His initial improvisations presented as playful, melodic, and heavily percussive displaying steady, organized rhythms and lively tempos. His final musical improvisation, however, changed significantly. It became increasingly chaotic, displayed sharp contrasting rhythms in a disorganized pattern and was punctuated by strong accentuated beats. Mid-way into this improvisation Josiah stopped abruptly and pointed directly to a Halloween face mask adjacent to him on the bed. He placed his finger over his mouth and with wide-eyed affect whispered, "we need to be very quiet... so we don't wake the bad man". He then proceeded to sing softly in an effort to avoid being captured by this "bad man" monster who wanted to "silence" his music.

As a music psychotherapist, I use my modality to help patients explore, express, and discover their internal worlds by inviting ongoing musical and verbal dialogues between their conscious and unconscious selves [29]. During our first session, I assessed that Josiah's impromptu musical dialogue between his conscious self and a fictional "bad man" monster may have been prompted by a need to safely and creatively explore, express, and process difficult thoughts and feelings surrounding his chronic illness, prolonged hospitalization, isolation, and family separation. What was most interesting to me during our first encounter was that in calling out to a higher power at the conclusion of the session, Josiah appeared to achieve some kind of resolution. By singing "loudly, all the way up to God" he had triumphantly silenced the "bad man", holding him captive. Essentially, Josiah had discovered comfort, personal strength, power, and self-agency by engaging in musical prayer.

Pre-transplant, my clinical work with Josiah was predominantly psychodynamic in that I continued to invite him to engage in musical dialogues between his conscious and unconscious selves. In these ongoing dialogues, he explored a variety of recurring themes in the music, including 'silence/sound', 'dominance/submission', 'danger/safety', 'fear/courage', 'separation/reunion', 'helplessness/empowerment', and 'salvation'.

Mid-way through his admission, Josiah was successfully transplanted, however, postoperative complications led to a cardiac arrest that resulted in anoxic brain injury and substantial decompensation. Following this event, the family was in crisis and the team reported uncertainty as to Josiah's neurological outcome.

For me, the shift was just as dramatic. In many ways, Josiah's musical journey paralleled his cardiac journey; his music had stopped abruptly, unexpectedly, and without warning, leaving in its wake a painfully uncomfortable silence. Clinical music therapists are trained to create space in the music for our patients because rests are just as important as the notes. But how could I begin to honor Josiah's notes when his voice as I knew it had been silenced?

As a result of this experience, my clinical practice evolved to become more flexible, innovative, and creative. I began by increasing communication with team members to help identify common goals and innovative solutions aimed at addressing a variety of barriers to care. Josiah displayed extreme spasticity in his lower extremities, which created limited mobility, and he had difficulty maintaining autonomic stability. This was most evident during physical and occupational therapy sessions when he often became tachycardic and tachypneic. In these sessions, he also displayed visible and audible signs of distress and emotional dysregulation, including moaning, crying, contracted limbs, and a constricted, tearful affect.

In response to these barriers, I worked closely with the team to design individualized music therapy co-treatments. To encourage homeostasis during rehabilitation therapy sessions, I played improvised harmonies on the guitar, which emphasized regular, steady rhythms and slow tempos while singing improvised melodies with prolonged phrases or musical meter. This intervention known as *rhythmic entrainment* (a term used to describe the temporal locking process phenomenon in which two or more independent rhythmic processes synchronize with each other) [30] helped to stabilize Josiah's heart rate and respiration throughout sessions. Entrainment also proved a useful assessment tool for the team. The occupational therapist reported that she was able to more accurately assess his neurological capacity as a result of the musical accompaniment I provided that both activated and relaxed Josiah throughout our session. Because Josiah entrained easily to live music, the speech and language pathologist informed me that live music helped keep Josiah calm, which enabled her to successfully complete a visual, audial, and cognitive assessment to determine his altered baseline.

In physical therapy sessions, I used a sound and vibration intervention known as *vibroacoustic therapy* [31,32] to minimize pain and increase his limited range of motion. By placing a bass tuned buffalo drum near Josiah's lower extremities I was able to reduce his hypertonicity and spasticity [33]. Suddenly, the physical therapist was able to increase the passive range of motion and encourage active range of motion when Josiah was able to successfully reach for, grasp, hold, and shake a small bell in time to the music. As a result of increased integrative practice that targeted and treated both psychosocial and physiological symptoms of distress, Josiah's autonomic stability and emotional regulation slowly improved over time.

A final collaboration with pastoral care led to a co-treatment that provided Josiah's family the opportunity to give voice to overwhelming feelings of fear and anxiety. I played simple chord intervals (e.g., two sounds differing in pitch) on the guitar and sang an improvised melody to create a musical environment that was secure, contained, and predictable while the chaplain led the family in prayer. This technique known as *vocal holding* consists of the intentional use of playing two alternating chords on a harmonic instrument in combination with improvised singing in order to create a consistent and stable environment [34]. Initially, Josiah's mother expressed doubt and confusion surrounding the event, "Why would God let this happen?" Throughout the music her demeanor shifted. Toward the end of the session she presented as calm and hopeful, reporting, "I can't be upset at God ... God has a plan. Even though it's bad, and it's dark ...We going to get through this. God's going to pull us through." In a way we had come full circle; once again, Josiah and his family were seeking comfort, empowerment, and strength in musical prayer.

At this point in the session, Josiah, who had been sleeping in a bed adjacent to our prayer circle, opened his eyes and his mother moved bedside to take his hand. Softly, she began to sing his favorite song, "Oh, the itsy, bitsy spider, went up the water spout..." I quietly fingered chords on my guitar to accompany her as she continued to sing, "Down came the rain, and washed the spider out..." Slowly, family members gathered around the bed holding hands, encircling Josiah as he held her gaze. "Out came the sun, and dried up all the rain..." Josiah opened his mouth slowly, hesitantly groping as his mother sang the last line, "and the itsy, bitsy spider went up the spout ah ... " Josiah completed the song, penetrating the silence with his voice at last, "...gin".

My favorite thing about music therapy is that it is inherently collaborative. Unlike conversation, music happens concurrently offering participants an "I" and "Thou" [35] experience through "We" engagement [36]. 'We' engagement, however, can sometimes limit opportunities to unite 'us' in clinical practice. By expanding our practice to include multiple voices, we participate in a richer, more dynamic symphony. Ultimately, an integrated practice promotes true harmony in healthcare.

6. Yoga Therapy and Meditation: An Integrative Partnership with Patients and Families

The chemotherapy charge nurse texted, "Please come to the Infusion Center to meet a new patient who wants to talk to you about yoga therapy and meditation during her cancer treatment".

The patient, Stacey, had recently celebrated her 18th birthday. Soon after, she had felt a lump near her right armpit. The staggering diagnosis of stage IV breast cancer with metastases to the liver and spine literally took her breath away. Today was the first of an anticipated 180-day chemotherapy treatment plan to be delivered once every three weeks.

As I approached the infusion area, I paused to center myself so I could be fully present with Stacey—allowing her to be heard, to be seen; holding her in compassionate, loving space. Elizabeth Kubler-Ross said, "Telling your story often and in detail is primal to the grieving process. You must get it out. Grief must be witnessed to be healed [37] (p. 63)".

I washed my hands, focusing on my own breath: "Take three deep belly breaths, relax into the exhalation, allow your awareness to rest on the present moment". I continued to practice this deep breathing, and soon Stacey mirrored the gentle rise and fall of my abdomen. Her breathing slowed as I guided her through a 15-min meditation. She said she felt calmer and I saw on the monitor her systolic blood pressure had dropped 15 points. I showed her various breathing techniques to practice at home and during treatments to help manage anxiety and discomfort, and we began to create a plan for a daily meditation practice that was based on her personal preferences.

As a Yoga Therapist in Integrative Oncology, I work closely with Psycho-Oncology and Palliative Care. The cornerstone of our team's integrative approach is to partner with patients and families, providing attentive, empathic clinical care to address the needs of mind, body, and spirit. I was the first of our team to meet Stacey and immediately suggested she consult our Psychologist and Palliative Nurse Practitioner for help managing anxiety and prospective chemotherapy induced peripheral neuropathy. During her half-year of treatment, our team met regularly to discuss her case, and I supported my colleagues' behavioral and pharmaceutical interventions by customizing weekly sessions of conscious breathing, meditation, and mindful movement to address her evolving physical and emotional needs.

Mind-body interventions are important self-regulation practices that support psychosocial therapies by fostering general mental well-being, calmness, clarity, and concentration [38–40]. They promote sleep, and can ease anxiety and depression [41,42]. Mindfulness meditation, in particular, helps manage anxiety and improve quality of life [43]. It also helps patients reframe their relationship with pain by teaching them to rest in the present moment and observe sensations and thoughts without judgment. Jon Kabat-Zinn, the founder of Mindfulness Based Stress Reduction (MBSR), wrote, "It's possible to befriend your pain or your fear...rather than feeling that you can't get anywhere until this thing that bothers you is cut out or walled off or shut down" [44].

There is substantial evidence to support the efficacy of mind-body therapies in the outpatient clinical setting. At its June 2018 annual conference, the American Society of Clinical Oncology (ASCO) endorsed yoga and meditation as adjuvant therapy during conventional breast cancer treatment and survivorship to mitigate the sequelae of acute and late treatment side effects, including anxiety, mood disorder, depression, and to improve quality of life [45].

At the end of her treatment Stacey was declared with *no evidence of disease* and told us that our integrative care had "saved her life" by teaching her how to manage her fear and anxiety, and to help her keep physically active during her difficult treatment. In her mother's words, "Stacey's medical oncologists may have eradicated the disease and put her in remission, but her integrative support team gave her back a life worth living".

It is imperative that we, as integrative therapists, spearhead the effort to create a paradigm shift in the way our healthcare system treats our patients and their loved ones. Mind-body therapies are evidence-based, drug free, cost effective, and available to everyone regardless of cultural background and socioeconomic status. Let us listen closely to our patients and their families, see the elephant in its entirety, and commit to treating the individual, not the disease.

7. Results: Barriers to Integrative Therapy Practice

The above vignettes clearly illustrate how integrative therapies address the mental, emotional, functional, spiritual, social, and community domains of the patient, thereby improving the overall patient experience while supporting standard medical treatment outcomes. Despite the overwhelming evidence that points to the effectiveness of integrative healthcare, these writers encountered areas for further consideration.

7.1. Funding

Currently, in conventional medical settings, integrative therapy positions are funded in a variety of ways. While many creative arts therapy positions are typically donor funded, at this institution, art and music therapy and pastoral care positions are billed to the cost of room and board. Yoga therapy is funded by a private donor, and acupuncture services in the pediatric emergency department are currently not separately reimbursed. It remains clear that additional cost analysis research is needed to find sustainable solutions to increased integrative programming.

7.2. Misses in Appropriation, Placement, Classification, and Understanding

7.2.1. Misappropriation

In conventional medical settings, mind-body practices are often misplaced, misunderstood, and misclassified. This leads to a misappropriation of services, impaired practice and, ultimately, identity confusion regarding the role integrative therapists play within the treatment team. For this reason, clarifying the scope of practice and managing staff and family expectations is paramount.

7.2.2. Misplacement/Misclassification

Misplacement of integrative therapists creates confusion within the interdisciplinary team. Therapists are difficult to locate, often possessing job titles or embedded in departments unrelated to their discipline. For example, a pain specialist may have a hard time locating a mind-body therapist when he/she is identified on his/her identification badge as a recreational therapist and managed by a child life department.

7.2.3. Misunderstanding

Integrative therapists are trained to facilitate and process the expression of anxiety and fear that accompany medical encounters that are interwoven with pain symptomatology [46–49]. Not all healthcare providers understand the concrete benefits of mind-body interventions and may minimize the complementary benefits integrative therapies can provide. A better understanding of mind-body practices is necessary in order to achieve appropriate integration and promote a more holistic approach to care.

8. Discussion: Recommendations for Future Practice

Despite the aforementioned barriers, these writers were able to identify a number of innovative solutions to minimize siloed practice and help break down existing barriers. Through workshops, targeted in-services, interdisciplinary rounding, co-treatments, lectures, grand rounds, and hospital-wide educational forums, including conferences and workshops, medical professionals are provided with opportunities to learn and experience firsthand the benefits of integrative therapies, including art, music, yoga, pastoral care, and acupuncture.

Innovative Solutions to Promote Increased Integrative Practice

The advancement of integrative health care in a major academic hospital takes time and strategy to promote complementary practice. Below are suggested actions steps to help increase visibility, awareness, and accessibility to integrative services. The recommendations listed are from these writers' personal accounts and experiences of successful implementation of hospital-wide programs and initiatives.

- Create a customized website with a dedicated email address to promote understanding and classification of integrative therapies.
- Design and distribute educational brochures and marketing materials to staff detailing services and appropriate referral criteria.
- Facilitate weekly in-services for interdisciplinary staff, fellows, residents, medical students, and physicians that lead to better integration of mind-body services in treatment plans. This

practice also generates potential funding for additional positions, including expanding services to outpatient or satellite clinics.
- Obtain funding through grant support from established national organizations, such as the American Academy of Pediatrics, Virginia Apgar Academy, American Art Therapy Association, private donors, and foundations to support educational workshops and research.
- Conduct workshops, lectures, and grand rounds for nurses, students, residents, and faculty members, thereby gaining more acceptance and understanding from providers across the hospital on integrative therapists' role in medicine.
- Publish and present locally, nationally, and internationally on integrative therapy research and practices.
- Create an integrative rotation elective as part of residency training to educate and promote utilization of complementary practices located throughout the hospital.
- Involve integrative therapy students in the creation and co-facilitation of expressive therapy pilot programs for outpatient clinics, which increases complementary services to more patients and families in need.

9. Conclusions

A cultural shift in this conventional medical setting is growing as a result of increased visibility, education, understanding, and collaboration, but the need for increased integration of mind-body practices still remains. Barriers to true integrative health care include limited funding, misappropriation of services, misclassification, misunderstanding, and continued siloed practice. To affect global change, it is incumbent for all mind-body clinicians in conventional medical settings to join this cultural revolution. This publication is just the first step. A restructuring of conventional medical frameworks is necessary in order to see and treat the whole patient. From revolutionary paradigm shifts and innovative practices to eradicating siloed services, integrative, complementary "wholistic" health is the future.

Organizations that begin to successfully integrate humanistic medicine with evidence-based mind-body practices empower patients to become active partners in their treatment. Such integrative practice reduces harm, sustains ethical and legal professional standards, gives purposeful direction to therapeutic interventions, and enhances the efficacy of conventional treatment plans. It is the future of good medicine. This is the elephant that we can all see and heal.

Author Contributions: Conceptualization, M.H. and S.M.B.; Methodology, M.H. and S.M.B.; Writing—Original Draft Preparation, M.H., S.M.B., L.L., L.S.G. and S.-L.T.; Writing—Review & Editing, M.H., S.M.B., and L.L.; Visualization, M.H. and S.M.B.; Supervision, S.-L.T.; Project Administration, M.H. and S.M.B.

Funding: This research has received no external funding.

Conflicts of Interest: The authors declare no conflict of interest.

References

1. Saxe, J.G. *The Poems of John Godfrey Saxe*; University of Michigan: Ann Arbor, MI, USA, 2009.
2. Wen, J.; Shulman, K. Can team-based care improve patient satisfaction? A systematic review of randomized controlled trials. *PLoS ONE* **2014**, *9*, 7. [CrossRef] [PubMed]
3. Mitchell, P.; Matthew, W.; Golden, R.; McNellis, B.; Okun, S.; Webb, C.E.; Rohrbach, V.; Von Kohorn, I. Core Principles and Values of Effective Team-Based Health Care. Available online: https://nam.edu/wp-content/uploads/2015/06/VSRT-Team-Based-Care-Principles-Values.pdf (accessed on 9 November 2018).
4. Nolte, J. Enhancing Interdisciplinary Collaboration in Primary Healthcare in Canada. Available online: http://tools.hhrrhs.ca/index.php?option=com_mtree&task=att_download&link_id=5305&cf_id=68&lang=e (accessed on 9 November 2018).
5. National Center for Complementary and Integrative Health. Available online: https://nccih.nih.gov/health/integrative-health#integrative (accessed on 12 May 2018).

6. National Center for Complementary and Integrative Health. Available online: https://nccih.nih.gov/health/mindbody (accessed on 12 May 2018).
7. Tsai, S.-L.; Reynoso, E.; Shin, D.W.; Tsung, J. Acupuncture as a nonpharmacologic treatment for pain in a pediatric emergency department. *Pediatr. Emerg. Care* **2018**. under review. [CrossRef] [PubMed]
8. Deng, L. *Chinese Acupuncture and Moxibustion*, 3rd ed.; Foreign Languages Press: Beijing, China, 2010.
9. NIH Consensus Conference. Acupuncture. *JAMA* **1998**, *280*, 1518–1524. [CrossRef]
10. Han, J.S. Acupuncture and endorphins. *Neurosci. Lett.* **2004**, *361*, 258–261. [CrossRef] [PubMed]
11. Maeda, Y.; Kim, H.; Kettner, N.; Kim, J.; Cina, S.; Malatesta, C.; Gerber, J.; McManus, C.; Ong-Sutherland, R.; Libby, A.; et al. Rewiring the primary somatosensory cortex in carpal tunnel syndrome with acupuncture. *Brain* **2017**, *140*, 914–927. [CrossRef] [PubMed]
12. Langevin, H.M.; Bouffard, N.A.; Badger, G.J.; Churchill, D.L.; Howe, A.K. Subcutaneous tissue fibroblast cytoskeletal remodeling induced by acupuncture: Evidence for a mechanotransduction-based mechanism. *J. Cell. Physiol.* **2006**, *207*, 767–774. [CrossRef] [PubMed]
13. Li, Q.Q.; Shi, G.X.; Xu, Q.; Wang, J.; Liu, C.Z.; Wang, L.P. Acupuncture effect and central autonomic regulation. *Evid. Based Complement. Altern. Med.* **2013**, *2013*, 267959. [CrossRef] [PubMed]
14. Reindl, T.; Geilen, W.; Hartmann, R.; Wiebelitz, K.R.; Kan, G.; Wilhelm, I.; Lugauer, S.; Behrens, C.; Weiberlenn, T.; Gottschling, S.; et al. Acupuncture against chemotherapy-induced nausea and vomiting in pediatric oncology. Interim results of a multicenter crossover study. *Support Care Cancer* **2006**, *14*, 172–176. [CrossRef] [PubMed]
15. Dundee, J.W.; Ghaly, R.G.; Fitzpatrick, K.T.; Abram, W.P.; Lynch, G.A. Acupuncture prophylaxis of cancer chemotherapy-induced sickness. *J. R. Soc. Med.* **1989**, *82*, 268–271. [CrossRef] [PubMed]
16. Ezzo, J.M.; Richardson, M.A.; Vickers, A.; Allen, C.; Dibble, S.L.; Issell, B.F.; Lao, L.; Pearl, M.; Ramirez, G.; Shen, J.; et al. Acupuncture-point stimulation for chemotherapy-induced nausea or vomiting. *Cochrane Database Syst. Rev.* **2006**, CD002285. [CrossRef]
17. Tsai, S.L.; McDaniel, D.; Taromina, K.; Lee, M.T. Acupuncture for Sickle Cell Pain Management in a Pediatric Emergency Department, Hematology Clinic, and Inpatient Unit. *Med. Acupunct.* **2015**, *27*, 510–514. [CrossRef]
18. CDC Guideline for Prescribing Opioids for Chronic Pain—United States, 2016 [press release]. MMWR Recomm Rep; 2016. Available online: https://www.cdc.gov/mmwr/volumes/65/rr/rr6501e1.htm (accessed on 9 November 2018).
19. FDA. *Education Blueprint for Health Care Providers Involved in the Management or Support of Patients with Pain (May 2017)*; FDA: Silver Spring, MD, USA, 2017.
20. Charon, R. What to Do with Stories: The Sciences of Narrative Medicine. *Can. Fam. Phys.* **2007**, *53*, 1265–1267.
21. Kelly, J.A.; May, C.S.; Maurer, S. Assessment of the Spiritual Needs of Primary Caregivers of Children with Life-Limiting Illnesses Is Valuable Yet Inconsistently Performed in the Hospital. *J. Palliat. Med.* **2016**, *19*, 763–766. [CrossRef] [PubMed]
22. McNutt, J. Art therapy as a form of visual narrative in oncology care. In *Art Therapy and Healthcare*; Malchiodi, C.A., Ed.; Guilford Press: New York, NY, USA, 2012; pp. 127–135.
23. Favara-Scacco, C. Art therapy as perseus' shield for children with cancer. In *Art Therapy and Cancer Care*; Waller, D., Sibbett, C., Eds.; Open University Press: Berkshire, UK, 2005; pp. 119–127.
24. Council, T. Medical art therapy with children. In *Handbook of Art Therapy*, 2nd ed.; Malchiodi, C.A., Ed.; Guilford Publications: New York, NY, USA, 2012; pp. 222–240.
25. Aguilar, B.A. The efficacy of art therapy in pediatric oncology patients: An integrative literature review. *J. Pediatr. Nurs.* **2017**, *36*, 173–178. [CrossRef] [PubMed]
26. Varni, J.W.; Limbers, C.; Burwinkle, T.M. Literature review: Health-related quality of life measurement in pediatric oncology: Hearing the voices of the children. *J. Pediatr. Psychol.* **2007**, *32*, 1151–1163. [CrossRef] [PubMed]
27. Nainis, N.; Paice, J.A.; Ratner, J.; Wirth, J.H.; Lai, J.; Shott, S. Relieving symptoms in cancer: Innovative use of art therapy. *J. Pain Symptom Manag.* **2006**, *31*, 162–169. [CrossRef] [PubMed]
28. American Music Therapy Association. Available online: https://www.musictherapy.org (accessed on 9 November 2018).
29. Austin, D. The Role of Improvised Music in Psychodynamic Music Therapy with Adults. *Music Ther.* **1996**, *14*, 29–43. [CrossRef]

30. Thaut, M.H.; McIntosh, G.C.; Hoemberg, V. Neurobiological foundations of neurologic music therapy: Rhythmic entrainment and the motor system. *Front. Psychol.* **2014**, *5*, 1185. [CrossRef] [PubMed]
31. Kvam, M.H. The effect of vibroacoustic therapy. *Physiotherapy* **1997**, *83*, 290–295. [CrossRef]
32. Patrick, G. The Effects of Vibroacoustic Music on Symptom Reduction. *IEEE Eng. Med. Biol. Mag.* **1999**, *18*, 97–100. [CrossRef]
33. Boyd-Brewer, C.; McCaffrey, R. Vibroacoustic sound therapy improves pain management and more. *Holist. Nurs. Pract.* **2004**, *18*, 111–118. [CrossRef]
34. The Use of Vocal Holding Techniques with Adults Traumatized as Children. Available online: http://dianeaustin.com/pdfs/Traumaar.pdf (accessed on 9 November 2018).
35. Buber, M. *I and Thou*; Martino Publishing: Mansfield Centre, CT, USA, 2010.
36. Hall, M.M. Yes and: Discovering the Authentic Voice Through Integrated Improvisational Musical Play. Master's Thesis, New York University, New York, NY, USA, 2014.
37. Kubler-Ross, E.; Kessler, D. *On Grief and Grieving: Finding the Meaning of Grief Through the Five Stages of Loss*; Simon & Schuster UK Ltd.: London, UK, 2005.
38. Weitzner, M.A.; Meyers, C.A.; Stuebing, K.K.; Saleeba, A.K. Relationship between quality of life and mood in long-term survivors of breast cancer treated with mastectomy. *Support Care Cancer* **1997**, *5*, 241–248. [CrossRef] [PubMed]
39. Culos-Reed, S.N.; Mackenzie, M.J.; Sohl, S.J.; Jesse, M.T.; Zahavich, A.N.; Danhauer, S.C. Yoga & cancer interventions: A review of the clinical significance of patient reported outcomes for cancer survivors [serial online]. *Evid. Based Complement. Altern. Med.* **2012**, *2012*, 642576. [PubMed]
40. Lin, K.Y.; Hu, Y.T.; Chang, K.J.; Lin, H.F.; Tsauo, J.Y. Effects of yoga on psychological health, quality of life, and physical health of patients with cancer: A meta-analysis. *Evid. Based Complement. Altern. Med.* **2011**, *2011*, 659–876. [CrossRef] [PubMed]
41. Mustian, K.M.; Sprod, L.K.; Janelsins, M.; Peppone, L.J.; Palesh, O.G.; Chandwani, K.; Morrow, G.R. Multicenter, Randomized Controlled Trial of Yoga for Sleep Quality Among Cancer Survivors. *J. Clin. Oncol.* **2013**, *31*, 3233–3241. [CrossRef] [PubMed]
42. Taso, C.J.; Lin, H.S.; Lin, W.L.; Chen, S.; Huang, W.T.; Chen, S.W. The effect of yoga exercise on improving depression, anxiety, and fatigue in women with breast cancer: A randomized controlled trial. *J. Nurs. Res.* **2014**, *22*, 155–164. [CrossRef] [PubMed]
43. Kieviet-Stijnen, A.; Visser, A.; Garssen, B.; Hudig, W. Mindfulness-based stress reduction training for oncology patients: Patients' appraisal and changes in well-being. *Patient Educ. Couns.* **2008**, *72*, 436–442. [CrossRef] [PubMed]
44. The Healing Power of Mindfulness. Available online: https://www.mindful.org/the-healing-power-of-mindfulness/ (accessed on 29 May 2018).
45. Lyman, G.H.; Greenlee, H.; Bohlke, K.; Bao, T.; DeMichele, A.M.; Deng, G.E.; Fouladbakhsh, J.M.; Gil, B.; Hershman, D.L.; Mansfield, S.; et al. Integrative Therapies During and After Breast Cancer Treatment: ASCO Endorsement of the SIO Clinical Practice Guideline. *J. Clin. Oncol.* **2018**, *36*, 2647–2655.
46. Curry, A.N.; Kasser, T. Can coloring mandalas reduce anxiety? *Art Ther.* **2005**, *22*, 81–85. [CrossRef]
47. Lumley, M.A.; Cohen, J.L.; Borszcz, G.S.; Cano, A.; Radcliffe, A.M.; Porter, L.S.; Keefe, F.J. Pain and emotion: A biopsychosocial review of recent research. *J. Clin. Psychol.* **2011**, *67*, 942–968. [CrossRef] [PubMed]
48. University of California—Los Angeles. Putting Feelings into Words Produces Therapeutic Effects in the Brain. *Science Daily*, 22 June 2007. Available online: www.sciencedaily.com/releases/2007/06/070622090727.htm (accessed on 28 May 2018).
49. Landier, W.; Tse, A. Use of complementary and alternative medical interventions for the management of procedure related pain, anxiety, and distress in pediatric oncology: An integrative review. *J. Pediatr. Nurs.* **2010**, *25*, 566–579. [CrossRef] [PubMed]

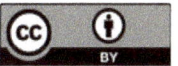

© 2018 by the authors. Licensee MDPI, Basel, Switzerland. This article is an open access article distributed under the terms and conditions of the Creative Commons Attribution (CC BY) license (http://creativecommons.org/licenses/by/4.0/).

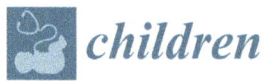

Brief Report

Implementing Integrative Nursing in a Pediatric Setting

Megan E. Voss * and Mary Jo Kreitzer

Center for Spirituality and Healing, University of Minnesota, Minneapolis, MN 55455, USA; kreit003@umn.edu
* Correspondence: vossx146@umn.edu; Tel.: +1-612-273-1801

Received: 29 June 2018; Accepted: 20 July 2018; Published: 31 July 2018

Abstract: Pediatric blood and marrow transplantation (BMT) is one of the most challenging allopathic treatments a patient and family can be faced with. A large Midwest academic health center, and leader in pediatric BMT, made the decision in 2013 to incorporate integrative nursing as the care delivery model. Nurses trained in advanced nursing practice and specialized in integrative health and healing performed a deep-dive needs assessment, national benchmarking, a comprehensive review of the literature, and ultimately designed a comprehensive integrative program for pediatric patients and their families undergoing BMT. Four years after implementation, this paper discusses lessons learned, strengths, challenges and next phases of the program, including a research agenda. The authors conclude that it is feasible, acceptable and sustainable to implement a nurse-led integrative program within an academic health center-based pediatric BMT program.

Keywords: pediatric integrative nursing; program development; pediatric blood and marrow transplant

1. Introduction

Integrative nursing has emerged as a framework for delivering sound patient care over the past five years. Principles closely aligned with the Institute for Healthcare Improvement's (IHI) Quadruple Aim can be used to help clinicians work with their patients to achieve better outcomes at lower costs, while at the same time tending to clinician well-being [1]. In the current healthcare environment, clinicians are consistently asked to do more with less. Nurses are caring for patients at much higher acuity levels than ever before, and often with higher nurse-to-patient ratios. Clinician burnout and early exit from the field are reaching alarming levels [2]. Integrative nursing as a care delivery model can be used as a strategy for mitigating the challenges faced by today's acute care nurses [3,4]. The aspirational vision of the pediatric blood and marrow transplantation (BMT) program's integrative model of care was to add an additional layer of supportive care that would palliate the patient and family on all dimensions: mind, body and spirit. The vision has remained closely aligned with the IHI Quadruple Aim. The goals of implementing integrative nursing are to improve the care experience of the patient and family, improve symptom management, and enhance the patient and family's capacity to cope. Additionally, in alignment with the IHI fourth aim, the program aspires to meet the self-care needs of staff from an organizational standpoint and to give providers and staff the tools they need to meet their individual responsibilities for self-care.

2. Methods

A team of advanced nursing practice leaders with specialty training in integrative health and healing performed a four-month long deep-dive needs assessment in order to develop a customized integrative program to complement the pediatric BMT program. Otto Scharmer's Theory U (Figure 1) served as the framework for the needs assessment. In this model of transformational change, there is a major focus on deeply listening to and understanding the needs of stakeholders in the organization;

in this case patients, families, staff and leaders, and to engage them in planning for the desired future [5]. Those five stages are outlined in Figure 1.

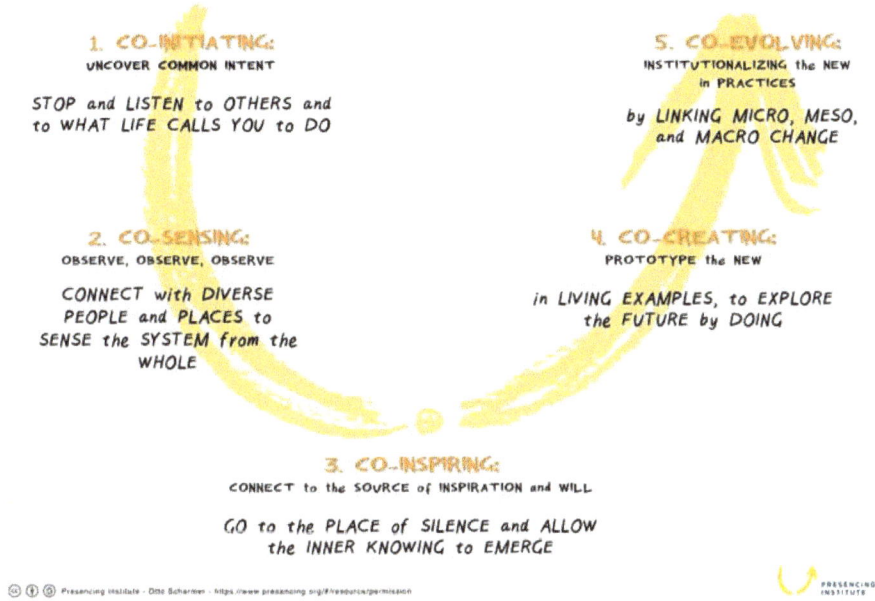

Figure 1. Theory U, reprinted with permission from [5].

2.1. Integrative Nursing as a Framework for Practice

The principles of integrative nursing (Table 1) informed the design, implementation and evaluation of the program. Integrative nursing is a whole person, whole system way of caring and healing that shapes and impacts patient care across the continuum. While the first text explicating the principles of integrative nursing was published in 2014, the concepts are timeless, are aligned with major nursing theorists, and date back to the philosophy, values and practices first introduced by Florence Nightingale in the 1800s [3,4].

Table 1. Principles of integrative nursing [3,6].

Human beings are whole systems inseparable from their environments.
Human beings have the innate capacity for health and well-being.
Nature has healing and restorative properties that contribute to health and well-being.
Integrative nursing is person-centered and relationship-based.
Integrative nursing practice is informed by evidence and uses the full range of therapeutic modalities to support/augment the healing process, moving from least intensive/invasive to more, depending on need and context.
Integrative nursing focuses on the health and well-being of caregivers as well as those they serve.

2.2. Program Design and Components

The pediatric BMT integrative therapy program was designed based on the outcomes of a four-month long needs assessment. The needs assessment included the following five components:

- Stakeholder dialogue—Interviews were conducted with clinical and administrative leadership as well as with frontline clinical staff.
- Shadowing practice—Current state of nursing and supportive care staff practice was observed to identify areas of opportunity.
- Prototyping—Experiential and educational sessions were conducted to engage staff and enhance their understanding of integrative modalities.
- Benchmarking—Other pediatric integrative therapy programs were examined through site visits, phone interviews, and extensive internet searches. These were reviewed for best practices.
- Staff survey—Nursing staff ($N = 32$) on the unit were surveyed to assess the knowledge, perceptions and comfort level with integrative modalities and care delivery.

Through this assessment, it was ascertained that the system overall had strong interest in and readiness for an integrative therapy program. The medical director was enthusiastically devoted to supporting this effort both clinically and financially. Many other pediatric hospitals around the nation have established integrative therapy programs; therefore, it was suddenly a market disadvantage to not offer what was becoming a standard of care in the eyes of patients and families [7]. While these strengths culminated to create a culture of momentum, there were still many challenges identified during the needs assessment.

2.2.1. Challenges

- Skepticism from staff—Due to historic start/stop efforts and initiatives that lacked structure, momentum and institutional support, staff doubted the likelihood of ever forming a sustainable, consistent and reliable integrative therapy program. There was distrust of the system and fatigue from working around system failures.
- Perceived barriers—Ranked by nursing staff in descending order: time, lack of skills, lack of knowledge, and comfort with integrative modalities.
- Inconsistencies in infrastructure—Processes, policies, procedure and methods of providing staff education had many variations across the board between the clinic and the hospital settings. These inconsistencies made it challenging to assess what existed, let alone what could be built.
- Lack of clinical expertise—The system did not employ any clinician with the level of training necessary to ensure that safe and effective integrative therapies were being utilized to the fullest potential to meet the needs of patients and families.

Ultimately, it was determined that a historic lack of cohesive institutional effort to form a comprehensive integrative therapy program led to the development of many variations in integrative therapy practices throughout the institution. While this demonstrates a high level of staff dedication to patient needs and adaptability, it also lends itself to inconsistency in standards of practice, policies, procedures and staff education. These types of efforts leave patients and families with minimal access to a consistent, reliable and safe set of services. Despite these challenges, several goals and a common vision emerged as part of the needs assessment process.

2.2.2. Vision

The vision was to create a world-class comprehensive integrative therapy program that would provide a seamless experience for pediatric BMT patients and families from the time of diagnosis through survivorship or bereavement. Additionally, the vision was to align the program with the organizational vision and mission and with national health care goals, including the Quadruple

Aim: improving the patient experience, the health of populations, reducing the cost of health care delivery, and improving care team well-being [2]. The program aimed to be viewed as a means to achieving essential health care outcomes by aligning fluidly with the challenges of today's health care environment. Integrative nursing is a key strategy in improving outcomes, enhancing patient/family satisfaction, and reducing the cost of care delivery, while at the same time improving its quality [3].

2.2.3. Goals

- Improve symptom management.
- Improve patient experience.
- Enhance patient and family resilience and capacity to cope.
- Provide patient and family with tools for incorporating integrative health practices before, during and after hospitalization.
- Improve care team well-being.
- Grow and support integrative health and healing research.
- Embed integrative approaches in every patient's care plan and every clinician's workflow.

2.2.4. Recommendations

The recommendations for achieving this vision and these goals were clear, yet extensive and arduous. To build a sustainable program, it would take years to accomplish every essential element. The following list of recommendations was developed five years ago following the initial needs assessment.

- Create an infrastructure and commit resources that are commensurate with the program vision and goals.

    ○ Hire or appoint an organizational lead.
    ○ Establish standards of care as well as policies and procedures that support those standards.
    ○ Create flowsheets and templates in the electronic medical record that not only allow for documentation of integrative approaches to care, but also allow for easy assessment of outcomes.

- Design a robust and comprehensive program evaluation strategy.
- Establish strong staff education and support.
- Offer access to a consistent set of therapeutic approaches that are evidenced-informed and focused on improved symptom management and quality of life.
- Expand patient and family education.
- Develop parent support resources to engage them in self-care and stress management, and to empower them to participate in comforting and caring for their child through the use of integrative approaches.
- Create an integrative health consult service for expertise, leadership and guidance to staff, patients and families.
- Establish an integrative health and healing research program focused on pediatric BMT patients' needs and clinical outcomes.

The program has three main components: care of patients and their families, staff well-being, and outcome evaluation. The components have been developed and implemented in that order. This order of evolution has been successful for several reasons. Nursing staff often does not recognize the need for self-care, does not identify burnout correctly or timely, or is reluctant to make changes. By implementing care of patients and families first, nurses and other frontline staff experienced secondary benefits of employing integrative strategies in the hospital setting. Nursing frequently received positive feedback from patients and families on the benefits they were experiencing from using integrative modalities.

2.2.5. Care Delivery Model

The framework for the nursing care delivery model comes from the integrative nursing work of Mary Jo Kreitzer and Mary Koithan [3]. The six principles of integrative nursing guide the practice of every nurse in the institution. Additionally, two doctoral prepared nurses with advanced nursing practice study in integrative health and healing lead the delivery of integrative therapy and integrative health consultation. Each new patient receives an integrative health consult with one of the integrative health doctor of nursing practice (DNP) nurses. These consults are triggered in the system to happen automatically for every patient. There is no fee associated with consultation or administration of integrative care. These services are offered to all patients regardless of insurance coverage or ability to pay. During this initial consultation, the patient and family's historical use of integrative therapies is discussed, an assessment of current or anticipated needs, symptoms and challenges is performed, as is a discussion of current skills, strengths and coping mechanisms. Safety and compatibility of integrative therapies with upcoming treatment regimen is discussed during this consult, and education is provided if a patient is currently using or desiring to use an integrative approach that might pose a safety risk during or immediately following the period of chemotherapy and radiation. Finally, a plan for integrative care during hospitalization is discussed and designed. Upon admission to the BMT unit, patients can choose to receive integrative services daily, as needed, or on a consultation basis only. The most common reasons patient engage in integrative therapies are for pain control, nausea, insomnia, anxiety and benefit of forming a therapeutic relationship with the clinician. Supplementary Materials Table S1 describes the integrative therapies that are offered consistently and reliably on the BMT unit.

2.3. Program Evaluation

Entering into the fifth year of the program, data has been gathered showing an uptick in integrative therapy utilization since year one. The authors hypothesize this could be due to several factors: (1) the first year of the program, there was only one full-time clinician dedicated to providing integrative services to patients and families. Currently, there are two-and-a-half full-time equivalent employees providing integrative services. (2) Patients and families affected by childhood cancer, and other rare diseases for which BMT is utilized as a treatment, are very well connected to one another. Patients and families now report having heard about the benefits of integrative therapies from people in their disease-specific communities before ever arriving to the facility. (3) Clinicians have indubitably become more skilled at applying integrative therapies to unique patient populations. Clinicians are skilled at assessing the root cause of a patient's symptom and applying the therapy that will modify the root cause rather than simply eliminating the symptom. For example, young children often experience nausea and/or vomiting before or after medication administration or in anticipation of chemotherapy. It is important to assess the characteristics of and the circumstances surrounding the nausea and/or vomiting. Often, it is anxiety or anticipatory anxiety that leads to sudden onset nausea and/or vomiting [8]. Mind/body techniques are more effective at mitigating the risk of emesis related to anxiety or a conditioned response to treatment than a pharmaceutical antiemetic [8]. Finally, (4) it is plausible that providers and staff recommend integrative therapies more often and demonstrate more confidence in integrative therapies now than they did four years ago. Once providers and staff began having first-hand observations and experiences with integrative therapies achieving positive results for their patients, they were more likely to recommend them.

The BMT program treats approximately 80 patients per year. Patients are engaged in treatment for a minimum of three to four months. Some patients remain in the system and seek in- and outpatient care intermittently for up to two years. Year one of the program, 51% of BMT patients engaged in integrative therapies. By year two, that number increased to 70%, and at the conclusion of year three, approximately 94% of patients participated in integrative therapies throughout their BMT experience. Patient and family engagement with the integrative therapy team ranges from a one-time consult to daily sessions of 30–60 min. The average patient is seen two or three times per week for approximately 30 min. Over the course of hundreds of integrative therapy sessions over the past four years, the program reports no adverse events. Practice guidelines and safety recommendations have been developed based on available literature, clinician experience, patient report, and occasionally "near misses".

2.4. Emerging Research Agenda

Establishing a research program was one of the eight original goals. This has been the most challenging goal to accomplish and was, by design, delayed for the first few years. Infrastructure needed to be built before clean data collection could occur. Now that a consistent set of services is offered by experienced clinicians, the program is ripe for an integrative research agenda. Several quality improvement surveys and one qualitative study have been completed and played an important role in shaping the research agenda. The first study published by the program examined themes around the usefulness of music therapy [9]. Table 2 outlines the research initiatives that are underway and projects that will be implemented over the next two years.

Table 2. Research agenda.

Study Concept	Description
Music therapy as a method to physical rehabilitation	Qualitative data has revealed that even when children are too physically ill or mentally reluctant to participate in physical rehabilitation therapies, many are still motivated to get out of bed and participate in music therapy. It is hypothesized that active participation in music therapy can help achieve physical rehabilitation goals in some patients [9].
Retrospective review of utilization and safety	Data mining will be done to assess the most common therapy used by each age group, adverse reactions in patients with safety considerations such as thrombocytopenia or impaired skin integrity, responses of pain, nausea and anxiety to integrative therapy, and average length and number of visits (inpatient and outpatient) each patient requests.
Self-assessment of change after the implementation of an integrative therapy plan of care	The self-assessment of change is a retrospective pre/post assessment that measures a variety of psychosocial indicators. The tool was designed specifically to capture change produced by integrative therapy.
Survivorship well-being for patients and families	Interactive online content based on the University of Minnesota's Wellbeing Model (Figure 2) will be developed and focused on teenagers and young adults. Virtual support groups will accompany content. Groups will be facilitated by a variety of healthcare professionals with an integrative lens. Data will be collected to assess the impact on overall well-being including indicators such as self-management, perceived stress, quality of life, anxiety, depression and resilience.
Microbiome	This study will examine the effects of chemotherapy and prolonged prophylactic antibiotic use on patients after engraftment and full recovery from pancytopenia. It will also look at the potential for the safe and judicial use of supplements to restore intestinal tissue integrity and the microbiome.
Staff self-care	Continuous data collection efforts have been and will continue to be underway assessing staff burnout and other components of well-being.

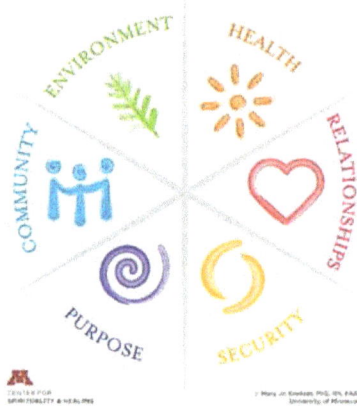

Figure 2. University of Minnesota's Wellbeing Model [6].

3. Results and Discussion

The integrative therapy program is entering into its fifth year of existence. It has grown and matured since the original design, but remains true to its initial mission, vision and goals. By all objective measures, the program has been deemed a success. Rates of patient engagement and utilization, increase in grant funding and institutional support, and provider and front-line clinician acceptance all speak to the accomplishments of the program over the past four years. The authors conclude that it is both feasible and acceptable to implement a nurse-led integrative program within an academic health center-based pediatric BMT program.

The success and sustainability of the program may be in large part due to nursing leadership. Nurses are uniquely positioned to assess and treat patients from a whole-person, whole-system framework. Nurses are by nature nurturing, caring and attuned to using their own self as a therapeutic intervention. Furthermore, by having advanced nursing practice consultation available, the model is more financially sustainable than a physician-centric integrative consult service. Patients receive competent assessment and continuity of care with nurses trained in integrative modalities accessible to them on a daily basis.

4. Conclusions

The work over the past few years has demonstrated that there is a strong clinical and business case for implementing integrative nursing within an acute-care pediatric setting. Patients and families are voicing a desire for this approach to care and there is increasing evidence that integrative approaches can improve clinical outcomes including symptom management [8]. If embedded into the ongoing delivery of care, the implementation of integrative nursing is both feasible and sustainable. It requires investment in education and leadership and perhaps most importantly a culture change that embraces a whole-person, whole-system approach to patient care.

Supplementary Materials: The following are available online at http://www.mdpi.com/2227-9067/5/8/103/s1, Table S1: Integrative therapy availability.

Author Contributions: M.J.K. has been an active advisor and mentor to the growth and development of the pediatric BMT integrative program since its conceptualization in 2012. M.E.V. began work on the pediatric BMT integrative program by joining the team that conducted the initial needs assessment under the guidance of M.J.K. and John E. Wager, executive medical director for pediatric BMT in 2013. M.E.V. continues to direct the program and its research efforts.

Funding: The pediatric BMT integrative therapy efforts and research have been funded in large part by the Children's Cancer Research Fund, a national nonprofit with a dual mission of curing cancer and simultaneously enhancing the quality of life of children battling cancer. The authors would like to express deep appreciation and gratitude for the support and dedication offered by the Children's Cancer Research Fund.

Acknowledgments: The authors would like to acknowledge the perpetual support of John E. Wagner, the executive medical director of the pediatric BMT program. Without his vision, leadership and support, this program would not exist. Without the constant administrative support of Janet Hegland, program director pediatric BMT, this program would not have made it off the ground. Hegland's leadership and dedication are appreciated. The other members of the original needs assessment team, Janet Tomaino and Rachel Trelstad Porter, the authors appreciate the initial work that helped to pave the path and plant the seeds of inspiration for this program. The insights and contributions of that group still play a daily role in the program evolution. Finally, the authors would like to thank all of the frontline staff working with pediatric BMT patients. The faculty, hospitalists, nurses, nurse practitioners, physicians' assistants, chaplains, social workers and support staff are the true essence of healing presence in the lives of these children.

Conflicts of Interest: The authors declare no conflict of interest.

References

1. Institute for Healthcare Improvement: IHI Home Page. Available online: http://www.ihi.org:80/ (accessed on 29 June 2018).
2. Clinician Resilience and Well-Being. National Academy of Medicine. Available online: https://nam.edu/initiatives/clinician-resilience-and-well-being/ (accessed on 29 June 2018).
3. Kreitzer, M.J.; Koithan, M. *Integrative Nursing*; Oxford University Press: New York, NY, USA, 2018.
4. Koithan, M.S.; Kreitzer, M.J.; Watson, J. Linking the unitary paradigm to policy through a synthesis of caring science and integrative nursing, linking the unitary paradigm to policy through a synthesis of caring science and integrative nursing. *Nurs. Sci. Q.* **2017**, *30*, 262–268. [CrossRef] [PubMed]
5. Presencing Institute—Theory U: Leading from the Future as It Emerges. Available online: https://www.presencing.org/#/aboutus/theory-u (accessed on 29 June 2018).
6. Integrative Nursing. Available online: https://www.csh.umn.edu/education/focus-areas/integrative-nursing (accessed on 6 July 2018).
7. Jacobs, S.S. Integrative therapy use for management of side effects and toxicities experienced by pediatric oncology patients. *Children* **2014**, *1*, 424–440. [CrossRef] [PubMed]
8. Roscoe, J.A.; Morrow, G.R.; Aapro, M.S.; Molassiotis, A.; Olver, I. Anticipatory nausea and vomiting. *Support. Care Cancer* **2011**, *19*, 1533–1538. [CrossRef] [PubMed]
9. Yates, G.J.; Beckmann, N.B.; Anderson, M.R.; Voss, M.E.; Silverman, M.J. Caregiver perceptions of music therapy for children hospitalized for a blood and marrow transplant: An interpretivist investigation. *Glob. Adv. Health Med.* **2018**. [CrossRef] [PubMed]

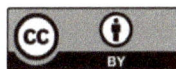

© 2018 by the authors. Licensee MDPI, Basel, Switzerland. This article is an open access article distributed under the terms and conditions of the Creative Commons Attribution (CC BY) license (http://creativecommons.org/licenses/by/4.0/).

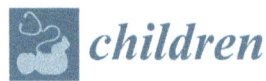

Article

Pediatric Integrative Medicine in Residency Program: Relationship between Lifestyle Behaviors and Burnout and Wellbeing Measures in First-Year Residents

Hilary McClafferty [1,*], Audrey J. Brooks [1,*], Mei-Kuang Chen [1], Michelle Brenner [2], Melanie Brown [3], Anna Esparham [4], Dana Gerstbacher [5], Brenda Goliaunu [6], John Mark [5], Joy Weydert [4], Ann Ming Yeh [5] and Victoria Maizes [1]

1. Department of Medicine, Arizona Center for Integrative Medicine, University of Arizona, Tucson, AZ 85724, USA; kuang@email.arizona.edu (M.-K.C.); vmaizes@email.arizona.edu (V.M.)
2. Department of Pediatrics, Eastern Virginia Medical School/Children's Hospital of the King's Daughters, Norfolk, VA 23507, USA; michelle.brenner@chkd.org
3. Department of Pediatrics, University of Chicago Comer Children's Hospital, Chicago, IL 60637, USA; Melanie.Brown@childrensmn.org
4. Department of Pediatrics, University of Kansas School of Medicine, Kansas City, KS 66160, USA; aeesparham@cmh.edu (A.E.); jweydert@kumc.edu (J.W.)
5. Department of Pediatrics, Stanford University School of Medicine, Palo Alto, CA 94304, USA; gerst1@stanford.edu (D.G.); jmark@stanford.edu (J.M.); annming@stanford.edu (A.M.Y.)
6. Department of Anesthesiology and Pain Management, Stanford University School of Medicine, Palo Alto, CA 94304, USA; bgolianu@stanford.edu
* Correspondence: hmcclafferty@email.arizona.edu (H.M.); brooksaj@email.arizona.edu (A.J.B.)

Received: 9 February 2018; Accepted: 17 April 2018; Published: 23 April 2018

Abstract: It is widely recognized that burnout is prevalent in medical culture and begins early in training. Studies show pediatricians and pediatric trainees experience burnout rates comparable to other specialties. Newly developed Accreditation Council for Graduate Medical Education (ACGME) core competencies in professionalism and personal development recognize the unacceptably high resident burnout rates and present an important opportunity for programs to improve residents experience throughout training. These competencies encourage healthy lifestyle practices and cultivation of self-awareness, self-regulation, empathy, mindfulness, and compassion—a paradigm shift from traditional medical training underpinned by a culture of unrealistic endurance and self-sacrifice. To date, few successful and sustainable programs in resident burnout prevention and wellness promotion have been described. The University of Arizona Center for Integrative Medicine Pediatric Integrative Medicine in Residency (PIMR) curriculum, developed in 2011, was designed in part to help pediatric programs meet new resident wellbeing requirements. The purpose of this paper is to detail levels of lifestyle behaviors, burnout, and wellbeing for the PIMR program's first-year residents (N = 203), and to examine the impact of lifestyle behaviors on burnout and wellbeing. The potential of the PIMR to provide interventions addressing gaps in lifestyle behaviors with recognized association to burnout is discussed.

Keywords: burnout; pediatrics; residents; preventive lifestyle behaviors; resilience

1. Introduction

Medical school and residency training are known for their scientific rigor and daunting hours of service [1,2]. Compounding burnout experienced in medical school, the life of a resident is dominated by exposure to significant human suffering, high levels of responsibility, lack of day-to-day control, steep learning curves, limited regeneration time, and chronic sleep deprivation. These realities, in conjunction with patient and family demands, subordinate ranking in the medical hierarchy, and other stressors predispose residents to high burnout prevalence [1,2].

Studies show that pediatricians and pediatric trainees experience burnout at rates comparable to other specialties, with higher prevalence in some high acuity pediatric subspecialties such as neonatology, intensive care, and hematology-oncology [3–6]. Across medical specialties and training levels, burnout has been associated with an increase in medical errors, lower adherence to best practices, substance abuse, self-medication, and poorer patient outcomes (for example, longer hospital stay), in addition to increased rates of clinician's depression, suicidal ideation, and completed suicide [7]. It has been widely reported that effective approaches must include changes at organizational, institutional, and individual levels to address the outdated culture of unrealistic endurance still pervasive in medicine [8].

Newly developed Accreditation Council for Graduate Medical Education (ACGME) core competencies in professionalism and personal development recognize the unacceptably high burnout rates in residents and present an important opportunity for programs to improve the experience of residents at all stages of training [9].

In addition to encouraging healthy lifestyle practices, the core competencies encourage cultivation of self-awareness, self-regulation skills, empathy, mindfulness, and compassion. They also highlight the need for innovation in clinical training and generate questions about how to best teach and measure success in these new areas. This endeavor provides important opportunities to introduce proactive approaches to burnout through a multidimensional model and development of educational curricula that emphasize and measure wellbeing at all phases of medical training.

To date, along with development of the new core competencies, purposeful steps taken by the ACGME include national symposia led by expert national faculty to identify actionable issues, new emphasis on education on physician wellbeing, and recommendations for annual measurement of resident burnout through its Clinical Learning Environmental Review (CLER) program which evaluates the quality of the program learning environment [10].

Despite these significant initiatives, few successful, sustainable programs in resident burnout prevention and wellness promotion have been described. Pediatricians are uniquely positioned to develop national initiatives for solution-based approaches to burnout, in part due to the timely initiation of the 2010 Pediatric Milestone Project, a collaboration between the ACGME and the American Board of Pediatrics (ABP) dedicated to development of revised core competencies. The University of Arizona Center for Integrative Medicine Pediatric Integrative Medicine in Residency (PIMR) curriculum was developed in 2011 and refined in 2012 to include a robust Self-Care unit, partly in response to the new priorities in the revised national pediatric training competencies targeting resident wellbeing outlined by the ACGME.

The 100-h curriculum is an interactive hybrid online-onsite program and has been described in detail in an earlier publication [11]. The program has been piloted since 2012 at the University of Arizona, Stanford University, the University of Kansas, the University of Chicago, and Eastern Virginia Medical School/Children's Hospital of the King's Daughters. The topics covered include: Self-; nutrition and physical activity; mind-body therapies; dietary supplements; whole systems of medicine; and clinical applications.

The curriculum was developed with the two-fold purpose of embedding foundational education in pediatric integrative medicine into residency training and introducing a 'train the trainer' model in teaching healthy lifestyle habits. In anticipation of high levels of burnout in incoming residents, the Self-Care unit was designed to provide an evidence-based 'blueprint' for learning about factors associated with lower burnout prevalence in medical trainees including: physical activity, sleep, stress management, mindfulness, and nutrition, thereby increasing resident knowledge about self-care and also providing a useful educational tool for residency programs to address new ACGME resident wellness competency requirements. An integrated evaluation arm measures resident burnout and lifestyle behaviors, and gathers feedback on perceived quality and relevance of the curriculum at four points (beginning, end Post Graduate Year (PGY) 1, end PGY2, end PGY3) of residency training.

We readily acknowledge that change is urgently needed on multiple levels to address the serious issues of preventing burnout and promoting wellbeing in medical trainees, ideally starting in pre-medical and medical students. We believe our study findings detailing the incoming resident levels of burnout, wellbeing, and lifestyle behaviors and examining the relationship between resident lifestyle habits and burnout and wellbeing measures reinforce this point and begin to explore areas of potential progress. The overarching purpose of this paper is to document the concerning state of burnout in early pediatric trainees and to examine the potential of the PIMR curriculum to provide interventions that address gaps in lifestyle behaviors with recognized association to burnout, and how they might be introduced into residency training.

2. Methods

Approval for the study was granted by the University of Arizona Institutional Review Board (Approval #12049200). First-year pediatric residents from five residencies participating in the PIMR program completed standardized wellbeing measures at the start of residency. The PIMR sites include academic and community-based programs led by pediatric faculty with fellowship training in integrative medicine, a field that blends conventional and evidence-based complementary medicine and prioritizes preventive health. Information about existing onsite physician wellness activities was collected and is presented. Data is being collected as part of a longitudinal study on resident wellbeing, burnout and lifestyle behaviors and the longitudinal impact of the PIMR curriculum.

2.1. Measures

Residents completed eight widely used, established scales assessing dimensions of well-being: perceived stress, depression symptoms, burnout (emotional exhaustion, depersonalization), life satisfaction, affect, mindfulness, emotional intelligence, and physician empathy (Table 1). A measure of lifestyle behaviors, the Arizona Lifestyle Inventory (ALI) [12], was also administered. The ALI was developed to assess changes in lifestyle behaviors in residents. The domains and items were identified from literature on evidence-based preventive services as well as other areas emphasized by integrative medicine practitioners. The items were reviewed by an expert panel of integrative medicine physicians and were revised based on their comments. The ALI primarily assesses the frequency of behaviors in the past seven days in the areas of diet/nutrition, exercise, mind-body/spiritual practices, social support activities, sleep, and work stress (see Table 2 for items by domain); areas known to mediate the relationships between stress reactivity and physical and mental health. The ALI also includes demographic variables, including hours worked, alcohol use, and health status questions, having a chronic medical condition, taking medication for a chronic medical condition, body mass index (BMI), taking prescription medication for stress or anxiety, days with pain in the past week, and days engaged in hobbies in the past week.

Site leaders completed a survey of onsite physician wellness activities in 2014 and 2016. Physician wellness activities included retreats, nutrition (healthy food options), empathy skills training, conflict resolution/communication skills training, stress management, physical activity options (e.g., exercise rooms), self-regulation skills training (e.g., mind-body skills training), and burnout prevention.

Table 1. Wellbeing measures.

Dimension	Measure	Description
Perceived stress	Perceived Stress Scale (PSS) [13]	10 items; scores 0–40
Depression symptoms	Center for Epidemiologic Studies—Depression Scale (CES-D) [14]	20 items; scores range from 0–60; score of 16 or higher indicates clinical syndrome
Burnout	Maslach Burnout Inventory (MBI) [15,16]	22 items; 3 subscales emotional exhaustion (EE), depersonalization (DEP), personal accomplishment (PA)
Life satisfaction	Satisfaction with Life Scale (SWLS) [17,18]	5 items; higher total scores indicate greater life satisfaction
Affect	Positive and Negative Affect Scale (PANAS) [19]	20 items; 2 subscales positive affect (POS), negative affect (NEG); higher score more positive, more negative affect
Mindfulness	Freiberg Mindfulness Inventory (FMI) [20]	14 items, higher score more mindful
Emotional Intelligence	Interpersonal Reactivity Index (IRI) [21]	21 items; 3 subscales perspective taking (PT), empathic concern (EC), personal distress (PD); higher scores greater perspective taking, empathic concern, personal distress
Empathy [a]	Jefferson Empathy Scale (JES) [22]	20 items, higher score greater empathy
Lifestyle Behaviors	Arizona Lifestyle Inventory [12]	35 items measuring frequency of diet/nutrition, exercise, mind-body/spiritual practices, social support activities, sleep, hobbies, alcohol consumption behaviors

[a] JES not collected in 2012 class.

2.2. Data Collection and Statistical Analysis

Data were collected directly from the residents online using an individualized link to an internet-based survey website (Survey Monkey, San Mateo, CA, USA) in the first trimester of the first year of residency. Prior to accessing the assessments, residents voluntarily completed an online informed consent form. Statistical analyses were conducted using SPSS v. 24.0 (IBM Corp. Released 2016. IBM SPSS Statistics for Windows, Version 24.0. Armonk, NY, USA).

Descriptive statistics are presented for the wellbeing measures and lifestyle behaviors. A burnout risk group variable was created utilizing medicine norms [15] as follows: high burnout consists of individuals scoring in the high range on both emotional exhaustion and depersonalization; low burnout group includes individuals scoring in the low range on both scales; remaining individuals were categorized as moderate burnout. One-way analysis of variance (ANOVA) with post hoc Tukey tests were conducted to compare wellbeing measures and lifestyle behaviors among burnout groups.

A series of multiple regression analyses were performed to examine the relationship between the lifestyle behavior domains and each of the wellbeing measures. For the lifestyle behaviors, due to variation in response format for some items, scale total scores were calculated utilizing two procedures. For scales where all items were rated on a 0–7 scale (number of days of carrying out the specific lifestyle behavior in the past seven days) the scale scores were formed using mean scores of the items in the same domain. For items where there was variation in response format, such as exercise, social support activities, and alcohol use, items were standardized first and then the means of the z-scores were used as the scale scores. Items were reverse-scored where indicated. With the exception of the work stress scale, higher scores indicate engaging in more of the behaviors in that domain. Higher scores on the work stress scale indicate a greater level of work stress. The correlation between the wellbeing measures and gender and marital status were examined. If the correlation was statistically significant, gender and/or marital status was included in the model. The initial regression models included all lifestyle variables and demographic variables, as indicated. A final regression analysis was performed dropping non-significant predictors ($p > 0.05$).

3. Results

3.1. Sample

The sample consisted of 203 first-year residents from four incoming classes (2012, $n = 15$; 2013, $n = 88$; 2014, $n = 59$; 2015, $n = 41$) at five pediatric residency programs participating in the PIMR program: (1) University of Arizona ($n = 41$); (2) University of Chicago ($n = 56$); (3) Eastern Virginia Medical School/Children's Hospital of the King's Daughters ($n = 55$); (4) University of Kansas Medical Center ($n = 26$); and (5) Stanford University ($n = 25$). The survey response rate across the cohorts was 63% and ranged between 45–88% across the residency programs. The sample was predominantly female (76%), white (71%) or Asian (13%), and non-Hispanic (94%) with an average age of 28 years old (range 24–39 years old). Half of the sample was married or cohabitating (50%) and 12% had children. The majority of residents were US Doctors of Medicine (76%), followed by foreign medical graduates (13%) and US Doctors of Osteopathic Medicine (11%). Residents completed the online surveys at the beginning of PGY1. In terms of health status, 25% ($n = 50$) reported a chronic medical condition and 19% ($n = 38$) reported taking medication for a chronic medical condition. The most common medical conditions reported were psychological (depression, anxiety, and/or attention deficit hyperactivity disorder; $n = 15$), asthma ($n = 12$) and allergies ($n = 9$). More than two-thirds (68.2%; $n = 135/198$) had a normal BMI, while 23% ($n = 46$) fell in the overweight range and 5% were in the obese range ($n = 10$). Residents reported experiencing pain an average of 1.3 days in the past seven days (range 0–7). Almost half of the residents (47%; $n = 95$) reported experiencing at least one day of pain. Few residents reported taking prescription medication for stress or anxiety ($n = 16$; 8%). Alcohol consumption averaged 2.8 drinks in the past 7 days, with a maximum of 15 drinks in the past week. Three residents reported smoking cigarettes (2%). In terms of hours worked in the past week, 92% ($n = 186$) reported working 80 h or less with 59% ($n = 119$) working 61–80 h.

3.2. Wellbeing Measures

Descriptive statistics for the wellbeing measures are presented in Table 2. The average perceived stress score (16) for this resident sample was slightly higher than normed sample data for the general public (11.9–14.7), but was consistent with ranges for healthcare students (15.5–16.7) [23]. The average depression score (12.9) was within the non-depressed range, with 70% of the sample scoring in this range. However, 30% scored over 16, the cut-off score indicating a risk for clinical depression [14,24]. Over half the sample (55%) scored in the low emotional exhaustion range. Less than half (42%) scored in the low depersonalization range. Twenty percent of residents scored in the high emotional exhaustion range and 32% scored in the high depersonalization range. Fifteen percent scored in the high burnout range on both the emotional exhaustion and depersonalization scales. The average score on personal accomplishment (29.5) was in the low range (high risk for burnout) [15]. The average life satisfaction score was 26.4 (in the satisfied range) with 68.9% scoring in the satisfied to extremely satisfied range [17,18]. The mean positive affect (35.2) and negative affect scores (20.6) were slightly better than the mid-point (30) on the Positive and Negative Affect Schedule (PANAS) scale and consistent with what was observed in incoming family medicine residents in the Integrative Medicine in Residency (IMR) program [25].

The average mindfulness score (35.4) was slightly higher than a general sample [20]. Residents in the current sample scored lower on perspective taking and empathic concern and higher on personal distress than a study of incoming internal medicine residents [26]. The average empathy score in this resident sample (110.75) is lower than means obtained in the Jefferson Empathy Scale (JES) validation study with both resident and medical student samples (118) [22].

Table 2. Measures of wellbeing—descriptive statistics.

Wellbeing Measures	N	n	Mean (SD)/% Yes	Range	Norm Data
Perceived stress	190		16.0 (5.9)	2–31	11.9–14.7 [1]
CES-D depression	190		12.9 (9.2)	0–42	
Non-depressed		132	69.5%		<16 non-depressed
Clinical depression risk		58	30.5%		≥16
MBI—Emotional exhaustion	203		18.1 (9.0)	0–54	19–26 average
Low emotional exhaustion		112	55.2%		
Moderate emotional exhaustion		50	24.6%		
High emotional exhaustion		41	20.2%		
MBI—Depersonalization	203		7.4 (4.9)	0–30	6–9 average
Low depersonalization		85	41.9%		
Moderate depersonalization		54	26.6%		
High depersonalization		64	31.5%		
MBI—Burnout risk group					
Low risk		70	34.5%		
Moderate risk		102	50.2%		
High risk		31	15.3%		
MBI—Personal accomplishment	203		29.5 (6.3)	12–48	39–34 average
Satisfaction with life	203		26.4 (5.8)	5–35	26–30 satisfied
PANAS Positive	174		35.2 (6.4)	10–50	35.3 [2]
PANAS Negative	174		20.6 (6.0)	10–42	19.6 [3]
Mindfulness	191		35.4 (7.1)	16–54	34.52 [3], 31.17 [4]
IRI Empathic concern	190		21.5 (4.0)	11–28	22.2 [5]
IRI Personal distress	190		10.4 (4.9)	0–25	8.9 [5]
IRI Perspective taking	189		18.3 (4.3)	2–28	20.6 [5]
Jefferson empathy	174		110.7 (14.2)	79–140	118 [6]

[1] General public validation sample; [2] Post Graduate Year (PGY1) Family medicine residents; [3] General sample; [4] Clinical sample; [5] PGY1 Internal medicine residents; [6] Resident and medical student mean, SD: standard deviation.

3.3. Lifestyle Behaviors

Descriptive statistics for the lifestyle behavior items by domain are presented in Table 3. Eating breakfast was the most frequent behavior (mean = 5.7 days), while eating 5 servings of fruits and vegetables was the least frequent (mean = 3.3 days). Most did not drink sugary beverages (60%). Residents reported an average of 2 days of at least 10 min moderate exercise and 1.6 days of 10 min of vigorous exercise. More than half of residents reported either 1–2 days (42%) or 3–4 days (28%) of 30 min of moderate exercise. Most residents (83%) reported sedentary behavior less than 70% on an average day. Residents reported engaging in an activity to manage stress an average of 3.3 days. The most frequent practice was prayer (mean 2.3 days). The least frequent practice was progressive muscle relaxation (mean = 0.2 days). While residents reported spending time in nurturing relationships with family or friends most days (mean = 4.8 days), much less time was spent socializing with friends (mean = 2.1 days). Most residents (74%) reported feeling a sense of belonging to a group. While getting 7–9 h of sleep (mean = 3.4 days) or waking feeling rested (mean = 3 days) averages were somewhat low, trouble staying asleep was not a frequent issue (mean = 1.4 days). Residents reported enjoying work an average of 4.6 days and feeling overwhelmed 2.6 days per week.

Table 3. Lifestyle behaviors—descriptive statistics.

Domain/Items	N	n	Mean/%	SD	Range
Diet/Nutrition					
5 Servings fruits & vegetables	203		3.3	2.2	0–7
Eat calcium rich foods	203		4.9	2.0	0–7
Eat breakfast	200		5.7	1.9	0–7
Eat home cooked dinner	203		4.2	2.0	0–7
Drank caffeinated beverages *	203		5.6	2.2	0–7
Sugary fluid drinks average day *	202		0.6	0.9	0–5
0		122	60.4%		
1		61	30.2%		
2		8	3.9%		
3		9	4.5%		
4		1	0.5%		
5 or more		1	0.5%		
Servings high fiber average day	203		2.1	1.3	0–5
0		15	7.4%		
1		51	25.1%		
2		67	33.0%		
3		43	21.2%		
4		14	6.9%		
5 or more		13	6.4%		
Vegetarian	188		0.07	0.25	0–1
Yes		13	6.9%		
Exercise					
Vigorous physical activity ≥ 10 min	202		1.6	1.8	0–7
Moderate physical activity ≥ 10 min	202		2.0	2.0	0–7
Moderate physical activity ≥ 30 min	187				
None		28	15.0%		
1–2 days		78	41.7%		
3–4 days		53	28.3%		
5–6 days		21	11.2%		
Everyday		7	3.7%		
Percent sedentary average day *	198				
Less than 5%		4	2.0%		
6–10%		8	4.0%		
11–20%		12	6.1%		
21–30%		19	9.6%		
31–40%		25	12.6%		
41–50%		36	18.2%		
51–60%		29	14.6%		
61–70%		31	15.7%		
71–80%		25	12.6%		
81–90%		9	4.5%		
91–100%		0	0%		
Mind-Body/Spiritual Practices					
Activity to relax or manage stress	202		3.3	2.4	0–7
Prayer	202		2.3	2.8	0–7
Spiritual ritual non-prayer	202		0.6	1.7	0–7
Personal reflection	201		1.5	2.2	0–7
Breathing for stress reduction	202		0.5	1.3	0–7
Progressive muscle relaxation	191		0.2	0.8	0–7
Social Support Activities					
Spend time family/friends	203		4.8	2.3	0–7
Receive healthy touch	203		4.4	2.6	0–7
Socialize with friends	202		2.1	1.6	0–7
Sense of belonging groups	203				
Yes		150	73.9%		
Not sure		20	9.9%		
No		33	16.3%		
Number groups belong	203		1.9	1.2	0–6
Sleep					
Get 7–9 h of sleep	203		3.4	2.2	0–7
Wake feeling rested	201		3.0	2.1	0–7
Trouble staying asleep *	201		1.4	2.0	0–7

Table 3. Cont.

Domain/Items	N	n	Mean/%	SD	Range
Hobbies	202		2.1	2.3	0–7
Number of Alcohol Drinks	200		2.8	3.0	0–15
Work					
Enjoy work *	203		4.6	1.9	0–7
Feel overwhelmed by work	203		2.6	2.2	0–7

* Items reverse-scored when creating scales.

3.4. Differences between Burnout Risk Groups on Wellbeing and Lifestyle Behaviors

In the analyses examining the impact of burnout risk level on wellbeing, all of the models were statistically significant ($p < 0.006$; Table 4). In comparing the burnout risk groups, the low burnout risk group experienced significantly greater wellbeing than the high-risk group ($p < 0.05$) in all of the models. Specifically, the low burnout risk group experienced less perceived stress, depression, negative affect, and personal distress and greater satisfaction with life, positive affect, mindfulness, empathic concern, perspective taking, and empathy than the high-risk burnout group ($p < 0.05$). Differences between the moderate burnout risk group and the high burnout risk group were also observed for perceived stress, depression, negative affect, satisfaction with life, positive affect, mindfulness, perspective taking and empathy ($p < 0.05$), with the moderate risk group experiencing greater wellbeing than the high-risk group. The low burnout risk group was significantly different from the moderate burnout risk group, experiencing less perceived stress, depression, and negative affect and greater positive affect, empathic concern, and empathy ($p < 0.05$). All post hoc group comparisons were statistically significant in the perceived stress, depression, negative affect, positive affect, and empathy analyses, indicating that wellbeing decreased significantly as burnout risk increased.

Table 4. Results of one-way variance analysis (ANOVA) for Burnout Group and wellbeing—means and standard deviations.

Wellbeing Measures	Total N *	Low Risk n = 70		Moderate Risk n = 102		High Risk n = 31		p-Value
		Mean	SD	Mean	SD	Mean	SD	
Perceived Stress	190	12.6 [a,c]	5.1	16.4 [b]	4.9	22.7	4.4	<0.001
CES-D Total	190	8.1 [a,c]	5.7	12.6 [b]	8.0	25.2	8.3	<0.001
Satisfaction with Life	203	27.9 [a]	4.3	27.0 [b]	5.3	21.1	7.4	<0.001
PANAS Positive	174	38.0 [a,c]	4.5	35.4 [b]	6.4	28.6	4.6	<0.001
PANAS Negative	174	17.5 [a,c]	4.6	20.5 [b]	5.2	27.8	4.9	<0.001
FMI Mindfulness	191	37.6 [a]	6.9	35.1 [b]	7.1	31.6	6.4	0.001
IRI Empathic Concern	190	22.8 [a,c]	3.7	21.2	3.9	19.7	3.9	0.001
IRI Perspective Taking	189	19.5 [a]	4.1	18.2 [b]	3.8	15.5	5.2	<0.001
IRI Personal Distress	190	9.3 [a]	4.7	10.4	4.8	12.7	4.7	0.006
Jefferson Empathy	174	115.8 [a,c]	13.0	110.6 [b]	13.2	99.2	14.1	<0.001
Lifestyle Behaviors								
Diet/Nutrition	203	0.084	0.51	0.043 [b]	0.40	−0.20	0.62	0.048
Exercise [d]	203	0.045	0.7	0.053	0.7	−0.25	0.6	0.095
Mind-body/Spiritual Practices	203	1.6	1.2	1.4	1.0	1.1	1.1	0.13
Social Support Activities [d]	203	0.018 [a]	0.7	0.075 [b]	0.6	−0.30	0.7	0.012
Sleep	203	4.4 [a]	1.5	4.1 [b]	1.4	2.9	1.3	<0.001
Hobbies	202	2.3	2.6	2.0	2.1	1.8	2.1	0.56
Alcohol drinks	200	2.5	2.7	3.2	2.9	2.5	3.6	0.32
Work Stress	203	1.7 [a,c]	1.1	2.6 [b]	1.5	4.2	1.6	<0.001

* N varied by measure. Post hoc Tukey tests: [a] low-risk vs. high-risk group, $p < 0.05$; [b] moderate-risk vs. high-risk group, $p < 0.05$; [c] low-risk vs. moderate-risk group, $p < 0.05$; [d] means for exercise and social relationships are z-scores, therefore the group mean is zero. Means greater than 0 indicate higher frequency than the group mean, while negative means indicate a frequency lower than the group mean.

For the lifestyle behaviors, the diet/nutrition, social relationships, sleep and work stress models were statistically significant ($p < 0.05$; Table 4). The post hoc group comparisons between the low-risk and high-risk groups or moderate-risk and high-risk groups, were statistically significant ($p < 0.05$) in these models. The low-risk and moderate-risk groups reported engaging in a greater frequency of social behaviors and quality sleep than the high-risk group. For diet/nutrition, the high-risk group reported a lower frequency of healthy eating behaviors than the moderate risk group. In the work stress model, the post hoc comparisons were significantly different between all burnout groups, indicating an increase in work stress as burnout risk increased ($p < 0.05$). There was no difference between the burnout risk groups for exercise, mind-body/spiritual practices, hobbies or alcohol use.

3.5. Relationship between Lifestyle Behaviors and Wellbeing Measures

Gender was significantly correlated with empathic concern and empathy and, therefore, included in those regression models. Marital status was correlated with life satisfaction and included in that regression model. The various combinations of lifestyle behaviors contributed 6% to 49% of the variance in the tested models (R^2), depending on the wellbeing measure examined (see Tables 5 and 6). Work stress was a statistically significant predictor in all but one regression model, empathic concern. Greater work stress was associated with increased perceived stress, depression, emotional exhaustion, depersonalization, negative affect, personal distress, and lower personal accomplishment, life satisfaction, positive affect, mindfulness, perspective taking, and empathy. The second-strongest predictor across the wellbeing models was exercise. A higher frequency of engaging in exercise was associated with less perceived stress, depression, negative affect, and personal distress, and higher levels of personal accomplishment, positive affect, mindfulness, perspective taking, and empathy. A higher frequency of engaging in social support activities was associated with higher life satisfaction, mindfulness, and empathic concern and less depression. More quality sleep was associated with less perceived stress, depression, emotional exhaustion, and negative affect. A greater frequency of healthy eating behaviors was associated with lower levels of depersonalization and higher life satisfaction. While a higher frequency of engaging in hobbies was associated with decreased personal distress, it was also associated with less mindfulness. Mind-body/spiritual practices were associated with increased mindfulness only. Alcohol use was non-significant in all the models. Gender was associated with empathic concern and empathy, with females having greater empathic concern and empathy, while marital status was non-significant.

Table 5. Lifestyle behavior predictors, R^2 and betas on measures of wellbeing [a].

Wellbeing Measure	Model Adjusted R^2	Model p-Value	β	t	p-Value
Perceived stress	0.39	<0.001			
Work stress			0.50	7.95	<0.001
Exercise			−0.19	−3.35	0.001
Sleep			−0.16	−2.45	0.015
CES-D Total	0.49	<0.001			
Work			0.47	7.80	<0.001
Sleep			−0.23	−3.93	<0.001
Social			−0.18	−3.14	0.002
Exercise			−0.13	−2.38	0.018
MBI emotional exhaustion	0.40	<0.001			
Work stress			0.56	9.52	<0.001
Sleep			−0.17	−2.94	0.004
MBI Depersonalization	0.16	<0.001			
Work stress			0.34	5.21	<0.001
Diet			−0.20	−3.09	0.002
MBI personal accomplishment	0.18	<0.001			
Work Stress			−0.34	−5.32	<0.001
Exercise			0.23	3.64	<0.001
Satisfaction with life [b]	0.26	<0.001			
Work stress			−0.36	−5.65	<0.001
Social			0.21	3.29	0.001
Diet			0.16	2.60	0.010

Table 5. Cont.

Wellbeing Measure	Model Adjusted R^2	Model p-Value	β	t	p-Value
PANAS positive	0.31	<0.001			
Work stress			−0.46	−7.29	<0.001
Exercise			0.27	4.25	<0.001
PANAS negative	0.26	<0.001			
Work stress			0.37	5.05	<0.001
Exercise			−0.17	−2.64	0.009
Sleep			−0.17	−2.34	0.021
Mindfulness	0.20	<0.001			
Work stress			−0.27	−3.95	<0.001
Exercise			0.25	3.66	<0.001
Social			0.15	2.18	0.031
Hobbies			−0.16	−2.27	0.024
Mind-body			0.14	2.01	0.046
IRI empathic concern [c]	0.06	0.001			
Gender			0.20	2.77	0.006
Social			0.17	2.41	0.017
IRI perspective taking	0.064	0.001			
Work stress			−0.20	−2.76	0.006
Exercise			0.18	2.47	0.014
IRI Personal distress	0.078	<0.001			
Exercise			−0.21	−2.94	0.004
Work stress			0.20	2.78	0.006
Hobbies			−0.15	−1.97	0.050
Jefferson empathy [c]	0.17	<0.001			
Gender			0.29	4.11	<0.001
Exercise			0.26	3.72	<0.001
Work stress			−0.17	−2.47	0.009

[a] Only statistically significant ($p < 0.05$) predictors in final model are presented. b Due to the correlation with marital status, marital status was included in the initial model. However, it was non-significant and was dropped from the final model. Married/cohabitating is coded as 1, single as 0. [c] Due to the correlation with gender, gender was included in the model. Gender is coded 1 for male, 2 for female.

Table 6. Lifestyle behavior predictors and relationship to wellbeing measures.

Lifestyle Behavior	PSS	CES-D	MBI-EE	MBI-DEP	MBI-PA	SWLS	PANAS Positive	PANAS Negative	FMI	IRI EC	IRI PT	IRI PD	JES
Work Stress	↑	↑	↑	↑			↓	↑	↓		↓	↑	↓
Exercise	↓	↓		↑			↑	↓	↑		↑	↓	↑
Social Support		↓				↑				↑	↑		
Sleep	↓	↓	↓					↓					
Diet/Nutrition				↓		↑							
Hobbies										↓		↓	↑
Gender										↑			↑
Mind-body/Spiritual								↓					
Alcohol drinks													

↑ Positive relationship between wellness behavior and wellbeing measure; ↓ Negative relationship between wellness behavior and wellbeing measure.

3.6. On-Site Physician Wellness Activities

Wellness retreats were the most frequent type of wellness activity offered, with all sites hosting wellness-focused retreats over the three-year period (see Figure 1). These retreats varied in content-based on-site faculty preferences and available resources. Most were held off-site in a private setting and provided opportunity for small group discussions and peer support, informational seminars, and experiential learning. The next-most frequently reported activity was increased nutrition options for residents, available initially at four sites, and at all sites by 2016. Physical activity options (mainly access to gyms) increased from two sites in 2014 to four sites by 2016. Burnout prevention activities increased from one site in 2014 to four sites; and by 2016, other wellness activities (empathy skills training, self-regulation skills, conflict resolution/communication, and stress management) were offered at three of the five sites.

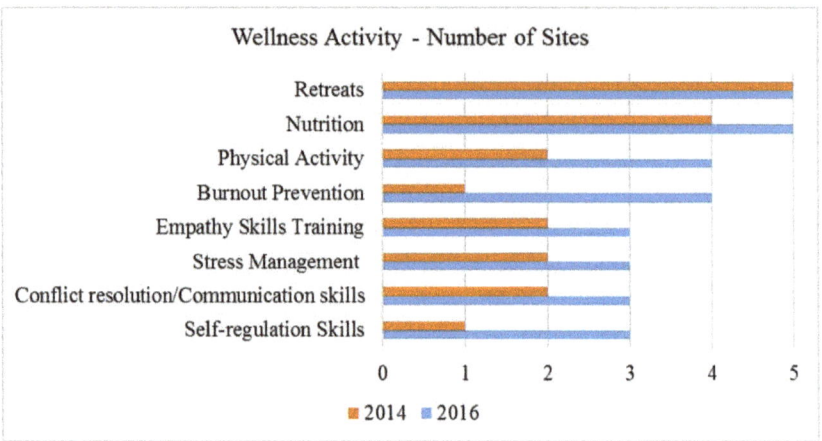

Figure 1. On-site physician wellness activities—number of sites by year.

4. Discussion

It is well established that burnout is prevalent in medical trainees and takes a steep toll on mental and physical health [2]. This highlights the need for reform of the current medical education model, and the paradox of recruiting medical students for both their academic strength and empathic qualities. A combination that may predispose talented trainees to distress during the rigors of conventional medical training. Addressing and preventing burnout from the very earliest stages of medical school training is necessary, because burnout impacts patient care, quality of patient counseling, and prevalence of medical errors [7]. The etiology of burnout is complex, involving a variety of factors at the organizational, institutional, and individual levels, requiring coordinated, systems-level solutions [8]. Surveys show that burnout rates in pediatric trainees mirror national prevalence, emphasizing the urgent need for change at the earliest stages of pediatric training in addition to preventive steps and education during medical school to avoid the recurring pitfall of receiving first-year residents already in serious stages of burnout [4,6].

To highlight this point, our study findings demonstrate that a substantial proportion of first-year pediatric residents in the PIMR pilot study began residency with higher levels of burnout and depression and poorer emotional intelligence and empathy than comparison samples, mirroring national trends [6]. Fifteen percent of residents in the study were high risk (high on both emotional exhaustion and depersonalization), 50% were in the moderate risk (high or moderate in either emotional exhaustion or depersonalization), and 35% were at low risk. In addition, with respect to depression, 30% scored in the clinical depression risk range. This is considerably higher than a study of residents and medical students that found 11% of first year residents were in the clinical depression risk range [27].

In the cohort, as burnout risk increases, overall wellbeing, empathy and emotional intelligence decreases. Residents with high burnout risk also reported more days of experiencing work stress, and had lower wellbeing, social support, stress management behaviors, emotional intelligence, and empathy than residents in the low and moderate risk groups. Overall, work stress was the strongest predictor of burnout, wellbeing, and emotional intelligence in our sample, significant in all models except empathic concern. The sense of feeling overwhelmed and lack of work enjoyment appears to permeate all areas of the resident's life, increasing burnout and decreasing wellbeing, emotional intelligence, mindfulness, and empathy.

Residents in the high-risk burnout group reported lower frequencies of healthy eating, social support activities, and quality sleep than their peers. One in four residents were living with a chronic illness, and 28% of residents entering the PIMR program were either overweight (23%) or obese (5%), highlighting the links between chronic stress and upregulation of inflammatory cytokines, depression, and other related comorbidities [28–30].

Exercise was a strong predictor of wellbeing and emotional intelligence, associated with less stress and depression, greater personal accomplishment, affect, mindfulness, emotional intelligence and empathy, although not distinguishing between burnout groups. Inadequate sleep was associated with emotional exhaustion, as well as stress, depression, and negative affect, similar to the burnout risk models. Social support activities were associated with less depression and greater life satisfaction, mindfulness, and empathic concern, although contrary to the burnout models, they were not associated with the burnout measures. Higher quality diet/nutrition behaviors were associated with less depersonalization and greater life satisfaction. Female gender was associated with greater empathic concern and empathy.

In our study, mind-body spiritual practices were not associated with any of the burnout, wellbeing, or emotional intelligence measures. One reason for these findings may be due to the low frequency of engagement in these behaviors in this sample. The narrow range may have limited the ability to detect an association to the burnout, wellbeing, and emotional intelligence variables. Fortunately, some residency programs are beginning to teach these behaviors, and future studies will be able to examine the role of mind-body practices in prevention of burnout.

In summary, a majority of residents in the study were at either moderate or high risk of burnout, not meeting basic recommendations for healthy lifestyle habits, and stood a 1 in 4 chance of being overweight or obese. Our findings are consistent with other surveys that document high levels of burnout in graduating US medical students [31], and mirror studies demonstrating lack of regular physical activity in residents [32,33], and published reports of lower levels of stress and burnout in medical students who exercised regularly [34–36]. While the percentage of overweight residents was lower in our sample (23%) when compared to a study of first year residents from multiple specialties (34%) [37], the rate of obese residents in our sample of pediatric residents was higher (5% vs. 0%). In addition to the protective lifestyle behaviors mentioned, the remaining wellness activities (empathy skills training, self-regulation skills, conflict resolution/communication, stress management) were offered at 3 of the 5 sites. Ideally, these would serve to help moderate perceived work stress and help build connections at work, cultivating social resilience, which has been shown to be protective against burnout in medical training [38].

National surveys have shown that organizational and institutional measures to reduce and prevent burnout are effective [39,40], and a prudent financial investment [41]. Despite these findings, and widespread recognition of burnout's mental and physical toll, few programs offer approaches to promote self-care activities associated with lower burnout prevalence [34,42–44].

The PIMR program addresses these gaps in two important ways. First, by embedding a curriculum on protective lifestyle behaviors into residency training, the concept of self-care is acknowledged and normalized. Second, engagement of a critical mass of residents and faculty instructors participating in and teaching these activities drives broader culture change within individual organizations. In our study, this is borne out by the increase in program wellness activities over time. Perhaps most notable is the increase from only 1 site offering burnout prevention activities in 2014 to 4 sites with burnout prevention activities in 2016. Newly revised ACGME competencies mandating specific attention to resident wellbeing will hopefully provide critical leverage to move this initiative forward [9].

Furthermore, promotion of healthy lifestyle behaviors in residents aligns with developing themes in the medical literature suggesting that trainees with healthier lifestyle habits are more likely to counsel patients on healthy lifestyle habits, and to do so more effectively than their less healthy colleagues [45–47]. This point has special relevance in pediatric trainees, who have the potential to encourage a lifetime of healthy habits in their young patients.

Limitations

One of the main limitations of this study is the limited generalizability of the findings. The five participating residencies were not randomly selected but volunteered to participate to pilot a new integrative medicine curriculum. Given that there are nearly 200 pediatric residencies nationwide, it is not possible to determine the representativeness of these 5 sites. In addition, the response rate was 63% across the sites, with variation in the response rate between the sites, also limiting our ability to generalize our findings. Data was collected during the first trimester of residency and does not reflect the full measure of residency stressors that accumulate throughout residency.

A second limitation is our primary emphasis on lifestyle behaviors as potential mediators/moderators in the relationship between stress and burnout and its consequent effects. Individual factors that can mediate the impact of stress, such as cognitive appraisals, coping styles and strategies, self-efficacy expectations, grit, optimism, resiliency, hardiness, and social competence were not assessed. System level factors were also not assessed. These include current rotations, prior experience, and levels of faculty support and burnout and how this influences resident burnout, all areas of active study. The newly developed lifestyle behavior instrument used in this study may not have fully captured the lifestyle behaviors most critical to wellbeing. Further, the lifestyle behaviors were captured retrospectively, thus it was not possible to confirm the accuracy of the self-reported lifestyle behaviors with other methods, such as daily recording of the behavior. Lastly, the study utilized online self-report surveys which may be subject to recall bias and social desirability influences.

Future directions could address efforts to increase the reach of the PIMR program by increasing the number of enrolled sites and residents, thereby increasing reach and diversity. Another strategy might include a more tailored rollout of self-care curriculum modules designed to educate leaders and encourage a culture of wellness and engagement within the top levels of organizations [48].

5. Conclusions

Accruing research suggests that first-year residents enter training with high levels of burnout, emphasizing the need for effective solutions to address burnout in medical education. Burnout prevalence in our study supported these findings. Furthermore, high burnout risk was associated with a decrease in overall wellbeing, increased work stress, inadequate sleep, fewer social support activities, and poorer diet quality. New mandates from the ACGME to promote resident wellbeing are encouraging, yet few educational programs currently exist to meet these requirements. National surveys show that organizational measures designed to reduce burnout have proven effective. The PIMR program offers an innovative curriculum that residency programs can use to target protective lifestyle behaviors correlated with decreased burnout measures. These include physical activity, sleep, nutrition, and stress management/coping skills. Within the PIMR program, education about these behaviors is delivered in a train the trainer educational model that will ideally equip residents to become more effective role models and counselors to their young patients.

Author Contributions: H.M. and A.J.B. conceived and designed the study; H.M., A.J.B., M.-K.C., M.B., M.B., A.E., D.G., B.G., J.M., J.W., and A.M.Y. participated in study design and data collection; H.M., A.J.B. and M.-K.C. analyzed and interpreted the data; H.M. and A.J.B. wrote the body of the paper, and all authors contributed substantially to individual sections and editing of drafts.

Acknowledgments: Sincere thanks to all the residents and faculty participating in the PIMR pilot program, as well as to all faculty involved in the early adopter phase including: Maria Mascarenhas and Miriam Stewart, Children's Hospital of Philadelphia; Carmen Herrera, University of New Mexico; Alexandra Russell, Vanderbilt University; Rukmani Vasan, University of Southern California; Marian Eckert, Kinderkrankenhaus St. Marien; Elena Ladas, Columbia University; Hillary Franke, University of Arizona; J. Paige Frazer, Eastern Virginia Medical School, Children's Hospital of the King's Daughters. Thanks also go to Paula Cook, Research Specialist, and Rhonda Hallquist, Instructional Web Developer, for their many contributions. And a special thanks to Emily Sherbrooke, IMR/PIMR Program Coordinator Sr.; and to Janice Curtis, Administrative Associate, for their administrative support and expert help in manuscript preparation. Funding was received from the David and Lura Lovell Foundation, the Weil Foundation, the Gerald J. and Rosalie E. Kahn Family Foundation, Inc., the John F. Long Foundation, the Resnick Foundation, and the Sampson Foundation.

Conflicts of Interest: The authors declare no conflict of interest.

References

1. Dyrbye, L.N.; West, C.P.; Satele, D.; Boone, S.; Tan, L.; Sloan, J.; Shanafelt, T.D. Burnout among US medical students, residents, and early career physicians relative to the general US population. *Acad. Med.* **2014**, *89*, 443–451. [CrossRef] [PubMed]
2. Dyrbye, L.; Shanafelt, T. A narrative review on burnout experienced by medical students and residents. *Med. Educ.* **2016**, *50*, 132–149. [CrossRef] [PubMed]
3. McClafferty, H.; Brown, O.W. Physician health and wellness. *Pediatrics* **2014**, *134*, 830–835. [CrossRef] [PubMed]
4. Pantaleoni, J.L.; Augustine, E.M.; Sourkes, B.M.; Bachrach, L.K. Burnout in pediatric residents over a 2-year period: A longitudinal study. *Acad. Pediatr.* **2014**, *14*, 167–172. [CrossRef] [PubMed]
5. Mahan, J.D. Burnout in pediatric residents and physicians: A call to action. *Pediatrics* **2017**, *139*, e20164233. [CrossRef] [PubMed]
6. Baer, T.E.; Feraco, A.M.; Sagalowsky, S.T.; Williams, D.; Litman, H.J.; Vinci, R.J. Pediatric resident burnout and attitudes toward patients. *Pediatrics* **2017**, *139*, e20162163. [CrossRef] [PubMed]
7. Jennings, M.L.; Slavin, S.J. Resident wellness matters: Optimizing resident education and wellness through the learning environment. *Acad. Med.* **2015**, *90*, 1246–1250. [CrossRef] [PubMed]
8. Shanafelt, T.D.; Dyrbye, L.N.; West, C.P. Addressing physician burnout: The way forward. *JAMA* **2017**, *317*, 901–902. [CrossRef] [PubMed]
9. Accreditation Council for Graduate Medical Education (ACGME). Revised Common Program Requirements, Section VI, The Learning and Working Environment. Available online: https://www.acgmecommon.org/press_release (accessed on 2 March 2017).
10. Accreditation Council for Graduate Medical Education (ACGME). Physician Wellbeing. Available online: http://www.acgme.org/What-We-Do/Initiatives/Physician-Well-Being (accessed on 3 February 2017).
11. McClafferty, H.; Dodds, S.; Brooks, A.J.; Brenner, M.; Brown, M.; Frazer, P.; Mark, J.; Weydert, J.; Wilcox, G.; Lebensohn, P.; Maizes, V. Pediatric integrative medicine in residency (PIMR): Description of a new online educational curriculum. *Children* **2015**, *2*, 98–107. [CrossRef] [PubMed]
12. Lebensohn, P.; Brooks, A.J.; Chen, M.K. A multi-dimensional integrative health measure to assess wellness behaviors—The Arizona lifestyle inventory. In Proceedings of the International Conference to Promote Resilience, Empathy and Well-Being in Health Care Professions (CENTILE 2017), Washington, DC, USA, 22–25 October 2017.
13. Cohen, S.; Kamarck, T.; Mermelstein, R. A global measure of perceived stress. *J. Health Soc. Behav.* **1983**, *24*, 385–396. [CrossRef] [PubMed]
14. Radloff, L.S. The CES-D scale: A self-report depression scale for research in the general population. *Appl. Psychol. Meas.* **1977**, *1*, 385–401. [CrossRef]
15. Maslach, C.; Jackson, S.E.; Leiter, M.P. *Maslach Burnout Inventory*, 3rd ed.; Consulting Psychologists Press: Palo Alto, CA, USA, 1996.
16. Maslach, C.; Jackson, S.E.; Leiter, M. *Maslach Burnout Inventory Manual*, 4th ed.; Mind Garden Inc.: Menlo Park, CA, USA, 2016.
17. Diener, E.; Emmons, R.A.; Larsen, R.J.; Griffin, S. The satisfaction with life scale. *J. Pers. Assess.* **1985**, *49*, 71–75. [CrossRef] [PubMed]
18. Pavot, W.; Diener, E. Review of the satisfaction with life scale. *Psychol. Assess.* **1993**, *5*, 164–172. [CrossRef]
19. Watson, D.; Clark, L.A.; Tellegen, A. Development and validation of brief measures of positive and negative affect: The PANAS scales. *J. Pers. Soc. Psychol.* **1988**, *54*, 1063–1070. [CrossRef] [PubMed]
20. Walach, H.; Buchheld, N.; Buttenmüller, V.; Kleinknecht, N.; Schmidt, S. Measuring mindfulness—The Freiburg mindfulness inventory (FMI). *Pers. Individ. Dif.* **2006**, *40*, 1543–1555. [CrossRef]
21. Davis, M.H. Measuring individual differences in empathy: Evidence for a multidimensional approach. *J. Pers. Soc. Psychol.* **1983**, *44*, 113–126. [CrossRef]
22. Hojat, M.; Mangione, S.; Nasca, T.J.; Cohen, M.J.M.; Gonnella, J.S.; Erdmann, J.B.; Veloski, J.; Magee, M. The Jefferson scale of physician empathy: Development and preliminary psychometric data. *Educ. Psychol. Meas.* **2001**, *61*, 349–365. [CrossRef]

23. Birks, Y.; McKendree, J.; Watt, I. Emotional intelligence and perceived stress in healthcare students: A multi-institutional, multi-professional survey. *BMC Med. Educ.* **2009**, *9*, 61. [CrossRef] [PubMed]
24. Weissman, M.M.; Sholomskas, D.; Pottenger, M.; Prusoff, B.A.; Locke, B.Z. Assessing depressive symptoms in five psychiatric populations: A validation study. *Am. J. Epidemiol.* **1977**, *106*, 203–214. [CrossRef] [PubMed]
25. Lebensohn, P.; Dodds, S.; Brooks, A.J.; Cook, P.; Schneider, C.D.; Woytowicz, J.; Maizes, V. A longitudinal study of well-being, burnout and emotional intelligence in family medicine residents. In Proceedings of the International Research Congress on Integrative Medicine and Health, Miami, FL, USA, 13–16 May 2014.
26. Bellini, L.M.; Shea, J.A. Mood change and empathy decline persist during three years of internal medicine training. *Acad. Med.* **2005**, *80*, 164–167. [CrossRef] [PubMed]
27. Goebert, D.; Thompson, D.; Takeshita, J.; Beach, C.; Bryson, P.; Ephgrave, K.; Kent, A.; Kunkel, M.; Schechter, J.; Tate, J. Depressive symptoms in medical students and residents: A multischool study. *Acad. Med.* **2009**, *84*, 236–241. [CrossRef] [PubMed]
28. Park, Y.-M.; Zhang, J.; Steck, S.E.; Cohen, M.J.M.; Gonnella, J.S.; Erdmann, J.B.; Veloski, J.; Magee, M. Obesity mediates the association between Mediterranean diet consumption and insulin resistance and inflammation in US Adults. *J. Nutr.* **2017**, *147*, 563–571. [CrossRef] [PubMed]
29. Chao, A.M.; Jastreboff, A.M.; White, M.A.; Grilo, C.M.; Sinha, R. Stress, cortisol, and other appetite-related hormones: Prospective prediction of 6-month changes in food cravings and weight. *Obesity* **2017**, *25*, 713–720. [CrossRef] [PubMed]
30. Razzoli, M.; Pearson, C.; Crow, S.; Bartolomucci, A. Stress, overeating, and obesity: Insights from human studies and preclinical models. *Neurosci. Biobehav. Rev.* **2017**, *76*, 154–162. [CrossRef] [PubMed]
31. Dyrbye, L.N.; Moutier, C.; Durning, S.J.; Massie, F.S., Jr.; Power, D.V.; Eacker, A.; Harper, W.; Thomas, M.R.; Satele, D.; Sloan, J.A.; Shanafelt, T.D. The problems program directors inherit: Medical student distress at the time of graduation. *Med. Teach.* **2011**, *33*, 756–758. [CrossRef] [PubMed]
32. Daneshvar, F.; Weinreich, M.; Daneshvar, D.; Sperling, M.; Salmane, C.; Yacoub, H.; Gabriels, J.; McGinn, T.; Smith, M.C. Cardiorespiratory fitness in internal medicine residents: Are future physicians becoming deconditioned? *J. Grad. Med. Educ.* **2017**, *9*, 97–101. [CrossRef] [PubMed]
33. Williams, A.S.; Williams, C.D.; Cronk, N.J.; Kruse, R.L.; Ringdahl, E.N.; Koopman, R.J. Understanding the exercise habits of residents and attending physicians: A mixed methodology study. *Fam. Med.* **2015**, *47*, 118–123. [PubMed]
34. Dyrbye, L.N.; Satele, D.; Shanafelt, T.D. Healthy exercise habits are associated with lower risk of burnout and higher quality of life among US medical students. *Acad. Med.* **2017**, *92*, 1006–1011. [CrossRef] [PubMed]
35. Olson, S.M.; Odo, N.U.; Duran, A.M.; Pereira, A.G.; Mandel, J.H. Burnout and physical activity in Minnesota internal medicine resident physicians. *J. Grad. Med. Educ.* **2014**, *6*, 669–674. [CrossRef] [PubMed]
36. Frank, E.; Tong, E.; Lobelo, F.; Carrera, J.; Duperly, J. Physical activity levels and counseling practices of US medical students. *Med. Sci. Sports Exerc.* **2008**, *40*, 413–421. [CrossRef] [PubMed]
37. Leventer-Roberts, M.; Zonfrillo, M.R.; Yu, S.; Dziura, J.D.; Spiro, D.M. Overweight physicians during residency: A cross-sectional and longitudinal study. *J. Grad. Med. Educ.* **2013**, *5*, 405–411. [CrossRef] [PubMed]
38. McKenna, K.M.; Hashimoto, D.A.; Maguire, M.S.; Bynum, W.E. The missing link: Connection is the key to resilience in medical education. *Acad. Med.* **2016**, *91*, 1197–1199. [CrossRef] [PubMed]
39. West, C.P.; Dyrbye, L.N.; Erwin, P.J.; Shanafelt, T.D. Interventions to prevent and reduce physician burnout: A systematic review and meta-analysis. *Lancet* **2016**, *388*, 2272–2281. [CrossRef]
40. Panagioti, M.; Panagopoulou, E.; Bower, P. Controlled interventions to reduce burnout in physicians: A systematic review and meta-analysis. *JAMA Intern. Med.* **2017**, *177*, 195–205. [CrossRef] [PubMed]
41. Shanafelt, T.; Goh, J.; Sinsky, C. The business case for investing in physician well-being. *JAMA Intern. Med.* **2017**, *177*, 1826–1832. [CrossRef] [PubMed]
42. Heinen, I.; Bullinger, M.; Kocalevent, R.D. Perceived stress in first year medical students—Associations with personal resources and emotional distress. *BMC Med. Educ.* **2017**, *17*, 4. [CrossRef] [PubMed]
43. Thompson, G.; McBride, R.B.; Hosford, C.C.; Halaas, G. Resilience among medical students: The role of coping style and social support. *Teach. Learn. Med.* **2016**, *28*, 174–182. [CrossRef] [PubMed]
44. Ward, S.; Outram, S. Medicine: In need of culture change. *Intern. Med. J.* **2016**, *46*, 112–116. [CrossRef] [PubMed]
45. Howe, A.; Smajdor, A.; Stockl, A. Towards an understanding of resilience and its relevance to medical training. *Med. Educ.* **2012**, *46*, 349–356. [CrossRef] [PubMed]

46. Frank, E.; Rothenberg, R.; Lewis, C.; Belodoff, B.F. Correlates of physicians' prevention-related practices. Findings from the Women Physicians' Health Study. *Arch. Fam. Med.* **2000**, *9*, 359–367. [CrossRef] [PubMed]
47. Frank, E.; Breyan, J.; Elon, L. Physician disclosure of healthy personal behaviors improves credibility and ability to motivate. *Arch. Fam. Med.* **2000**, *9*, 287–290. [CrossRef] [PubMed]
48. McClafferty, H.; Ricker, M.; Brooks, A.J.; Lebensohn, P. Cracking the nut: Wellbeing in training, increasing resilience in both individuals & across healthcare organizations. In Proceedings of the International Conference to Promote Resilience, Empathy and Well-Being in Health Care Professions (CENTILE 2017), Washington, DC, USA, 22–25 October 2017.

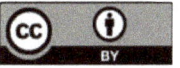

© 2018 by the authors. Licensee MDPI, Basel, Switzerland. This article is an open access article distributed under the terms and conditions of the Creative Commons Attribution (CC BY) license (http://creativecommons.org/licenses/by/4.0/).

MDPI
St. Alban-Anlage 66
4052 Basel
Switzerland
Tel. +41 61 683 77 34
Fax +41 61 302 89 18
www.mdpi.com

Children Editorial Office
E-mail: children@mdpi.com
www.mdpi.com/journal/children

www.ingramcontent.com/pod-product-compliance
Lightning Source LLC
LaVergne TN
LVHW071947080526
838202LV00064B/6693